EAT A BAGEL OR A BURGER . . .
BUT MAKE SMART CHOICES
AND INFORMED DECISIONS
WITH THE BEST REFERENCE BOOK
FOR TODAY'S CARBO-CONSCIOUS CONSUMER

It's simple, painless, and effective: counting carbohydrates to meet your daily dietary needs. And if you're serious about watching your carbohydrates, you want all the information in one place. Whether you're working out, training for a specific sport, bodybuilding, weight-watching, or following a doctor's diet, here is the only book a carbohydrate-conscious consumer needs.

Go for the grams with Corinne T. Netzer's up-to-date classic, chock-full of the information you need to restrict *or* boost the carbohydrates in your daily eating plan. America's #1 expert on the nutritional content of food gives you comprehensive carbohydrate counts for a wide variety of foods, including fresh and frozen produce, meats and dairy products, breads, grains and pastas, sweets, brand-name and fast foods, and more. The choice is yours!

**THE
CORINNE T. NETZER
CARBOHYDRATE
COUNTER**

THE CORINNE T. NETZER CARBOHYDRATE COUNTER

Corinne T. Netzer

Revised Edition

A Dell Book

Published by
Dell Publishing
a division of
Bantam Doubleday Dell Publishing Group, Inc.
1540 Broadway
New York, New York 10036

ISBN: 0-440-22550-7

Printed in the United States of America

Published simultaneously in Canada

April 1998

10 9 8 7 6 5 4

OPM

Introduction

The Carbohydrate Counter is the largest compilation of carbo grams available under one cover. No matter what your aim or interest in carbohydrates might be, the information on all the foods—whether generic or brand name, fresh or frozen, even a fast-food favorite—can be found here.

Because this book is alphabetized, there is no index. I have tried to cross-reference as many items as possible; however, space does not allow this in every instance. If you do not find the item you are seeking in one place, please look for it under a category—e.g., if you don't find "apple pie" under "Apple," look for it under "Pie."

If you are making comparisons, remember to compare only foods that are similar in measure. Eight ounces is not necessarily equivalent to one eight-ounce cup. Eight ounces is a measure of how much the food weighs, while an eight-ounce cup is a measure of how much space the food occupies. For example, a cup of popcorn weighs about an ounce; thus, eight ounces of popcorn would fill quite a few cups.

The data contained herein are derived from information supplied by the various food producers, processors, distributors, and food chains, and from the United States Department of Agriculture. As we go to press, this information is the most complete and accurate available.

Good luck and good eating.

C.T.N.

Abbreviations & Symbols in This Book

"	inch
<	less than
approx.	approximately
cont.	container
diam.	diameter
lb.	pound(s)
pkg.	package(s)
pkt.	packet(s)
oz.	ounce(s)
tbsp.	tablespoon(s)
tsp.	teaspoon(s)
*	prepared according to basic package directions

Note: Brand-name foods and restaurants listed in italics denote registered trademarks.

THE
CORINNE T. NETZER
CARBOHYDRATE
COUNTER

A

FOOD AND MEASURE	CARBOHYDRATE GRAMS

A la king sauce mix *(Durkee)*, 1 cup* 8.0
Abalone, meat only, raw, 4 oz. 6.8
Abruzzese sausage *(Boar's Head Cinghiale)*, 1 oz. . . . . <1.0
Acerola, fresh:
untrimmed, 1 lb. 27.9
trimmed, ½ cup 3.8
1 medium, approx. .2 oz. 4
Acerola juice, 8 fl. oz. 12.0
Ackee, trimmed, 1 oz. 1.6
Acorn:
raw, in shell, 1 lb. 114.6
raw, shelled, 1 oz. 11.8
dried, shelled, 1 oz. 15.2
Acorn flour, full-fat, 1 oz. 15.2
Acorn squash:
raw:
   (Frieda's), ¾ cup, 3 oz. 9.0
   untrimmed, 1 lb. 35.9
   1 medium, 4″ diam., approx. 1.3 lb. 44.9
baked, cubed, ½ cup 14.9
boiled, mashed, ½ cup 10.7
Adobo *(Durkee)*, ¼ tsp. 0
Adzuki beans:
dry *(Arrowhead Mills)*, ¼ cup 29.0
dry, boiled, ½ cup 28.5
canned *(Eden* Organic Aduki)*, ½ cup 19.0
canned, sweetened, ½ cup 81.4
Agar, see "Seaweed"
Albacore, see "Tuna, canned"
Alcapurrius, frozen *(Goya)*, 1 piece 26.0
Alfalfa sprouts, 1 cup, except as noted:
(Arrowhead Mills) 4.0
(Jonathan's) 3.0
1 lb. 17.1
with dill, garlic, or onion *(Jonathan's)* 3.0

Alfalfa sprouts *(cont.)*
with radish sprouts *(Jonathan's)* 4.0
Alfredo entree, frozen, see "Entree mixes, frozen" and
    specific entree listings
Alfredo sauce:
(Five Brothers), ¼ cup 2.0
(Progresso), ½ cup 5.0
cheese, three *(Lawry's),* 3 tbsp. 0
with mushrooms *(Five Brothers),* ¼ cup 3.0
refrigerated, ¼ cup:
    (Contadina/Contadina Light) 5.0
    (Di Giorno) 2.0
    (Di Giorno Reduced Fat) 16.0
Alfredo sauce mix:
(Knorr), ⅓ pkg. 7.0
(Spice Islands), ½ pkg. 3.0
Alfredo seasoning mix *(Lawry's),* 1½ tbsp. 4.0
Algae, see "Seaweed"
All-purpose seasoning *(Aromat),* ¼ tsp. 0
Allspice:
(McCormick), ¼ tsp. 3
1 tbsp. 4.3
1 tsp. 1.4
Almond, shelled, except as noted:
(Dole), 1 oz. 5.0
(Planters), 1 oz. 5.0
dried:
    in shell, 4 oz. 9.3
    1 oz. 5.8
    blanched, 1 oz. 5.3
    sliced or diced, 1 cup packed 19.2
    slivered, 1 cup 27.5
dry-roasted, 1 oz. 6.9
dry-roasted, kernels, 1 cup 33.4
honey-roasted, 1 oz. 7.9
honey-roasted *(Planters),* 1 oz. 7.0
oil-roasted, 1 oz. or approx. 22 kernels 4.5
oil-roasted, kernels, 1 cup 24.9
slivered *(Paradise/White Swan),* ¼ cup, 1.1 oz. 3.0
slivered *(Planters Gold Measure),* 2-oz. pkg. 11.0
tamari-roasted *(Eden),* 1 oz. 8.0
toasted, 1 oz. 6.5

Almond butter, crunchy or creamy:
(Roaster Fresh/Roaster Fresh Unsalted), 1 oz. 6.0
honey cinnamon, 1 tbsp. 4.3
salted or unsalted, 1 tbsp. 3.4
Almond meal, partially defatted, 1 oz. 8.2
Almond paste:
(Solo), 2 tbsp. 19.0
1 oz. 12.4
Almond powder:
full-fat, 1 cup 14.5
partially defatted, 1 cup 20.7
Alum *(Durkee),* 1/4 tsp. 0
Amaranth:
raw, untrimmed, 1 lb. 17.2
raw, trimmed, 1/2 cup 6
boiled, drained, 1/2 cup 2.7
Amaranth, whole-grain:
1 oz. 18.8
1/2 cup 64.5
Amaranth entree, canned *(Health Valley* Fast Menu), 1 cup 31.0
Amaranth flour *(Arrowhead Mills),* 1/4 cup 25.0
Amaranth seed *(Arrowhead Mills),* 1/4 cup 29.0
Amberjack, without added ingredients 0
Anaheim chili, see "Pepper, chili"
Anasazi beans *(Arrowhead Mills),* 1/4 cup 27.0
Anchovy, fresh or canned in oil 0
Anchovy paste *(Reese),* 1 tbsp. 0
Angel-hair pasta:
dry, see "Pasta"
refrigerated *(Contadina),* 1 1/4 cups 43.0
refrigerated *(Di Giorno),* 2 oz. 31.0
Angel-hair pasta entree, frozen:
(Lean Cuisine), 10 oz. 48.0
(Smart Ones), 9 oz. 29.0
with sausage *(Marie Callender's),* 1 cup, 8 oz. 43.0
Angel-hair pasta mix:
chicken broccoli *(Lipton Pasta & Sauce),* 1/3 cup or 1 cup* 43.0
with herbs *(Pasta Roni),* approx. 1 cup* 42.0
lemon and butter *(Pasta Roni),* approx. 1 cup* 48.0
Parmesan *(Lipton* Pasta & Sauce), 1/3 cup or 1 cup* 41.0
Parmesan *(Pasta Roni),* approx. 1 cup* 40.0

Anise seed:
1 tbsp. 3.4
1 tsp. 1.1
Antelope, without added ingredients 0
Apio root, see "Celeriac"
Appaloosa beans, dried *(Frieda's),* ½ cup 22.0
Apple:
fresh:
    (Dole), 1 apple 18.0
    (Frieda's Lady Apple), 5 oz. 21.0
    with peel, 2¾″ apple 21.1
    with peel, sliced, ½ cup 8.4
    peeled, 2¾″ apple 19.0
    peeled, sliced, ½ cup 8.2
fresh, cooked, peeled, sliced, boiled, ½ cup 11.7
fresh, cooked, peeled, sliced, microwaved, ½ cup 12.3
canned, ½ cup, except as noted:
    baked, Dutch *(Lucky Leaf/Musselman's)* 41.0
    baked *(Seneca* Extra Large), 1 apple 18.0
    baked *(Seneca* Large), 1 apple 16.0
    escalloped *(White House)* 35.0
    fried *(Apple Time/Lucky Leaf)* 43.0
    sliced *(Comstock),* ⅓ cup 7.0
    sliced *(Lucky Leaf/Musselman's)* 12.0
    sliced *(Musselman's* Home Style) 43.0
    sliced *(Seneca* Sweetened) 13.0
    sliced *(Seneca* Unsweetened) 11.0
    sliced *(White House)* 22.0
    spiced whole *(Comstock),* 1 apple 8.0
    spiced rings *(Comstock),* 2 rings 7.0
    spiced rings *(Lucky Leaf/Musselman's),* 1.1-oz. ring 9.0
    spiced rings *(S&W),* 2 rings 7.0
    spiced rings *(White House),* ½-oz. ring 5.0
dried:
    (Sonoma), 1.4 oz. 29.0
    chips *(Smart Snackers),* .75 oz. 18.0
    chips, all varieties *(Seneca),* 1 oz. 20.0
    sliced *(Del Monte),* ⅓ cup, 1.4 oz. 23.0
    sulfured, uncooked, 2 oz. 37.4
Apple, escalloped:
canned, see "Apple"
frozen *(Stouffer's* Side Dish), 6 oz. 37.0

Apple-almond crisp, freeze-dried *(AlpineAire)*, 1½ cups ... 44.0
Apple butter, 1 tbsp.:
(Apple Time/Lucky Leaf/Musselman's) 8.0
(Dutch Girl/Mary Ellen) 9.0
(Eden) 5.0
(R.W. Knudsen) 9.0
(Smucker's/Simply Fruit) 11.0
(White House) 9.0
spread *(Apple Time)* 6.0
spread *(New Morning)* 6.0
Apple cider, see "Apple juice"
Apple drink blends, 8 fl. oz., except as noted:
berry *(Dole Burst)*, 16 fl. oz. 61.0
black cherry–white grape *(Veryfine Quenchers)* 30.0
cranberry:
    (Dole), 10 fl. oz. 40.0
    (Tree Top), 10 fl. oz. 51.0
    (Tree Top), 11.5 fl. oz. 58.0
    tangerine *(Veryfine Quenchers)* 31.0
peach-kiwi *(Veryfine Quenchers)* 33.0
peach-plum *(Veryfine Quenchers)* 32.0
pear–passion fruit *(Veryfine Quenchers)* 31.0
punch *(Minute Maid)* 33.0
raspberry *(Tree Top)*, 10 fl. oz. 47.0
raspberry *(Tree Top)*, 11.5 fl. oz. 54.0
raspberry-blackberry *(Tropicana Twister)* 32.0
raspberry-blackberry *(Tropicana Twister)*, 11.5 fl. oz. 44.0
raspberry-cherry *(Veryfine Quenchers)* 31.0
raspberry-lime *(Veryfine Quenchers)* 30.0
strawberry-banana *(Veryfine Quenchers)* 30.0
frozen*:
    berry *(Dole Burst)* 31.0
    berry-cherry *(Schwan's Vita-Sun)* 24.0
    cranberry *(Schwan's Vita-Sun)* 25.0
Apple dumpling, frozen *(Pepperidge Farm)*, 1 piece 44.0
Apple flauta *(Schwan's)*, 1 piece 22.0
Apple fritter, frozen *(Mrs. Paul's)*, 2 pieces 36.0
Apple fruit roll, see "Fruit snack"
Apple juice, 8 fl. oz., except as noted:
(After the Fall) 22.0
(Apple & Eve) 26.0
(Apple Time/Lincoln/Lucky Leaf/Speas Farm Regular/Cider) 31.0

Apple juice *(cont.)*
(*Apple Time/Lucky Leaf/Musselman's*), 5.5 fl. oz. 20.0
(*Dole*), 10 fl. oz. 39.0
(*Goya*) 30.0
(*Heinke's* Natural/Organic/Gravenstein) 30.0
(*R.W. Knudsen* Clear/Aseptic) 28.0
(*R.W. Knudsen* Natural/Organic/Gravenstein) 30.0
(*Minute Maid* Box), 8.45 fl. oz. 29.0
(*Mott's* Natural) 29.0
(*Musselman's* Regular/Natural/Cider) 31.0
(*Musselman's* Premium Natural) 33.0
(*Red Cheek*) 29.0
(*S&W*) 30.0
(*Santa Cruz* Organic) 30.0
(*Season's Best*), 11.5 fl. oz. 40.0
(*Seneca*) 28.0
(*Snapple*), 10 fl. oz. 36.0
(*Tree Top/Tree Top* Box/Country Style/Cider) 29.0
(*Tree Top*), 5.5 fl. oz. 20.0
(*Tree Top*), 10 fl. oz. 36.0
(*Tree Top*), 11.5 fl. oz. 42.0
(*Tree Top* Fiber Rich) 36.0
(*Tree Top* Not from Concentrate) 30.0
(*Veryfine*) 35.0
(*Veryfine*), 11.5 fl. oz. 43.0
(*White House*) 30.0
cider (*Lincoln*) 31.0
cider, sparkling (*Apple Time/Lucky Leaf/Musselman's*) 36.0
spiced (*Apple & Eve* Cider & Spice) . . . .•. 26.0
frozen (*Seneca*), 2 oz. 29.0
frozen*:
    (*R.W. Knudsen*) 30.0
    (*Minute Maid*) 28.0
    (*Schwan's*) 30.0
    (*Tree Top*) 29.0
    cider (*Schwan's Vita-Sun*) 24.0
Apple juice blends, 8 fl. oz., except as noted:
all blends, except cherry cider (*R.W. Knudsen*) 30.0
apricot (*After the Fall*) 22.0
apricot (*Tree Top* Fiber Rich) 40.0
boysenberry (*Heinke's*) 30.0
cherry (*After the Fall*) 30.0

cherry cider *(R.W. Knudsen)* 33.0
cranberry:
    (Apple & Eve) 30.0
    (R.W. Knudsen Aseptic) 29.0
    frozen* *(Tree Top)* 32.0
grape:
    (Apple & Eve), 8.45 fl. oz. 32.0
    (Juicy Juice) 30.0
    (Tree Top), 5.5 fl. oz. 22.0
    (Tree Top), 8.45 fl. oz. 34.0
    (Tree Top), 10 fl. oz. 40.0
    (Tree Top), 11.5 fl. oz. 46.0
    frozen* *(Tree Top)* 32.0
orange-banana *(Tree Top Fiber Rich)* 41.0
pear:
    (Tree Top) 29.0
    (Tree Top), 5.5 fl. oz. 20.0
    (Tree Top), 8.45 fl. oz. 31.0
    (Tree Top), 10 fl. oz. 36.0
    frozen* *(Tree Top)* 29.0
raspberry:
    (After the Fall) 23.0
    (Heinke's) 30.0
    (Tree Top), 5.5 fl. oz. 19.0
    (Tree Top), 8.45 fl. oz. 29.0
    (Tree Top), 11.5 fl. oz. 40.0
    frozen* *(Tree Top)* 28.0
strawberry *(After the Fall)* 24.0
Apple pastry (see also specific pastry listings), 1 piece:
pocket *(Tastykake)* 40.0
puffs *(Entenmann's)* 36.0
squares, frozen *(Pepperidge Farm)* 27.0
Apple syrup *(R.W. Knudsen)*, ¼ cup 38.0
Applesauce, ½ cup, except as noted:
(Apple Time Regular/Granny Smith/Red Delicious/McIntosh) 22.0
(Apple Time/Lucky Leaf/Musselman's Lite) 13.0
(Eden) 15.0
(Lincoln) 22.0
(Lucky Leaf), 4-oz. jar 21.0
(Lucky Leaf Regular/Chunky/Delicious) 22.0
(Lucky Leaf Regular/Cinnamon), 6-oz. jar 30.0
(Lucky Leaf Cinnamon) 25.0

Applesauce *(cont.)*

(Mott's)	28.0
(Mott's Chunky)	26.0
(Mott's Cinnamon)	29.0
(Musselman's Chunky/Cinnamon)	25.0
(Musselman's Regular/Cinnamon), 4 oz.	21.0
(Musselman's), 6 oz.	30.0
(Musselman's Cinnamon), 6 oz.	31.0
(Musselman's Regular/Delicious/McIntosh/Premium)	22.0
(S&W Gravenstein)	21.0
(Seneca Regular/Cinnamon/McIntosh/Golden Delicious)	24.0
(Tree Top Original/Cinnamon)	25.0
(Tree Top Original/Cinnamon), 4-oz. cont.	21.0
(White House)	23.0
(White House Cinnamon)	25.0

unsweetened/natural:

(Apple Time), 4 oz.	12.0
(Apple Time/Lincoln)	13.0
(Lucky Leaf), 6 oz.	18.0
(Lucky Leaf Regular/Cinnamon)	13.0
(Musselman's Regular/Cinnamon), 4 oz.	12.0
(Musselman's), 6 oz.	18.0
(S&W Gravenstein)	13.0
(Santa Cruz Regular/Gravenstein)	15.0
(Seneca)	14.0
(Tree Top)	18.0
(Tree Top), 4-oz. cont.	16.0
(White House)	15.0

Applesauce blends, 4 oz.:

all blends *(Santa Cruz)*	15.0
with apricot *(Musselman's Fruit 'N Sauce)*	24.0
with cherry *(Musselman's Fruit 'N Sauce)*	20.0
with peach *(Musselman's Fruit 'N Sauce)*	22.0

Apricot:

fresh:

3 medium, 12 per lb.	11.8
pitted *(Dole),* ½ cup	9.0
pitted, halves, ½ cup	8.6

canned, ½ cup:

(Del Monte Lite)	16.0
in juice	15.3
in juice *(Libby's* Lite)	13.0

in heavy syrup, with skin 27.7
in heavy syrup *(Del Monte)* 26.0
in heavy syrup *(S&W)* 26.0
dried:
    (Dole Sun Giant), 6 pieces, 1.4 oz. 22.0
    (Sonoma), 1.4 oz. 31.0
    sulfured, 2 oz. 35.0
    sun-dried *(Del Monte),* ⅓ cup, 1.4 oz. 25.0
frozen, sweetened, ½ cup 30.4
Apricot fruit roll, see "Fruit snack"
Apricot juice *(Ceres),* 8 fl. oz. 30.0
Apricot nectar, 8 fl. oz., except as noted:
(Goya) 38.0
(R.W. Knudsen) 30.0
(Libby's/Kern's) 36.0
(Libby's/Kern's), 11.5 fl. oz. 52.0
(S&W) 35.0
(S&W), 12 fl. oz. 53.0
(Santa Cruz) 30.0
pineapple *(Kern's),* 11.5 fl. oz. 53.0
Arby's, 1 serving:
breakfast items:
    bacon, 2 strips 0
    biscuit, plain 34.0
    blueberry muffin 35.0
    cinnamon-nut Danish 60.0
    croissant, plain 25.0
    egg portion 5
    French-Toastix, 6 pieces 52.0
    ham or sausage 0
    Swiss cheese, ½ oz. 5
    table syrup 25.0
chicken fingers, 2 pieces 20.0
sandwiches, chicken:
    breaded fillet 46.0
    Cordon Bleu 46.0
    grilled, BBQ 47.0
    grilled, deluxe 41.0
    roast, club 37.0
    roast, deluxe, light 33.0
    roast, deluxe, sesame seed bun 36.0
    roast, Santa Fe 35.0

Arby's (cont.)

sandwich, fish fillet 50.0
sandwich, Ham 'n Cheese or Ham 'n Cheese melt 34.0

sandwiches, roast beef:
   Arby's Melt with cheddar 36.0
   Arby-Q 48.0
   Bac'n Cheddar deluxe 38.0
   Beef 'n Cheddar 40.0
   deluxe, light 33.0
   giant 43.0
   junior 35.0
   regular 33.0
   super 50.0

sandwiches, sub roll:
   French dip 40.0
   hot Ham 'n Swiss 43.0
   Italian sub 46.0
   Philly Beef 'n Swiss 48.0
   roast beef sub 44.0
   triple cheese melt 46.0
   turkey sub 47.0

sandwich, turkey, roast, deluxe, light 33.0

salads:
   garden 12.0
   roast chicken 12.0
   side 4.0

soups:
   Boston clam chowder 18.0
   broccoli, cream of 15.0
   cheese, Wisconsin 20.0
   chicken noodle, old fashion 11.0
   chili, timberline 17.0
   potato with bacon 23.0
   vegetable, mixed, lumberjack 10.0

potatoes:
   baked, plain, 11.5 oz. 82.0
   baked, with margarine and sour cream 85.0
   baked, Broccoli 'n Cheddar 89.0
   baked, deluxe 86.0
   cakes, 2 pieces 20.0
   fries, curly 38.0
   fries, curly, cheddar 40.0

fries, french 30.0
sauces and dressings:
    Arby's Sauce 4.0
    barbecue sauce 1.0
    beef stock au jus 7.0
    blue cheese dressing 2.0
    buttermilk ranch dressing, reduced calorie 12.0
    cheddar sauce 1.0
    honey French dressing 18.0
    honey mayonnaise, reduced calorie 1.0
    Horsey Sauce 2.0
    Italian dressing, reduced calorie 3.0
    Italian sub sauce 1.0
    ketchup 4.0
    mayonnaise 0
    mayonnaise, light 5
    Parmesan cheese sauce 2.0
    ranch dressing, red 5.0
    tartar sauce 0
    Thousand Island dressing 7.0
desserts:
    apple turnover 48.0
    cheesecake, plain 23.0
    cherry turnover 46.0
    chocolate chip cookie 16.0
    Polar Swirl:
        Butterfinger 62.0
        Heath 76.0
        Oreo 66.0
        Snickers 73.0
        peanut butter cup 61.0
    shake, chocolate 76.0
    shake, jamocha 62.0
    shake, vanilla 50.0
Arrowhead:
raw, untrimmed, 1 lb. 68.8
raw, 2⅝" corm 2.4
boiled, 1" corm 1.9
Arrowroot *(Durkee),* ¼ tsp. 0
Arrowroot flour, 1 cup 112.8

Artichoke, globe:

fresh:

    (Dole), 1 medium 13.0

    raw, untrimmed, 1 lb. 19.1

    boiled, 10.6-oz. choke 13.4

    hearts, boiled, drained, 1/2 cup 9.4

canned or in jars:

    bottoms *(S&W),* 3 pieces 4.0

    hearts *(S&W),* 3 pieces 5.0

    hearts, in brine or marinated, see "Artichoke appetizer"

frozen, hearts, 9-oz. pkg. 19.8

frozen, hearts *(Birds Eye),* 1/2 cup 8.0

Artichoke, Jerusalem, see "Jerusalem artichoke"

Artichoke appetizer, marinated:

(Contorno Caponata di Carciofi), 1/3 cup 7.0

(Progresso), 1/3 cup 6.0

in brine *(Goya),* 4.5 oz. 13.0

in brine *(Progresso),* 2 pieces 6.0

marinated *(Progresso),* 2 pieces with liquid 2.0

in olive oil *(Goya),* 3 oz. 5.6

quarters *(S&W),* 2 pieces 2.0

Artichoke dip *(Victoria),* 2 tbsp. 2.0

Arugula, trimmed:

(Frieda's), 3.5 oz. 4.0

1 oz. 1.0

1/2 cup 4.0

Asian pear *(Frieda's),* 5 oz. 15.0

Asparagus, 1/2 cup, except as noted:

fresh:

    raw *(Dole),* 5 spears 5.0

    raw, untrimmed, 1 lb. 8.9

    raw, 4 spears, 3.8 oz. 2.6

    boiled, 4 spears, 1/2"-diam. base 2.5

    boiled, drained, cuts 3.8

canned:

    (S&W Blended), 6 pieces 4.0

    (S&W Colossal), 3 pieces 3.0

    (Seneca) 3.0

    (Stokely/Stokely No Salt) 3.0

    all varieties *(Del Monte)* 3.0

    spears, extra large *(LeSueur),* 4.5 oz. 3.0

    spears, regular or extra long *(Green Giant),* 4.5 oz. 3.0

cuts *(Green Giant/Green Giant* 50% Less Sodium) 3.0
frozen:
    boiled, 4 spears, approx. 2.1 oz. 2.9
    boiled, cuts and spears, 4 oz. 5.5
    cuts *(Green Giant Harvest Fresh)*, ²/₃ cup 4.0
    spears *(Birds Eye)*, 3 oz. 4.0
Asparagus, pickled *(Hogue Farms)*, 3 spears, 1.1 oz. 1.0
Asparagus beans, see "Winged beans"
Atemoya *(Frieda's)*, 3.5 oz. 24.0
Au jus gravy, ¼ cup:
(Franco-American) 2.0
(Heinz Homestyle) 2.0
mix* *(Durkee/French's)* 1.0
mix* *(Knorr)* 3.0
Au jus seasoning mix *(Durkee/French's* Roasting Bag),
    ⅛ pkg. 2.0
Aubergine, see "Eggplant"
Australian blue squash, see "Blue squash"
Avocado, California:
(Dole), ⅕ medium, 1.1 oz. 2.0
1 medium, approx. 8 oz. 12.0
trimmed, 1 oz. 2.0
pureed, ½ cup 8.0
Avocado, cocktail *(Frieda's)*, 1 piece, 1.4 oz. 3.0
Avocado dip, 2 tbsp.:
(Kraft) 4.0
(Nalley) 3.0

B

FOOD AND MEASURE   **CARBOHYDRATE GRAMS**

Baba ghanouj *(Cedar's)*, 2 tbsp. 5.0
Bacalaito, mix *(Goya)*, 3 tbsp. 19.0
Bacon, cooked:
4.5 oz. (yield from 1 lb. raw) 8
2 slices 0
Bacon, Canadian:
unheated, 1-oz. slice 5
grilled, 4.9 oz. (yield from 6-oz. pkg. unheated) 1.9
Bacon, Irish, back *(Shannon Traditional)*, 2 slices, 2 oz. 1.0
Bacon, turkey, see "Turkey bacon"
"Bacon," vegetarian, frozen, 2 strips:
(Morningstar Farms Breakfast Strips) 2.0
(Worthington Stripples) 2.0
Bacon bits:
real, 1 tbsp. 0
imitation:
   (Bac'n Pieces) 1½ tbsp. 2.0
   *(Bac*Os)*, 1 tbsp. 2.0
   (Durkee), 1 tbsp. 2.0
Bacon dip, 2 tbsp.:
cheese, see "Cheese dip"
horseradish:
   (Heluva Good) 2.0
   (Heluva Good Free) 4.0
   (Kraft) 3.0
   (Kraft Premium) 2.0
onion:
   (Breakstone's) 2.0
   (Knudsen Premium) 2.0
   (Kraft Premium) 2.0
   (Nalley) 2.0
Bagel, 1 piece:
plain:
   (Awrey's), 2.6 oz. 40.0
   (Awrey's), 4 oz. 56.0

(Thomas')	33.0
blueberry *(Awrey's)*, 4 oz.	60.0
cinnamon raisin:	
(Awrey's), 2.6 oz.	42.0
(Awrey's), 4 oz.	58.0
(Thomas')	34.0
egg *(Thomas')*	33.0
mini *(Awrey's)*	22.0
multi-grain *(Thomas')*	33.0
onion *(Thomas')*	33.0
Bagel, frozen, 1 piece, except as noted:	
plain:	
(Lender's)	30.0
(Lender's Bagelettes), 2 pieces	28.0
(Lender's Big 'N Crusty)	43.0
blueberry *(Lender's)*	38.0
cinnamon raisin:	
(Lender's)	39.0
(Lender's Big 'N Crusty)	47.0
(Sara Lee)	45.0
egg *(Lender's)*	30.0
egg *(Lender's Big 'N Crusty)*	44.0
garlic *(Lender's)*	29.0
oat bran *(Lender's)*	36.0
onion *(Lender's)*	30.0
onion *(Lender's Big 'N Crusty)*	43.0
poppy *(Lender's)*	30.0
pumpernickel *(Lender's)*	31.0
rye *(Lender's)*	30.0
sesame *(Lender's)*	29.0
soft *(Lender's* Original)	37.0
Bagel chips, 1 oz.:	
cheese, three *(Pepperidge Farm)*	16.0
onion and garlic *(Pepperidge Farm)*	18.0
onion multigrain *(Pepperidge Farm)*	19.0
Bagel sandwich, see specific listings	
Baked beans (see also specific bean listings), ½ cup, except as noted:	
(Allens)	29.0
(Campbell's New England Style/Old Fashioned)	32.0
(Friend's)	32.0
(Grandma Brown's)	28.0

Baked beans *(cont.)*
(*Heartland* Iron Kettle) 29.0
(*Open Range* Ranch Beans) 23.0
(*S&W* Brick Oven) 32.0
(*Van Camp's* Fat Free) 28.5
(*Van Camp's* Original) 29.0
with bacon (*Grandma Brown's* Saucepan) 26.0
with bacon and brown sugar:
    (*Bush's* Homestyle Sauce) 28.0
    (*Bush's* Original) 29.0
    (*Campbell's*) 29.0
    (*S&W*) 31.0
    and onion (*B&M*) 36.0
barbecue:
    (*B&M*) 33.0
    (*Campbell's/Campbell's* Old Fashioned) 29.0
    (*Green Giant/Joan of Arc*) 28.0
    Texas style (*S&W*) 25.0
brown sugar (*Van Camp's*) 31.0
with franks, see "Beans and franks"
hickory, sweet, and bacon (*Van Camp's*) 32.0
honey:
    (*B&M*) 30.0
    (*Health Valley/Health Valley* No Salt) 24.0
    bacon (*Green Giant/Joan of Arc*) 34.0
    mustard (*S&W*) 31.0
maple sugar (*S&W*) 29.0
Mexican style, see "Mexican beans"
with onion:
    (*Bush's*) 26.0
    (*Green Giant/Joan of Arc*) 28.0
    sautéed (*Van Camp's* Southern Style) 35.0
with pork:
    (*B&M*) 33.0
    (*Campbell's*) 24.0
    (*Crest Top*) 21.0
    (*Green Giant/Joan of Arc*) 20.0
    (*Hunt's*) 27.0
    (*Stokely* Sugar) 29.0
    (*Stokely* Tomato) 26.0
    (*Van Camp's*) 23.0
    (*Wagon Master/Trappey's*) 21.0

(Wagon Master/Trappey's 42 oz.) 23.0
with jalapeño (Trappey's) 24.0
peas (East Texas Fair Peas 'n Pork) 19.0
vegetarian:
   (B&M) 31.0
   (Eden Organic) 27.0
   (Heinz) 27.0
   (Stokely) 26.0
   (Van Camp's) 23.0
   4 oz. 23.3
   brown sugar sauce (Stokely) 29.0
Baking mix, all purpose (Arrowhead Mills), ¼ cup 30.0
Baking powder:
(Calumet), ¼ tsp. 0
(Davis), 1 tsp. 2.0
Baking soda (Tone's), 1 tsp. 0
Baklava:
wheat (Cedar's), 1.3-oz. piece 20.0
white (Cedar's), 1-3-oz. piece 18.0
Balsam pear, ½ cup, except as noted:
(Frieda's Bittermelon), 1 cup, 3 oz. 3.0
leafy tips, raw 8
leafy tips, boiled 2.0
pods, raw, ½" pieces 1.7
pods, boiled, drained, ½" pieces 2.7
Bamboo shoots:
fresh:
   raw, untrimmed, 1 lb. 6.8
   raw, ½" slices, ½ cup 4.0
   boiled, drained, ½" slices, ½ cup 1.2
canned, drained:
   (Chun King), 2 tbsp. 1.0
   (La Choy), 2 tbsp. 1.0
   ½ cup 2.1
Banana:
fresh:
   (Dole), 1 medium 29.0
   (Frieda's Burro/Nino/Manzano), 4.9 oz. 33.0
   untrimmed, 1 lb. 69.1
   1 medium, 8¾" long 26.7
   mashed, ½ cup 26.4
dehydrated, ¼ cup 22.1

Banana *(cont.)*
dried *(Frieda's)*, 1 piece 33.0
dried *(Sonoma)*, 2 pieces 33.0
Banana, baking, see "Plantain"
Banana, red:
(Frieda's), 5 oz. 33.0
1 medium, 7¼" long 30.7
sliced, ½ cup 17.6
Banana drink *(After the Fall* Casablanca), 8 fl. oz. 19.0
Banana milk drink:
chilled, low-fat *(Nestlé Quik)*, 1 cup 30.0
mix *(Nestlé Quik)*, 2 tbsp. 22.0
Banana nectar, 11.5-fl.-oz. can:
(Libby's/Kern's) 47.0
blend *(Libby's* Quanabana) 50.0
blend, pineapple *(Kern's)* 52.0
Banana squash *(Frieda's)*, ¾ cup, 3 oz. 7.0
Bananaberry shake *(Nestlé Killer)*, 14 oz. 66.0
Barbecue beans, see "Baked beans"
Barbecue dip *(Heluva Good)*, 2 tbsp. 2.0
Barbecue sauce, 2 tbsp., except as noted:
(Heinz Thick & Rich) 9.0
(Heinz Thick & Rich Old Fashioned) 10.0
(Hunt's Original) 9.0
(Hunt's Original Light) 6.0
(Hunt's Original Bold) 11.0
(Hunt's Open Range Original) 9.0
(Hunt's Open Range Premier) 13.0
(KC Masterpiece Original) 11.0
(Kraft Char-Grill) 12.0
(Kraft Original) 10.0
(Kraft Original Extra Rich) 12.0
(Kraft Thick'N Spicy Original) 12.0
(Lea & Perrins Original/Bold & Spicy) 13.0
(Maull's) 10.0
(Mississippi) 16.0
(Open Pit Original) 11.0
(Woody's Cook-In') 4.0
all varieties *(Healthy Choice)* 6.0
all varieties *(Stubb's Legendary)* 6.0
Buffalo wing *(Heinz)* 4.0
Cajun *(Luzianne)* 19.0

Dijon, mild *(Hunt's)* 9.0
Dijon and honey *(Lawry's)* 12.0
garlic *(Kraft)* 9.0
garlic and herb *(Lea & Perrins)* 9.0
hickory:
   (Hunt's Bold) 11.0
   (Open Pit) 11.0
   (Open Pit Thick and Tangy) 12.0
hickory and brown sugar *(Hunt's)* 18.0
hickory smoke:
   (Kraft) 10.0
   (Kraft Thick'N Spicy) 12.0
   (Open Pit) 11.0
   hot *(Kraft* Hot) 9.0
   with onion bits *(Kraft)* 11.0
honey:
   (Heinz Thick & Rich) 11.0
   (Kraft) 13.0
   (Kraft Thick'N Spicy) 13.0
honey Dijon *(KC Masterpiece)* 10.0
honey hickory *(Hunt's)* 12.0
honey mustard *(Hunt's)* 11.5
honey and spice *(Open Pit* Thick and Tangy) 11.0
hot *(Kraft)* 9.0
hot *(Open Pit)* 11.0
hot and spicy *(Hunt's)* 11.5
hot and spicy *(Master Choice)*, 1 tbsp. 7.0
Italian *(Porino's)* 7.0
Italian seasonings *(Kraft)* 10.0
jalapeño *(Maull's)* 12.0
Kansas City style:
   (Kraft) 11.0
   (Kraft Thick'N Spicy) 13.0
   (Maull's) 15.0
mesquite:
   (Hunt's) 9.0
   (Open Pit) 11.0
   smoke *(Kraft)* 9.0
   smoke *(Kraft Thick'N Spicy)* 12.0
mild *(Hunt's)* 10.0
onion:
   (Open Pit) 11.0

Barbecue sauce, onion *(cont.)*
   (Open Pit Thick and Tangy) 12.0
   bits *(Kraft)* 11.0
   bits *(Maull's)* 9.0
Oriental *(House of Tsang* Hong Kong), 1 tsp. 2.0
Oriental, pork *(House of Tsang)* 20.0
salsa style *(Kraft)* 9.0
smoky *(Hunt's Open Range)* 9.0
smoky *(Maull's)* 10.0
sweet:
   (Maull's Sweet-N-Mild) 12.0
   (Maull's Sweet-N-Smokey) 13.0
   (Open Pit) 12.0
sweet and sour *(Lawry's)* 20.0
sweet and sour *(Open Pit)* 10.0
teriyaki *(Hunt's)* 11.0
teriyaki *(Kraft)* 12.0
tropical *(World Harbors Maui Mountain)* 17.0
Barbecue seasoning *(Durkee)*, ¼ tsp. 0
Barley:
uncooked, 1 cup 155.5
pearled, uncooked:
   (Arrowhead Mills), ¼ cup 37.0
   (Goya), ¼ cup 24.0
   (Quaker Scotch Quick), ⅓ cup 37.0
   medium *(Quaker* Scotch), ¼ cup 37.0
pearled, cooked, 1 cup 44.3
Barley flakes *(Arrowhead Mills)*, ⅓ cup 28.0
Barley flour *(Arrowhead Mills)*, ¼ cup 19.0
Barley malt syrup *(Eden* Organic), 1 tbsp. 14.0
Barley pilaf mix *(Near East)*, 1 cup* 41.0
Basil:
fresh:
   1 oz. 1.2
   5 medium leaves 1
   chopped, 2 tbsp. 2
dried:
   (McCormick), ¼ tsp. 1
   leaf *(Tone's)*, ¼ tsp. 0
   ground, 1 tbsp. 2.7
   ground, 1 tsp. 9
frozen *(Seabrook)*, 1 tbsp., ¼ oz. 3

Baskin-Robbins:
ice cream, deluxe:

Baby Ruth, ½ cup	18.0
Baby Ruth, regular scoop	32.0
banana nut, ½ cup	15.0
banana nut, regular scoop	26.0
banana strawberry, ½ cup	17.0
banana strawberry, regular scoop	30.0
Baseball nut, ½ cup	16.0
Baseball nut, regular scoop	31.0
black walnut, ½ cup	13.0
black walnut, regular scoop	23.0
blackberry, Oregon, ½ cup	15.0
butter pecan, ½ cup	13.0
butter pecan, regular scoop	23.0
Butterfinger, ½ cup	21.0
Butterfinger, regular scoop	39.0
caramel chocolate crunch, ½ cup	19.0
caramel chocolate crunch, regular scoop	33.0
cheesecake, blueberry, ½ cup	18.0
cheesecake, cherry, ½ cup	20.0
cheesecake, New York, ½ cup	17.0
cheesecake, strawberry, ½ cup	19.0
cheesecake, strawberry, regular scoop	34.0
cherries jubilee, ½ cup	16.0
cherries jubilee, regular scoop	29.0
chocolate, ½ cup	18.0
chocolate, regular scoop	31.0
chocolate, triple passion, ½ cup	21.0
chocolate, triple passion, regular scoop	34.0
chocolate, world class, ½ cup	18.0
chocolate, world class, regular scoop	32.0
chocolate almond, ½ cup	17.0
chocolate almond, regular scoop	30.0
chocolate cake, German, ½ cup	20.0
chocolate chip, ½ cup	15.0
chocolate chip, regular scoop	26.0
chocolate chip cookie dough, ½ cup	20.0
chocolate chip cookie dough, regular scoop	35.0
chocolate fudge, ½ cup	20.0
chocolate fudge, regular scoop	34.0
chocolate mousse royale, ½ cup	20.0

Baskin-Robbins, ice cream, deluxe *(cont.)*

chocolate mousse royale, regular scoop	35.0
chocolate raspberry truffle, ½ cup	20.0
chocolate raspberry truffle, regular scoop	36.0
chocolate ribbon, ½ cup	17.0
chocolate ribbon, regular scoop	30.0
Choc O The Irish, ½ cup	17.0
Choc O The Irish, regular scoop	30.0
Chocoholic's Resolution, ½ cup	21.0
Chocoholic's Resolution, regular scoop	37.0
Chunk A Cherry Burnin' Love, ½ cup	16.0
Chunk A Cherry Burnin' Love, regular scoop	29.0
coconut, ½ cup	14.0
coconut, regular scoop	24.0
coconut, nutty, ½ cup	15.0
coconut, nutty, regular scoop	27.0
cookies 'n cream, ½ cup	16.0
cookies 'n cream, regular scoop	29.0
Everyone's Favorite Candy Bar, ½ cup	22.0
Fudge, Here Comes the, ½ cup	20.0
fudge brownie, ½ cup	19.0
fudge brownie, regular scoop	35.0
gold medal ribbon, ½ cup	20.0
gold medal ribbon, regular scoop	35.0
Heath Bar, ½ cup	19.0
Heath Bar, regular scoop	33.0
jamoca, ½ cup	14.0
jamoca, regular scoop	25.0
jamoca, almond fudge, ½ cup	17.0
jamoca, almond fudge, regular scoop	30.0
Kahlua and chocolate cream, ½ cup	16.0
lemon custard, ½ cup	16.0
lemon custard, regular scoop	29.0
mint, chocolate chip, ½ cup	15.0
mint, chocolate chip, regular scoop	26.0
mint, Martian, ½ cup	19.0
mint, Martian, regular scoop	30.0
Mississippi mudd, ½ cup	22.0
Naughty New Year's Resolution, ½ cup	22.0
Nutty or Nice, ½ cup	20.0
Nutty or Nice, regular scoop	36.0
peach, ½ cup	16.0

peach, regular scoop 28.0
peanut butter, *Reese's*, ½ cup 17.0
peanut butter, *Reese's*, regular scoop 39.0
peanut butter 'n chocolate, ½ cup 16.0
peanut butter 'n chocolate, regular scoop 29.0
pecan caramel fudge, ½ cup 18.0
peppermint, ½ cup 18.0
peppermint, regular scoop 33.0
peppermint, winter wondermint, ½ cup 18.0
peppermint, winter wondermint, regular scoop 33.0
pink bubble gum, ½ cup 19.0
pink bubble gum, regular scoop 34.0
pistachio-almond, ½ cup 13.0
pistachio-almond, regular scoop 23.0
pralines 'n cream, ½ cup 19.0
pralines 'n cream, regular scoop 34.0
pumpkin pie, ½ cup 16.0
Quarterback Crunch, ½ cup 18.0
Quarterback Crunch, regular scoop 32.0
rocky road, ½ cup 19.0
rocky road, regular scoop 34.0
rum raisin, ½ cup 18.0
rum raisin, regular scoop 32.0
S'mores, ½ cup 23.0
S'mores, regular scoop 41.0
strawberry, very berry, ½ cup 16.0
strawberry shortcake, ½ cup 18.0
strawberry shortcake, regular scoop 32.0
toffee, English, ½ cup 19.0
toffee, English, regular scoop 34.0
vanilla, ½ cup 14.0
vanilla, regular scoop 24.0
vanilla, decorating, ½ cup 14.0
vanilla, decorating, regular scoop 24.0
vanilla, French, ½ cup 14.0
vanilla, French, regular scoop 25.0
white chocolate, winter, ½ cup 18.0
white chocolate, winter, regular scoop 31.0
ice cream, light, ½ cup:
  cherry cheesecake 20.0
  chocolate caramel nut 20.0
  espresso 'n cream 18.0

Baskin-Robbins, ice cream, light *(cont.)*
praline dream 18.0
ice cream, fat free, ½ cup:
caramel banana 24.0
cheesecake, berry innocent 24.0
chocolate marshmallow 26.0
chocolate vanilla twist 21.0
jamoca swirl 23.0
soft-serve, caramel praline or vanilla 25.0
ice cream, no sugar added, ½ cup:
berries 'n banana 15.0
Call Me Nuts 19.0
cherry cordial 19.0
jamoca Swiss almond 16.0
Mad About Chocolate 19.0
mint, thin 17.0
raspberry revelation 20.0
ices, sherbets, and sorbets:
daiquiri ice, ½ cup 27.0
daiquiri ice, regular scoop 33.0
grape ice, ½ cup 27.0
mandarin mimosa sorbet, ½ cup 26.0
margarita ice, ½ cup 28.0
The Mask Twist ice, ½ cup 29.0
orange sherbet, ½ cup 26.0
orange sherbet, regular scoop 34.0
peachy keen sorbet, ½ cup 24.0
rainbow sherbet, ½ cup 26.0
rainbow sherbet, regular scoop 34.0
raspberry sherbet, blue, ½ cup 25.0
raspberry sorbet, red, ½ cup 30.0
raspberry sorbet, red, regular scoop 34.0
raspberry-cranberry sorbet, Rudolph's red, ½ cup 30.0
raspberry-cranberry sorbet, Rudolph's red, regular scoop 34.0
raspberry lemonade sorbet, pink, ½ cup 29.0
strawberry island delight ice, ½ cup 26.0
novelties, 1 piece:
Cappy Blast bar, cappuccino 20.0
Cappy Blast bar, mocha cappuccino 21.0
chillyburger, regular or mint chocolate chip 27.0
sundae bar, jamoca almond fudge 28.0
sundae bar, peanut butter chocolate 22.0

sundae bar, pralines 'n cream 28.0
Tiny Toon bar, vanilla 8.0
yogurt, frozen (hard-packed), ½ cup:
brownie madness, Maui, low-fat 26.0
Caramelcopia 29.0
Have Your Cake, low-fat 22.0
Jumpin' Java Bean, nonfat 25.0
Last Mango In Paradise, nonfat 28.0
Praline, Perils of, low-fat 25.0
raspberry cheese Louise, low-fat 24.0
yogurt, frozen, low-fat, ½ cup:
blueberry 24.0
cheesecake 21.0
chocolate 23.0
vanilla 22.0
yogurt, frozen, nonfat, ½ cup:
black cherry 24.0
chocolate, Dutch 23.0
coconut 24.0
kahlua 21.0
maple walnut 22.0
peach 22.0
peppermint twist 22.0
piña colada 22.0
raspberry 22.0
strawberry 23.0
vanilla 16.0
yogurt, frozen, nonfat, reduced sugar, ½ cup:
apple pie 18.0
berry delight, triple 17.0
butter pecan 17.0
cafe mocha 17.0
cherry, wild 17.0
chocolate 15.0
strawberry patch 17.0
tropical 17.0
vanilla 18.0
Whata Banana 15.0
fountain drinks, 1 serving, except as noted:
blueberry strawberry smoothie 31.0
Cappy Blast 22.0
Capply Blast, nonfat 20.0

Baskin-Robbins, fountain drinks *(cont.)*
  chocolate, *Cappy Blast* 46.0
  chocolate, low-fat, *Cappy Blast*. 40.0
  chocolate shake, vanilla ice cream 64.0
  malt powder, 1 oz. 23.0
  orange banana smoothie 24.0
  piña colada, *Paradise Blast* 33.0
  piña colada, nonfat, *Paradise Blast* 31.0
  strawberry banana smoothie 39.0
  strawberry luau, *Paradise Blast* 32.0
  strawberry luau, low-fat, *Paradise Blast* 30.0
cones, 1 piece:
  cake cone. 4.0
  sugar cone 7.0
  waffle cone, large 14.0
  waffle cone, fresh baked 30.0
toppings:
  butterscotch, 2 oz. 47.0
  chocolate syrup, 2 tbsp. 22.0
  gummy bears, baby, 75 pieces 30.0
  hot fudge, 1 oz. 17.0
  hot fudge, no sugar added, 1 oz. 20.0
  praline caramel, 1 oz. 19.0
  sprinkles, 1/6 oz. 3.0
  strawberry, 1 oz. 14.0
  whipped cream, Rod's, 2 tsp. 1.0
Bass, all varieties, without added ingredients 0
Batter, seasoning *(House of Tsang Cantonese),* 4 tbsp. 29.0
Bay leaf, dried:
(McCormick), 1 leaf 1
(Tone's), 2 leaves 0
crumbled, 1 tbsp. 1.4
crumbled, 1 tsp. 3
Bean dip, 2 tbsp.:
(Chi-Chi's Fiesta) 4.0
(Frito-Lay) 6.0
(Marie's Fiesta) 2.0
(Old Dutch) 5.0
black bean *(Old El Paso)* 4.0
black bean, spicy *(Guiltless Gourmet)* 5.0
jalapeño *(Frito-Lay)* 5.0
pinto, spicy *(Guiltless Gourmet)* 6.0

Bean dip mix, black or Mexican *(Knorr),* 1 tsp. 2.0
Bean dishes, canned, see specific bean listings
Bean dishes, mix (see also specific bean listings):
Florentine, with bow ties *(Bean Cuisine),* ½ cup* 27.0
French, country, with gemelli *(Bean Cuisine),* ½ cup* 27.0
Italian *(Knorr Cup),* 1 pkg. 50.0
Bean entree, frozen, white, Parisian:
(Weight Watchers International Selections), 9.87-oz. pkg. . . 23.0
Bean loaf, frozen *(Natural Touch),* 1″ slice 13.0
Bean salad:
deli style *(S&W),* ½ cup 20.0
marinated *(S&W),* ½ cup 16.0
three:
  (Green Giant), ½ cup 20.0
  (Hanover), ⅓ cup 22.0
  (Seneca), ⅓ cup 13.0
Bean sauce, brown, spicy *(House of Tsang),* 1 tsp. 3.0
Bean sprouts (see also "Sprouts" and specific listings):
fresh *(Frieda's),* 1 oz. 1.9
canned *(Chun King),* 1 cup 1.5
canned *(La Choy),* 1 cup 1.0
Beans, see specific listings
Beans, mixed, canned *(Stokely* Chulent), ½ cup 19.0
Beans, refried, see "Refried beans"
Beans, snap or string, see "Green beans"
Beans and franks, 1 cup, except as noted:
(Hormel), 7½ oz. 32.0
(Kid's Kitchen), 7½ oz. 37.0
(Libby's Diner), 7¾ oz. 36.0
(Van Camp's Beanee Weenee Microwave) 29.0
(Van Camp's Beanee Weenee Original Large) 35.0
(Van Camp's Beanee Weenee Original Single Serve) 30.0
(Van Camp's Beanee Weenee Original Small) 40.0
baked *(Van Camp's Beanee Weenee)* 58.0
baked *(Van Camp's Beanee Weenee* Single Serve) 49.0
barbecue *(Van Camp's Beanee Weenee)* 36.0
chili *(Van Camp's Beanee Weenee* Chilee) 27.0
zesty *(Van Camp's Beanee Weenee)* 40.0
Beans and rice, see "Rice dishes, mix"
Béarnaise sauce mix *(Knorr),* 1/10 pkg. 2.0
Beechnut, dried:
in shell, 1 lb. 92.7

Beechnut *(cont.)*

shelled, 1 oz. 9.5

Beef, all cuts, without added ingredients 0

Beef, canned (see also "Beef entree, canned" and specific listings):

corned, 2 oz. 0

roast, with gravy *(Hormel)*, 2 oz. 1.0

roast, with gravy *(Libby's)*, ²/₃ cup 2.0

Beef, corned (see also "Beef, canned" and "Beef lunch meat"), brisket, cooked, 4 oz. 5

Beef, dried:

cured, 1 oz. 4

sliced *(Hormel)*, 1 oz. 1.0

sliced *(Hormel* 2.5-oz. pkg.), 1 oz. 1.0

Beef, frozen:

ground, patty, 1 patty:

    80% lean *(Schwan's)*, 4 oz. 0

    90% lean *(Schwan's)*, 3.75 oz. 0

    melt *(Schwan's)*, 4 oz. 4.0

    pizza *(Schwan's)*, 3.3 oz. 3.0

sirloin tips *(Schwan's)*, 4 oz. 2.0

steak:

    (Schwan's Big Sam), 6 oz. 1.0

    chopped *(Schwan's)*, 5.3-oz. piece 0

    cubed, breaded *(Schwan's)*, 4 oz. 10.0

    sirloin, top *(Schwan's)*, 9.3 oz. 0

    sirloin, tri tip *(Schwan's)*, 5 oz. 0

    sirloin ball tip *(Schwan's)*, 6 oz. 0

    sirloin filet *(Schwan's)*, 4 oz. 2.0

Beef, refrigerated:

ribeye, salted *(Hebrew National)*, 4 oz. 0

sliced, barbecue sauce with *(Lloyd's)*, ¼ cup 9.0

"Beef," vegetarian:

burger, see " 'Hamburger,' vegetarian"

canned:

    (Worthington Savory Slices), 3 slices 6.0

    (Worthington Prime Stakes), 1 piece 4.0

    (Worthington Vegetable Steaks), 2 slices 3.0

    stew *(Worthington* Country), 1 cup 20.0

frozen:

    (Worthington Meatless), ³/₈" slice 4.0

corned *(Worthington* Slices), 4 slices 5.0
smoked *(Worthington* Sliced), 6 slices 6.0
Beef dinner, frozen:
barbecue, mesquite *(Healthy Choice)*, 11 oz. 38.0
and broccoli:
   (Swanson), 1 pkg. 51.0
   (Swanson Hungry Man), 1 pkg. 73.0
   Beijing *(Healthy Choice)*, 12 oz. 45.0
chicken fried steak:
   (Banquet Extra Helping), 18.65 oz. 73.0
   (Marie Callender's), 15 oz. 69.0
   with gravy *(Swanson)*, 1 pkg. 44.0
and gravy *(Swanson)*, 1 pkg. 37.0
patty, charbroiled *(Freezer Queen* Meal), 9.5 oz. 17.0
and peppers Cantonese *(Healthy Choice)*, 11.5 oz. 32.0
pot roast:
   (Freezer Queen Meal), 9.2 oz. 20.0
   homestyle *(Schwan's)*, 1 pkg. 43.0
   Yankee *(The Budget Gourmet)*, 11 oz. 32.0
   Yankee *(Healthy Choice)*, 11 oz. 48.0
   Yankee *(Swanson)*, 1 pkg. 36.0
   Yankee *(Swanson Hungry Man)*, 1 pkg. 47.0
roast beef sandwich, smothered *(Swanson)*, 1 pkg. 46.0
Salisbury steak:
   (Banquet Extra Helping), 19 oz. 52.0
   (Freezer Queen Meal), 9.5 oz. 19.0
   (Healthy Choice), 11.5 oz. 48.0
   (Swanson), 1 pkg. 40.0
   (Swanson Hungry Man), 1 pkg. 45.0
   con queso *(Patio)*, 11 oz. 33.0
   sirloin *(The Budget Gourmet)*, 11 oz. 34.0
sirloin:
   (The Budget Gourmet Special Recipe), 11 oz. 36.0
   chopped, with gravy *(Swanson)*, 1 pkg. 34.0
   meatballs and gravy *(The Budget Gourmet)*, 11 oz. 35.0
   tips *(Swanson Hungry Man)*, 1 pkg. 49.0
   tips, with noodles *(Swanson)*, 1 pkg. 32.0
   in wine sauce *(The Budget Gourmet)*, 11 oz. 32.0
sliced, gravy and *(Freezer Queen* Meal), 9 oz. 18.0
steak patty, charbroiled *(Healthy Choice)*, 11 oz. 41.0
Stroganoff *(Healthy Choice)*, 11 oz. 44.0
teriyaki *(The Budget Gourmet)*, 11 oz. 53.0

Beef dinner *(cont.)*
teriyaki *(Schwan's)*, 10 oz. 63.0
tips *(Healthy Choice)*, 11¼ oz. 32.0
Beef entree, canned:
chow mein *(Chun King/La Choy* Bi-Pack), 1 cup 11.0
goulash *(Hormel)*, 7.5-oz. can 19.0
hash, see "Beef hash"
pepper, Oriental *(Chun King/La Choy* Bi-Pack), 1 cup 13.0
pepper, Oriental, with noodles *(La Choy* Bi-Pack), 1 cup . . . 17.5
pot roast *(Dinty Moore American Classics)*, 10 oz. 22.0
roast, with mashed potato *(Dinty Moore American·Classics)*,
    10 oz. 25.0
Salisbury steak *(Dinty Moore American Classics)*, 10 oz. . . . 22.0
stew:
    (Dinty Moore), 1 cup 16.0
    (Dinty Moore Can/Cup), 7.5 oz. 15.0
    (Dinty Moore American Classics), 10 oz. 21.0
    (Hormel Micro Cup), 7.5 oz. 15.0
    (Hunt's Homestyle), 1 cup 20.0
    (Libby's Diner), 7¾ oz. 19.0
    (Nalley), 7.5 oz. 18.0
    (Nalley Big Chunk), 1 cup 25.0
    (Nalley Homestyle), 1 cup 18.0
    burger *(Dinty Moore* Hearty Cup), 7.5 oz. 19.0
Beef entree, freeze-dried, 1 cup:
    peppers, onions, rice *(Mountain House)*. 32.0
stew *(Mountain House)* 24.0
Stroganoff, with noodles *(Mountain House)*. 28.0
teriyaki, with rice *(Mountain House)* 42.0
Beef entree, frozen:
casserole *(Schwan's)*, 1 cup. 34.0
chipped:
    (Banquet Topper), 4-oz. bag 8.0
    creamed *(Freezer Queen* Cook-in-Pouch), 4-oz. pkg. . . . 8.0
    creamed *(Schwan's)*, 1 cup 21.0
    creamed *(Stouffer's)*, 4.4 oz. 6.0
chopped, barbecue *(Schwan's* BBQ), ½ cup 17.0
enchilada, see "Enchilada entree"
goulash *(Schwan's)*, 1 cup 31.0
ground, with rice *(Goya)*, 1 pkg. 111.0
macaroni *(Healthy Choice)*, 8.5 oz. 34.0
mesquite, with rice *(Lean Cuisine* Cafe Classics), 9 oz. 38.0

noodles with *(Freezer Queen* Family), 1 cup, 8.5 oz. 26.0
Oriental *(The Budget Gourmet* Light), 9 oz. 31.0
Oriental *(Lean Cuisine)*, 9¼ oz. 33.0
patty:
    (Swanson Fun Feast), 1 pkg. 54.0
    charbroiled, gravy and *(Morton)*, 1 pkg. 25.0
    charbroiled, mushroom gravy and *(Freezer Queen*
      Family), ⅙ of 28-oz. pkg. 5.0
    gravy and *(Banquet* Homestyle), 9.5 oz. 21.0
    mushroom *(Banquet* Family), 1 patty, 4.7 oz. 7.0
    onion gravy and *(Banquet* Family), 1 patty, 4.7 oz. 7.0
    onion gravy and *(Freezer Queen* Family),
      ¼ of 28-oz. pkg. 6.0
and peppers, with rice *(Freezer Queen* Homestyle), 9 oz. . . . 30.0
pepper, Oriental *(La Choy)*, 1 cup, 7.4 oz. 29.5
pepper steak:
    (The Budget Gourmet), 10 oz. 39.0
    (Stouffer's), 10½ oz. 45.0
    (Weight Watchers), 10 oz. 33.0
    Oriental *(Healthy Choice)*, 9.5 oz. 34.0
pie or potpie:
    (Banquet), 7-oz. pie 38.0
    (Stouffer's), 10-oz. pie 36.0
    (Swanson), 1 pkg. 39.0
    (Swanson Hungry Man), 1 pkg. 71.0
    Yankee *(Marie Callender's)*, 10 oz. 57.0
    Yankee *(Marie Callender's)*, 1 cup, 7.5 oz. 53.0
pot roast:
    (Freezer Queen Deluxe Family), 1 cup, 8.5 oz. 20.0
    (Freezer Queen Homestyle), 9 oz. 20.0
    and gravy *(Marie Callender's)*, 1 cup 21.0
    with potatoes *(Lean Cuisine)*, 9 oz. 22.0
    with potatoes *(Stouffer's* Homestyle), 8⅞ oz. 29.0
roast *(Healthy Choice* Hearty Handfuls), 6.1 oz. 52.0
Salisbury steak:
    (Banquet Homestyle), 9.5 oz. 28.0
    gravy and *(Banquet* Family), 1 patty, 4.7 oz. 7.0
    gravy and *(Banquet* Toppers), 5-oz. bag 8.0
    gravy and *(Freezer Queen* Cook-in-Pouch), 5-oz. pkg. . . . 8.0
    gravy and *(Freezer Queen* Family), ⅙ of 28-oz. pkg. 4.0
    gravy and *(Morton)*, 1 pkg. 23.0
    gravy, mashed potato *(Swanson)*, 1 pkg. 23.0

Beef entree, frozen, Salisbury steak *(cont.)*

gravy and whipped potatoes *(Freezer Queen* Homestyle),
9 oz. 21.0

grilled *(Weight Watchers),* 8.5 oz. 24.0

sirloin *(The Budget Gourmet* Light), 9 oz. 28.0

with macaroni and cheese *(Lean Cuisine),* 9.5 oz. 28.0

with macaroni and cheese *(Stouffer's* Homestyle),
9⅝ oz. 27.0

sandwich, see "Beef sandwich"

shepherd's pie *(Schwan's),* 1 cup 22.0

shredded, with rice *(Goya),* 1 pkg. 118.0

sirloin:

cheddar melt *(The Budget Gourmet),* 9.4 oz. 29.0

in herb sauce *(The Budget Gourmet* Light), 9.5 oz. . . . 30.0

peppercorn *(Lean Cuisine* Cafe Classics), 8¾ oz. 25.0

roast supreme *(The Budget Gourmet),* 9 oz. 32.0

tips, and noodles *(Swanson),* 1 pkg. 20.0

tips, with vegetables *(The Budget Gourmet),* 10 oz. . . . 20.0

sliced:

(Banquet Country), 9 oz. 19.0

gravy and *(Banquet* Family), 2 slices, 5.6 oz. 7.0

gravy and *(Banquet* Topper), 4-oz. bag 5.0

gravy and *(Freezer Queen* Cook-in-Pouch), 4-oz. pkg. . . . 5.0

gravy and *(Freezer Queen* Family), ⅔ cup, 4.9 oz. 7.9

steak, chicken fried *(Banquet* Country), 10 oz. 39.0

steak, Philly *(Healthy Choice* Hearty Handfuls), 6.1 oz. 47.0

steak patty, grilled peppercorn *(Healthy Choice),* 9 oz. 26.0

stew:

(Banquet Family), 1 cup, 8.7 oz. 17.0

(Freezer Queen Family), 1 cup, 8.6 oz. 21.0

with rice *(Goya),* 1 pkg. 117.0

Stroganoff:

(The Budget Gourmet Light), 8.75 oz. 32.0

(Stouffer's), 9¾ oz. 30.0

and noodles *(Marie Callender's),* 1 cup 23.0

tips, Français *(Healthy Choice),* 9.5 oz. 40.0

tips and gravy *(Schwan's),* 1 cup 9.0

Beef entree mix:

pepper steak *(Chun King/La Choy* Dinner Classics), ⅕ pkg. . 7.0

Stroganoff *(Dinner Sensations),* 1 cup 27.0

Stroganoff *(Dinner Sensations),* 1 cup* 28.0

teriyaki *(Dinner Sensations),* ½ cup or 1 cup* 38.0

Beef entree mix, frozen, see "Entree mix, frozen"
Beef gravy, ¼ cup:
(Franco-American) 4.0
hearty *(Pepperidge Farm)* 4.0
savory *(Heinz Home Style)* 2.0
Beef hash, canned, 1 cup, except as noted:
(Broadcast Morning Classics Original) 22.0
corned beef:
    (Castleberry's) 25.0
    (Dinty Moore Cup), 7.5 oz. 19.0
    (Goya) 20.0
    (Libby's) 26.0
    (Mary Kitchen) 22.0
    (Mary Kitchen), 7.5 oz. 22.0
    (Nalley) 26.0
roast beef:
    (Libby's) 23.0
    (Mary Kitchen) 22.0
    (Mary Kitchen), 7.5 oz. 21.0
sausage flavor *(Broadcast Morning Classics)* 22.0
Beef hash, refrigerated, corned *(Jones Dairy Farm),* 2 oz. . 7.0
Beef jerky, see "Sausage stick"
Beef lunch meat (see also "Bologna," etc.), 2 oz., except as
    noted:
all varieties *(Boar's Head)* 0
all varieties *(Hormel/Hormel Light & Lean 97)* 0
corned, cooked *(Hebrew National)* 0
corned, round *(Healthy Deli)* 2.0
roast:
    (Oscar Mayer Deli-Thin), 4 slices, 1.8 oz. 1.0
    Italian *(Healthy Deli)* 1.0
    seasoned *(Healthy Deli)* 0
Beef pie, see "Beef entree, frozen"
Beef sandwich, frozen, 1 piece, except as noted:
barbecue *(Hormel Quick Meal)* 39.0
barbecue *(Hot Pockets),* 4.5-oz. piece 45.0
cheddar *(Hot Pockets),* 4.5-oz. piece 36.0
cheeseburger:
    (Hormel Quick Meal) 35.0
    (Micromagic), 4.2-oz. piece 33.0
    (White Castle), 2 pieces, 3.67 oz. 23.0
    bacon *(Hormel Quick Meal)* 34.0

Beef sandwich, cheeseburger *(cont.)*

    bacon *(Micromagic)*, 4-oz. piece 39.0

    chili *(Hormel Quick Meal)* 39.0

  fajita *(Hot Pockets)*, 4.5-oz. piece 39.0

  hamburger *(Hormel Quick Meal)* 34.0

  hamburger *(White Castle)*, 2 pieces, 3.17 oz. 23.0

  patty, with cheese *(Kid Cuisine Buckaroo)*, 8.5 oz. 58.0

  steak:

    biscuit *(Hormel Quick Meal)* 36.0

    cheese *(Deli Stuffs)*, 4.5-oz. piece 40.0

    mushroom *(Mrs. Paterson's Aussie Pie)* 39.0

    Philly, and cheese *(Croissant Pockets)*, 4.5-oz. piece . . . 40.0

Beef sauce, see "Steak sauce" and specific listings

Beef seasoning mix (see also specific listings):

ground *(Durkee Pouch)*, 1/4 pkg. 5.0

marinade *(Durkee Pouch)*, 1/10 pkg. 5

marinade *(Lawry's)*, 3/4 tsp. 1.0

Beef seasoning and coating mix:

pot roast *(McCormick Bag 'n Season)*, 1 tbsp. 1.0

spareribs *(McCormick Bag 'n Season)*, 1 tbsp. 6.0

Swiss steak *(McCormick Bag 'n Season)*, 1 tsp. 3.0

Beef spread, roast *(Underwood)*, 1/4 cup 0

Beef stew, see "Beef entree"

Beef stew seasoning:

(Adolph's Meal Makers), 1 tbsp. 4.0

(Durkee), 1/9 pkg. 3.0

(Durkee Roasting Bag), 1/10 pkg. 3.0

(Lawry's), 2 tsp. 5.0

Beer, 12 fl. oz.:

regular 13.2

light 4.8

Beet, fresh:

raw:

  untrimmed, 1 lb. 30.4

  2 medium, 2″ diam., approx. 8.6 oz. 15.6

  trimmed, sliced, 1/2 cup 6.5

boiled, drained, 2 medium, 2″ diam., approx. 3.5 oz. 10.0

boiled, drained, sliced, 1/2 cup 8.5

Beet, canned, 1/2 cup, except as noted:

all varieties, except Harvard *(Green Giant/Green Giant No
Salt)* 8.0

all varieties, except Harvard and pickled *(Seneca)* 7.0

whole:
- *(Stokely)*, 4.5 oz. 8.0
- baby *(LeSueur)* 8.0
- or sliced *(Del Monte)* 8.0
- sliced or julienne *(S&W)* 7.0

sliced *(Goya)* 9.0
sliced *(Stokely)* 8.0

Harvard:
- *(Green Giant)*, 1/3 cup 15.0
- *(Greenwood)* 27.0
- *(Seneca)* 21.0
- *(Stokely)*, 1/3 cup 19.0

pickled:
- *(S&W)*, 1 oz. 4.0
- *(Stokely* Can/Jar), 1 oz. 5.0
- all varieties *(Greenwood)*, 1.06 oz. 6.0
- all varieties *(Seneca)*, 2 tbsp. 4.0
- crinkle *(Del Monte)* 19.0

Beet greens, fresh:
raw, untrimmed, 1 lb. 10.1
raw, 1″ pieces, 1/2 cup 8
boiled, drained, 1″ pieces, 1 cup 3.9
Berliner, pork and beef, 1 oz. 7
Berries, mixed, frozen *(Big Valley* Burst O' Berries), 3/4 cup   16.0
Berry drink, 8 fl. oz., except as noted:
(After the Fall Oregon) 25.0
(Capri Sun Yo Yogi Berry), 6.75 fl. oz. 27.0
(Hi-C Boppin') 32.0
(Hi-C Boppin' Box) 34.0
(R.W. Knudsen Razzleberry) 33.0
(R.W. Knudsen Razzleberry Aseptic) 29.0
citrus *(Five Alive)* 30.0
nectar *(Santa Cruz)* 27.0

punch:
- *(Minute Maid)* 32.0
- *(Minute Maid* Box) 33.0
- *(Tropicana)* 32.0
- red *(Tree Top Juice Rivers* Box), 8.45 fl. oz. 31.0

frozen* *(Minute Maid* Punch) 31.0
Berry juice, 8 fl. oz.:
(Apple & Eve Nothin' But Juice) 29.0
(Ceres Youngberry) 30.0

Berry juice *(cont.)*
(*Heinke's* Berry Patch) 30.0
(*Juicy Juice*) 31.0
(*Veryfine* Juice-Ups) 34.0
Biryani paste *(Patak's),* 2 tbsp. 4.0
Biscuit, 1 piece, except as noted:
(*Arnold* Old Fashioned), 2 pieces 18.0
(*Awrey's* Country) 21.0
(*Awrey's* Round), 1 oz. 10.0
(*Awrey's* Round), 2 oz. 22.0
(*Awrey's* Round), 3 oz. 35.0
Biscuit, frozen, 1 piece:
cinnamon raisin, iced *(Schwan's)* 41.0
garlic and cheese *(Pepperidge Farm)* 24.0
Biscuit, refrigerated, 1 piece, except as noted:
(*Ballard Extra Lights Ovenready*), 3 pieces 29.0
(*Big Country Butter Tastin'*) 13.0
(*Grands! Butter Tastin'*) 23.0
(*Grands! Butter Tastin'* Reduced Fat) 27.0
(*Grands!* Homestyle) 24.0
baking powder *(1869 Brand)* 12.0
buttermilk:
   (*Ballard Extra Lights Ovenready*), 3 pieces 29.0
   (*Big Country*) 14.0
   (*1869 Brand*) 12.0
   (*Grands!*) 23.0
   (*Grands!* Reduced Fat) 27.0
cinnamon raisin *(Grands!)* 28.0
flaky *(Grands!)* 24.0
fluffy, extra *(Grands!)* 24.0
rich, extra *(Grands!)* 25.0
Southern style *(Big Country)* 14.0
Southern style *(Grands!)* 23.0
Biscuit mix:
(*Arrowhead Mills*), ¼ cup 23.0
(*Bisquick*), ⅓ cup 25.0
(*Bisquick* Reduced Fat), ⅓ cup 28.0
(*Gold Medal* Biscuit Mix), ⅓ cup 26.0
(*Gold Medal* Biscuit Mix), 2 biscuits* 27.0
buttermilk:
   (*Gladiola* Biscuit Mix), ⅓ cup 23.0
   (*Gladiola* Biscuit Mix), ⅓ cup* 24.0

   (Martha White Bismix), ½ cup 22.0
   (Martha White Bismix), ½ cup* 23.0
Biscuit sandwich, see "Sausage biscuit"
Bitter melon, see "Balsam pear"
Black beans:
canned, ½ cup:
   (Eden Organic) 18.0
   (Goya) 19.0
   (Green Giant/Joan of Arc) 18.0
   (Old El Paso) 17.0
   (Progresso) 17.0
   (S&W/S&W 50% Less Salt) 17.0
   (Stokely) 19.0
   (Sun-Vista) 20.0
   with ginger and lemon *(Eden* Organic) 21.0
   refried, see "Refried beans"
   seasoned *(Allens/Trappey's)* 20.0
dried:
   (Frieda's), ⅓ cup, 3 oz. 20.0
   (Goya), ¼ cup 23.0
   boiled, ½ cup 20.4
turtle soup, dried:
   (Arrowhead Mills), ¼ cup 28.0
   uncooked, ½ cup 58.2
   boiled, ½ cup 22.4
Black bean dip, see "Bean dip"
Black bean dishes, mix:
with fusilli *(Bean Cuisine)*, ½ cup* 27.0
Jamaican, and brown rice *(Fantastic* One Pot Meals), ⅜ cup 32.0
rice and, see "Rice dishes, mix"
zesty, and penne *(Fantastic* One Pot Meals), ⅜ cup 31.0
Black bean mix, instant *(Fantastic)*, ½ cup* 29.0
Black bean sauce, 1 tbsp.:
(Ka•Me) 2.0
garlic *(Lee Kum Kee)* 3.0
Blackberry:
fresh, trimmed, ½ cup 9.2
canned, ½ cup, except as noted:
   (Allens/Wolco), ⅔ cup 13.0
   in syrup *(Oregon)* 30.0
   in heavy syrup 29.6
   in heavy syrup *(Comstock)* 26.0

Blackberry *(cont.)*
frozen:
    (Schwan's), 1¼ cups 12.0
    (Stilwell), 1 cup 22.0
    unsweetened, ½ cup 11.8
Blackberry syrup *(Knott's Berry Farm)*, 2 tbsp. 30.0
Black-eyed peas, ½ cup:
fresh, see "Cowpeas"
canned, fresh shell:
    (Allens/East Texas Fair/Homefolks) 21.0
    (Goya Cowpeas*)* 17.0
    (Green Giant/Joan of Arc) 16.0
    (Stokely) 19.0
    (Sun-Vista) 15.0
    with jalapeños *(Homefolks)* 20.0
    with jalapeños *(Stubb's Harvest)* 20.0
    with snaps *(Allens/East Texas Fair/Homefolks)* 20.0
canned, dry:
    (Allens/East Texas Fair) 18.0
    with bacon *(Allens)* 20.0
    with bacon *(Trappey's)* 19.0
    with bacon and jalapeños *(Trappey's)* 19.0
frozen *(Stilwell)* 21.0
Blintz, frozen, 2 pieces:
apple *(Empire* Kosher*)* 36.0
blueberry *(Empire* Kosher*)* 36.0
cheese *(Empire* Kosher*)* 29.0
cherry *(Empire* Kosher*)* 38.0
potato *(Empire* Kosher*)* 32.0
Blood sausage, 1 oz. 4
Bloody Mary mixer:
(Mr & Mrs T), 8 fl. oz. 9.0
(V-8), 11.5 fl. oz. 13.0
rich and spicy *(Mr & Mrs T)*, 8 fl. oz. 12.0
Blue hake, frozen, loins *(Schwan's)*, 4 oz. 0
Blue hake entree, frozen, breaded *(Schwan's)*, 1 piece,
    3 oz. 9.0
Blue squash, Australian *(Frieda's)*, ¾ cup, 3 oz. 7.0
Blueberry:
fresh *(Diamond Blues)*, 1 dry pint, 5 oz. 19.0
fresh, ½ cup 10.2

canned, ½ cup, except as noted:

   in syrup *(Oregon)* 26.0

   in heavy syrup *(Comstock)* 26.0

   in heavy syrup *(Lucky Leaf/Musselman's)* 29.0

   in heavy syrup *(S&W* Wild Maine), ⅓ cup 16.0

dried *(Frieda's)*, ¼ cup, 1.4 oz. 33.0

dried *(Sonoma)*, ¼ cup 33.0

freeze-dried *(AlpineAire)*, 1 oz. 15.0

frozen:

   (Cascadian Farm Organic), 1 cup 12.0

   (Schwan's), ⅔ cup 17.0

   (Stilwell), 1 cup 21.0

   unsweetened, ½ cup 9.4

   sweetened, ½ cup 25.2

Blueberry juice *(After the Fall)*, 8 fl. oz. 25.0

Blueberry syrup:

(Knott's Berry Farm), 2 tbsp. 30.0

(R.W. Knudsen), ¼ cup 38.0

(S&W Reduced Cal), ¼ cup 15.0

Bluefish, without added ingredients 0

Boar, wild, without added ingredients 0

Bockwurst, raw, 1 oz. 1

Bok choy, see "Cabbage, Chinese"

Bologna (see also "Ham bologna," etc.), 2 oz., except as
  noted:

(Healthy Deli Regular/German 95% Fat Free) 3.0

(John Morrell) 4.0

(Oscar Mayer), 1-oz. slice 1.0

(Oscar Mayer Fat Free/Light), 1-oz. slice 2.0

(Oscar Mayer Wisconsin Ring) 2.0

all varieties *(Boar's Head/Boar's Head* 28% Lower Sodium) .. 0

beef:

   (Hebrew National/Hebrew National Lean) 0

   (Hebrew National Reduced Fat) 2.0

   (Oscar Mayer), 1-oz. slice 1.0

   (Oscar Mayer Light), 1-oz. slice 2.0

garlic *(Oscar Mayer)*, 1.5-oz. slice 1.0

"Bologna," vegetarian, frozen *(Worthington Bolono)*,
  3 slices 2.0

Bonito, meat only, raw, 4 oz. 5

Boston Market, 1 serving:
entrees:
    chicken, half, with skin 2.0
    chicken, quarter, dark meat, no skin 1.0
    chicken, quarter, dark meat, with skin 2.0
    chicken, quarter, white meat, no skin or wing 0
    chicken, quarter, white meat, with skin 2.0
    chicken potpie 78.0
    ham, with cinnamon apples 35.0
    meat loaf, and gravy 19.0
    meat loaf, and tomato sauce 32.0
    turkey breast, skinless 1.0
sandwiches:
    chicken 61.0
    chicken, with cheese and sauce 71.0
    chicken salad 63.0
    ham 66.0
    ham, with cheese and sauce 71.0
    ham and turkey club 64.0
    ham and turkey club, with cheese and sauce 79.0
    meat loaf 86.0
    meat loaf, with cheese 95.0
    turkey 61.0
    turkey, with cheese and sauce 68.0
salads:
    Caesar, 10 oz. 16.0
    Caesar, without dressing, 8 oz. 14.0
    Caesar, 4 oz. 6.0
    Caesar, chicken 16.0
    chicken, chunky 3.0
    coleslaw 32.0
    fruit[1] 17.0
    pasta, Mediterranean 16.0
    tortellini 29.0
side dishes, soup, and bread:
    apples, cinnamon 56.0
    baked beans, BBQ 53.0
    corn, buttered 39.0
    corn bread 33.0
    cranberry relish 84.0

[1]*Average; recipes vary from restaurant to restaurant.*

gravy, chicken, 1 oz. 2.0
macaroni and cheese 36.0
potatoes, mashed 25.0
potatoes, mashed, with gravy 27.0
potatoes, new 25.0
rice pilaf 32.0
soup, chicken 4.0
soup, chicken tortilla 19.0
spinach, creamed 13.0
squash, butternut 25.0
stuffing 44.0
vegetables, steamed 7.0
zucchini 10.0
desserts:
brownie 47.0
chocolate chip cookie 48.0
oatmeal raisin cookie 48.0
Bouillabaisse seasoning mix *(Knorr* Recipe), 1 tbsp. 3.0
Bouillon (see also "Broth concentrate"), 1 tsp., cube,
or pkt., except as noted:
beef *(Herb-Ox* Instant) 1.0
beef or chicken:
(Herb-Ox) 1.0
(Knorr) . . . . <1.0
(MBT/Wyler's Instant) 2.0
(MBT/Wyler's Low Sodium) 3.0
(Weight Watchers Instant) 2.0
(Wyler's/Steero/Steero Reduced Sodium) 1.0
chicken *(Herb-Ox* Instant) 0
fish *(Knorr)*, ½ cube 0
onion *(MBT* Instant) 3.0
vegetable:
(Herb-Ox) 0
(MBT Instant) 2.0
(Wyler's) 1.0
vegetarian *(Knorr)*, ½ cube 1.0
Bourguignonne seasoning *(Knorr)*, 1 tbsp. 6.0
Bow-tie dishes, mix:
and beans, with herb sauce *(Knorr)*, ⅔ cup 47.0
chicken primavera *(Lipton* Pasta & Sauce), ¾ cup 40.0
chicken primavera *(Lipton* Pasta & Sauce), 1 cup* 43.0
Italian cheese *(Lipton* Pasta & Sauce), ¾ cup 38.0

Bow-tie dishes, mix *(cont.)*
Italian cheese *(Lipton Pasta & Sauce)*, 1 cup* 41.0
Bow-tie entree, frozen:
and chicken *(Lean Cuisine Cafe Classics)*, 9.5 oz. 35.0
and creamy tomato sauce *(Lean Cuisine Lunch Classics)*,
   9.5 oz. 47.0
mushrooms Marsala *(Weight Watchers* International
   Selections)*, 9.65 oz. 36.0
Boysenberry, ½ cup:
fresh, see "Blackberry"
canned in heavy syrup *(Comstock)* 28.0
canned in heavy syrup 28.6
frozen, unsweetened 8.1
Boysenberry drink, 8 fl. oz.:
(Farmer's Market) 30.0
cider *(Heinke's)* 30.0
Boysenberry syrup *(Knott's Berry Farm)*, 2 tbsp. 30.0
Bran, see "Cereal" and specific grains
Bratwurst:
(Boar's Head), 4 oz. 0
(Jones Dairy Farm Dinner), 1 cooked link 0
(Schwan's), 3-oz. link 2.0
pork, cooked, 1 oz. 6
Braunschweiger, 2 oz., except as noted:
(Jones Dairy Farm Chub/Chunk) 1.0
(Oscar Mayer), 1-oz. slice 1.0
light *(Boar's Head)* 0
light *(Jones Dairy Farm* Chub/Chunk) 1.0
sliced *(Jones Dairy Farm)*, 1.2-oz. slice 1.0
sliced *(Jones Dairy Farm)*, 2 slices, 1.6 oz. 1.0
spread *(Oscar Mayer)* 1.0
with bacon *(Jones Dairy Farm* Chub) 1.0
with onion *(Jones Dairy Farm* Chub) 2.0
Brazil nuts:
in shell, 1 lb. 27.9
shelled, 1 oz., 6 large or 8 medium kernels 3.6
Bread, 1 slice, except as noted:
(Arnold/Arnold Bran'nola Country) 18.0
(Brownberry Bran'nola Original) 18.0
(Merita Autumn Grain) 14.0
apple honey wheat *(Brownberry)* 12.0
apple walnut *(Pepperidge Farm)* 14.0

bran:

    honey *(Pepperidge Farm)* 17.0

    light *(August Bros./Brownberry Bakery* Country), 2 slices 21.0

    whole *(Brownberry)* 12.0

buttermilk *(Arnold)* 18.0

cinnamon *(Brownberry)* 14.0

cinnamon *(Pepperidge Farm)* 14.0

cranberry *(Arnold)* 14.0

date nut *(Thomas')*, 1 oz. 16.0

French:

    (Arnold Francisco), 1 oz. 14.0

    (Pepperidge Farm), 1/9 loaf 25.0

    (Pepperidge Farm Sliced), 1/9 loaf 24.0

    twin *(Brownberry Francisco Intl.)* 18.0

golden, light *(Brownberry Bakery)*, 2 slices 20.0

golden swirl *(Pepperidge Farm* Vermont Maple) 15.0

Italian:

    (Arnold Francisco), 2 slices 23.0

    (Arnold Savoni's) 13.0

    (Wonder 20 oz.) 15.0

    brown and serve *(Pepperidge Farm)*, 1/9 loaf 24.0

    light *(Arnold/Brownberry Bakery)*, 2 slices 21.0

    light *(Wonder* 1 lb.) 18.0

    stick *(Arnold Francisco* 10 oz.), 1 oz. 14.0

    stick, sliced *(Arnold Francisco* 1 lb.) 15.0

    thick *(Brownberry Francisco Intl.)*, 2 slices 23.0

kamut, sprout *(Shiloh Farms* Egyptian) 18.0

mixed/multi grain:

    (Brownberry Hearth) 17.0

    (Roman Meal Round Top) 13.0

    (Roman Meal Sun) 12.0

    5, sprouted *(Shiloh Farms/Shiloh Farms* No Salt) 19.0

    7 *(Roman Meal)* 16.0

    7, hearty *(Pepperidge Farm)* 18.0

    7, light *(Pepperidge Farm)*, 3 slices 28.0

    7, light *(Roman Meal)*, 2 slices 19.0

    7, sprouted *(Breads for Life/Shiloh Farms)* 19.0

    7, white *(Arnold/Brownberry Bran'nola)* 18.0

    9 *(Pepperidge Farm)* 16.0

    12 *(Arnold Bran'nola)* 18.0

    12 *(Brownberry)*, 2 slices 20.0

    12 *(Roman Meal)* 12.0

Bread, mixed/multi grain *(cont.)*
    crunchy *(Pepperidge Farm)* 15.0
    nutty *(Arnold Bran'nola/Brownberry Bran'nola)* 18.0
    with oat bran *(Roman Meal)* 13.0
    sprouted *(Shiloh Farms Sandwich)* 17.0
    whole *(Pepperidge Farm 100%)* 15.0
  nut *(Brownberry Natural Health)* 13.0
  oat:
    (Brownberry Bran'nola) 18.0
    (Roman Meal) 13.0
    crunchy, hearty *(Pepperidge Farm)* 17.0
  oat bran, honey or honey nut *(Roman Meal)* 13.0
  oat bran, light *(Roman Meal)*, 2 slices 19.0
  oatmeal:
    (Brownberry Natural) 13.0
    (Pepperidge Farm) 15.0
    light *(Arnold/Brownberry Bakery)*, 2 slices 20.0
    light *(Pepperidge Farm)*, 3 slices 27.0
    soft *(Brownberry)* 14.0
    soft *(Pepperidge Farm)* 12.0
    thin *(Pepperidge Farm)* 11.0
  orange raisin *(Brownberry)* 14.0
  poppy seed, hazelnut *(Roman Meal)* 16.0
  potato:
    (Arnold Country) 18.0
    country *(Wonder 20 oz.)* 17.0
    hearty *(Pepperidge Farm Russet)* 18.0
  pumpernickel:
    (Arnold/Arnold August Bros. 1 lb./Arnold Levy's) 16.0
    (Arnold August Bros. 24 oz.) 19.0
    dark *(Pepperidge Farm)* 15.0
    party *(Pepperidge Farm)*, 8 slices 22.0
    rye *(Brownberry)* 14.0
  raisin:
    (Arnold Sunmaid) 14.0
    cinnamon *(Arnold/Brownberry)* 14.0
    cinnamon *(Pepperidge Farm)* 14.0
    walnut *(Brownberry)* 13.0
    whole wheat *(Shiloh Farms)*, 2 slices 30.0
  rye:
    (Arnold Deli) 16.0
    (Brownberry Hearth) 18.0

Dijon *(Arnold Real Jewish)* 16.0
Dijon, thin *(Pepperidge Farm)*, 2 slices 18.0
dill *(Arnold)* 16.0
dill *(Brownberry)* 15.0
hearty or soft *(Beefsteak)* 13.0
onion *(Arnold August Bros.)* 16.0
onion *(Pepperidge Farm)*........................ 15.0
onion, with seeds *(Arnold August Bros.)* 18.0
party *(Pepperidge Farm)*, 8 slices 22.0
seeded *(Arnold/Arnold August Bros.* 1 lb.) 16.0
seeded *(Brownberry* Natural) 15.0
seeded *(Levy's* Real Jewish) 16.0
seeded or unseeded *(Arnold August Bros.* 24 oz.) 18.0
seeded or unseeded *(Pepperidge Farm)* 15.0
soft *(Arnold* Country) 13.0
soft, light *(Arnold/Brownberry Bakery)*, 2 slices 20.0
soft, seeded or unseeded *(Arnold Bakery)* 15.0
thin *(Arnold Levy's Melba)*, 2 slices 19.0
unseeded *(Arnold August Bros.* 1 lb./*Arnold* Real Jewish
    1 lb.) 16.0
unseeded *(Arnold* Real Jewish 1 lb./*Brownberry* Natural) 15.0
unseeded *(Arnold Levy's* Real Jewish) 16.0
unseeded, thin *(Arnold August Bros.)*, 2 slices 19.0
unseeded, thin *(Brownberry)*, 2 slices 20.0
rye and pump *(Arnold August Bros.)* 18.0
sourdough:
   (Arnold August Bros.) 23.0
   (Arnold Francisco) 19.0
   brown and serve *(Arnold Francisco)*, 1 oz. 14.0
   light *(Arnold)*, 2 slices 20.0
   light *(Pepperidge Farm)*, 3 slices 27.0
   thick *(Brownberry Francisco Intl.)*............... 19.0
   whole grain *(Roman Meal)* 13.0
spelt *(Shiloh Farms)* 21.0
stick, sliced *(Arnold August Bros.)*, 2 slices 22.0
stick, sliced *(Brownberry Francisco)* 21.0
toast, Texas *(Arnold August Bros.)* 28.0
Vienna, light *(Pepperidge Farm)*, 3 slices 28.0
Vienna, thick *(Pepperidge Farm)* 12.0
wheat:
   (Arnold Brick Oven) 14.0
   (Arnold Brick Oven 8 oz.), 2 slices 20.0

Bread, wheat *(cont.)*

    (Arnold Brick Oven 1 lb.), 2 slices 21.0
    (Arnold Sunny Valley), 2 slices 20.0
    (Arnold/Brownberry Country/*Brownberry* Hearth) 18.0
    (Brownberry Natural) 17.0
    (Home Pride) 13.0
    (Pepperidge Farm/Pepperidge Farm Natural) 16.0
    (Pepperidge Farm Family) 13.0
    (Roman Meal Natural) 12.0
    (Shiloh Farms Homestyle), ½″ slice, 2 oz. 29.0
    (Wonder Lowfat), 2 slices 18.0
    cracked, thin *(Pepperidge Farm)* 12.0
    dark *(Arnold/Brownberry Bran'nola)* 12.0
    hearty *(Arnold/Brownberry Bran'nola)* 16.0
    light *(Pepperidge Farm),* 3 slices 28.0
    light *(Roman Meal),* 2 slices 20.0
    light, golden *(Arnold),* 2 slices 20.0
    light, hearty *(Roman Meal Light),* 2 slices 19.0
    sesame, hearty *(Pepperidge Farm)* 18.0
    soft *(Brownberry)* 14.0
    soft *(Brownberry* 16 oz.), 2 slices 21.0
    very thin *(Pepperidge Farm),* 3 slices 22.0
  wheat, whole:
    (Arnold Stoneground 1 lb. 4 oz.) 12.0
    (Arnold Stoneground 2 lb.), 2 slices 19.0
    (Merita 100%) 11.0
    (Roman Meal) 13.0
    (Shiloh Farms/Shiloh Farms No Salt), 2 slices 26.0
    (Wonder 24 oz.) 14.0
    light *(Roman Meal),* 2 slices 18.0
    soft or thin *(Pepperidge Farm)* 11.0
  wheatberry, honey:
    (Arnold) 16.0
    (Arnold Bran'nola) 19.0
    (Roman Meal) 13.0
    hearty *(Pepperidge Farm)* 18.0
    light *(Roman Meal),* 2 slices 15.0
  white:
    (Arnold Brick Oven) 16.0
    (Arnold Brick Oven 8 oz./1 lb.), 2 slices 24.0
    (Arnold Country) 19.0
    (Arnold Sunny Valley), 2 slices 21.0

(Brownberry Country) 19.0
(Brownberry Natural), 2 slices 24.0
(Home Pride) 14.0
(Wonder 12 oz.), 2 slices 21.0
(Wonder 1 lb.) 12.0
(Wonder 22 oz.), 2 slices 23.0
(Wonder Lowfat), 2 slices 18.0
hearty *(Pepperidge Farm/Pepperidge Farm* Country) 19.0
light *(Arnold/Brownberry Bakery)*, 2 slices 21.0
light *(Roman Meal)*, 2 slices 20.0
sandwich *(Pepperidge Farm)*, 2 slices 23.0
sandwich *(Roman Meal)*, 2 slices 21.0
soft *(Arnold* Country) 16.0
soft *(Brownberry)* 14.0
soft *(Brownberry* 16 oz.), 2 slices 21.0
toasting *(Pepperidge Farm)* 16.0
thin *(Pepperidge Farm/Pepperidge Farm* Large Family) . . 13.0
very thin *(Pepperidge Farm)*, 3 slices 14.0
Bread, brown, canned:
(B&M), ½″ slice 29.0
(S&W), ½″ slice, 1.6 oz. 21.0
raisin *(B&M)*, ½″ slice 29.0
Bread, frozen, ⅛ loaf, except as noted:
cheddar, two *(Pepperidge Farm)* 21.0
five cheese and garlic *(Schwan's)* 26.0
garlic *(Pepperidge Farm)* 14.0
garlic mozzarella *(Pepperidge Farm)* 21.0
garlic Parmesan *(Pepperidge Farm)* 19.0
garlic sourdough *(Pepperidge Farm)* 20.0
Monterey Jack/jalapeño cheese *(Pepperidge Farm)* 22.0
ready-to-bake, honey wheat *(Schwan's)*, ⅛ loaf 24.0
ready-to-bake, white *(Schwan's)*, ⅛ loaf 25.0
stuffed, cheese *(Schwan's)*, 3″ wedge 19.0
Bread, mountain, 1 piece:
six grain *(Cedar's)*, 2 oz. 35.0
wheat *(Cedar's)*, 2 oz. 34.0
white *(Cedar's)*, 2 oz. 35.0
white or whole wheat *(Cedar's* Mountainette), 1.1 oz. 26.0
Bread, pita/pocket, 1 piece, except as noted:
(Arnold), 2 oz. 29.0
(Arnold), 3 oz. 44.0
(Pepperidge Farm) 30.0

Bread, pita/pocket *(cont.)*
(Pepperidge Farm Mini), 1 oz. 15.0
(Thomas' Sahara), 2 oz. 31.0
(Thomas' Sahara), 3 oz. 48.0
(Thomas' Sahara Mini), 1 oz. 15.0
garlic *(Arnold)* 30.0
oat bran *(Thomas' Sahara)* 30.0
onion *(Arnold)* 28.0
onion *(Thomas' Sahara)* 31.0
salsa *(Thomas' Sahara)* 36.0
6 grain *(Cedar's),* ½ piece, 1.5 oz. 18.0
sourdough *(Thomas' Sahara)* 33.0
wheat:
    (Arnold 4″), 1 oz. 14.0
    (Arnold), 2 oz. 29.0
    (Arnold), 3 oz. 42.0
    (Thomas' Sahara), 2 oz. 28.0
    (Thomas' Sahara Mini), 1 oz. 14.0
    whole *(Cedar's),* ½ piece, 1.5 oz. 25.0
white *(Arnold* 4″), 1 oz. 15.0
white *(Cedar's),* ½ piece, 1.5 oz. 23.0
Bread, refrigerated, ready-to-bake, French
    (Pillsbury), ⅕ loaf 27.0
Bread, stuffed:
broccoli and cheese *(Stuffed Breads),* 6 oz. 54.0
pepperoni and cheese *(Stuffed Breads),* 6 oz. 45.0
Bread crumbs, ¼ cup or 1 oz., except as noted:
(Contadina), ⅓ cup 19.0
(Devonsheer/Old London) 20.0
(Progresso) 19.0
garlic and herb *(Progresso)* 18.0
Italian *(Devonsheer)* 19.0
Italian or lemon herb *(Progresso)* 20.0
Parmesan *(Progresso)* 17.0
seasoned *(Old London)* 19.0
tomato basil *(Progresso)* 22.0
Bread cubes, see "Stuffing"
Bread dough, see "Bread, frozen" and "Bread, refrigerated"
Bread mix (see also "Bread mix, sweet"):
beer *(Buckeye),* ¹⁄₁₄ pkg. 27.0
beer, whole wheat *(Buckeye),* ¹⁄₁₄ pkg. 26.0
cheddar cheese *(Dromedary),* ⅑ pkg. 25.0

corn bread:
   (Arrowhead Mills), ¼ cup 24.0
   (Ballard), ¹⁄₁₈ pkg. 21.0
   (Ballard), ¹⁄₁₈ loaf* 23.0
   (Buckeye), ¹⁄₁₆ pkg. 29.0
   (Dromedary), ¹⁄₁₀ pkg. 26.0
   buttermilk *(Martha White)*, ⅕ pkg. 23.0
   buttermilk *(Martha White)*, ⅕ loaf* 25.0
   buttermilk *(Martha White Cotton Pickin)*, ⅕ pkg. . . . 23.0
   chili fiesta *(Martha White)*, ⅙ pkg. 19.0
   chili fiesta *(Martha White)*, ⅙ loaf* 20.0
   golden honey *(Martha White)*, ⅙ pkg. 20.0
   golden honey *(Martha White)*, ⅙ loaf* 21.0
   Mexican *(Gladiola/Martha White)*, ⅙ pkg. 19.0
   Mexican *(Gladiola/Martha White)*, ⅙ loaf* 20.0
   white:
      (Gladiola), ⅙ pkg. 18.0
      (Gladiola), ⅙ loaf* 20.0
      (Martha White Light Crust), ⅙ pkg. 19.0
      (Martha White Light Crust), ⅙ loaf* 21.0
   yellow:
      (Gladiola), ⅙ pkg. 19.0
      (Gladiola), ⅙ loaf* 20.0
      (Martha White), ⅕ pkg. 24.0
      (Martha White), ⅕ loaf* 25.0
      (Martha White Light Crust), ⅙ pkg. 20.0
      (Martha White Light Crust), ⅙ loaf* 21.0
herb, Italian *(Dromedary)*, ⅑ pkg. 25.0
kamut *(Arrowhead Mills)*, ⅓ cup 31.0
multigrain *(Arrowhead Mills)*, ⅓ cup 31.0
oatmeal, honey *(Dromedary)*, ⅑ pkg. 27.0
rye *(Arrowhead Mills)*, ⅓ cup 33.0
sourdough *(Buckeye)*, ¹⁄₁₄ pkg. 27.0
sourdough *(Dromedary)*, ⅑ pkg. 27.0
spelt *(Arrowhead Mills)*, ⅓ cup 31.0
wheat, cracked *(Pillsbury* Bread Machine), ¹⁄₁₂ loaf* . . . 25.0
wheat, stoneground *(Dromedary)*, ⅑ pkg. 26.0
wheat, whole *(Arrowhead Mills)*, ⅓ cup 31.0
white *(Arrowhead Mills)*, ⅓ cup 31.0
white, country *(Dromedary)*, ⅑ pkg. 28.0
white, crusty *(Pillsbury* Bread Machine), ¹⁄₁₂ loaf* . . . 25.0

Bread mix, sweet:
(Buckeye), 1/16 pkg. 26.0
apple cinnamon *(Dromedary)*, 1/9 pkg. 27.0
apple cinnamon *(Pillsbury)*, 1/12 pkg. or 1/12 loaf* 30.0
banana *(Pillsbury)*, 1/12 pkg. or 1/12 loaf* 26.0
blueberry *(Pillsbury)*, 1/12 pkg. or 1/12 loaf* 29.0
carrot *(Pillsbury)*, 1/16 pkg. or 1/16 loaf* 22.0
cinnamon swirl *(Pillsbury)*, 1/12 pkg. or 1/12 loaf* 32.0
cranberry *(Pillsbury)*, 1/12 pkg. or 1/12 loaf* 30.0
date *(Pillsbury)*, 1/12 pkg. or 1/12 loaf* 32.0
gingerbread *(Dromedary)*, 1/6 pkg. 52.0
gingerbread *(Pillsbury)*, 1/8 loaf* 40.0
lemon poppyseed *(Pillsbury)*, 1/12 pkg. or 1/12 loaf* 27.0
nut *(Pillsbury)*, 1/12 pkg. or 1/12 loaf* 27.0
pumpkin *(Pillsbury)*, 1/12 pkg. 27.0
pumpkin *(Pillsbury)*, 1/12 loaf* 26.0

Bread snack:
crisps, cinnamon raisin swirl *(Pepperidge Farm)*, 1 oz. 19.0
crisps, garlic butter swirl *(Pepperidge Farm)*, 1 oz. 16.0
sticks, 9 pieces:
    cheese, three *(Pepperidge Farm)* 20.0
    pretzel *(Pepperidge Farm)* 23.0
    pumpernickel/sesame *(Pepperidge Farm)* 20.0

Breadfruit:
untrimmed, 1 lb. 96.0
1/4 small, approx. 3.5 oz. 26.0
trimmed, 1/2 cup 29.8

Breadfruit nut *(Goya Pana de Pepita)*, 4 nuts 7.0

Breadstick:
(Stella D'Oro Fat Free Traditional Original), 2 sticks 15.0
(Stella D'Oro Sodium Free), 1 stick 7.0
all varieties:
    (Awrey's), 2 sticks 16.0
    (Stella D'Oro Fat Free Original Deli), 5 sticks 12.0
    (Stella D'Oro Fat Free Grissini), 3 sticks 12.0
cheddar, thin *(Pepperidge Farm)*, 7 sticks 11.0
cheese, three *(Pepperidge Farm)*, 9 sticks 20.0
with cheese *(Handi-Snacks)*, 1 stick 11.0
garlic *(Stella D'Oro)*, 1 stick 7.0
garlic *(Stella D'Oro Fat Free Traditional)*, 2 sticks 14.0
onion *(Stella D'Oro)*, 1 stick 6.0
onion, thin *(Pepperidge Farm)*, 7 sticks 11.0

pretzel *(Pepperidge Farm)*, 9 sticks 23.0
pumpernickel *(Pepperidge Farm)*, 9 sticks 20.0
regular *(Stella D'Oro)*, 1 stick 7.0
sesame:
    (Pepperidge Farm), 9 sticks 20.0
    (Stella D'Oro), 1 stick 7.0
    (Stella D'Oro Low Fat Traditional), 2 sticks 14.0
    thin *(Pepperidge Farm)*, 7 sticks 11.0
wheat *(Stella D'Oro)*, 1 stick 6.0
Breadstick, refrigerated, 1 piece:
(Pepperidge Farm Brown and Serve) 28.0
(Pillsbury) 18.0
corn bread twist *(Pillsbury)* 18.0
Breakfast dishes, see specific listings
Breakfast syrup, see "Maple syrup" and "Pancake syrup"
Broad beans:
raw:
    (Frieda's Fava Beans), 1 oz. 1.9
    untrimmed, 1 lb. 51.5
    1 medium, .3 oz. 1.0
    trimmed, ½ cup 6.4
boiled, drained, 4 oz. 11.5
Broad beans, mature:
dried, ½ cup 21.9
dried, boiled, ½ cup 16.7
canned *(Progresso Fava Beans)*, ½ cup 20.0
canned, with liquid, ½ cup 15.9
Broccoli, fresh:
raw:
    untrimmed, 1 lb. 14.5
    untrimmed, 1 stalk, 8.7 oz. 7.9
    trimmed *(Dole)*, 1 stalk, 5.3 oz. 8.0
    chopped, ½ cup 2.3
boiled, drained, 1 stalk, 6.3 oz. 3.9
boiled, drained, chopped, ½ cup 9.1
Broccoli, frozen:
spears:
    10-oz. pkg. 15.2
    (Green Giant), 3 oz. 4.0
    (Green Giant Harvest Fresh), 3.5 oz. 4.0
    (Schwan's), 1 spear 3.0
    or baby spears *(Birds Eye)*, 3 oz. 4.0

Broccoli, frozen *(cont.)*

florets *(Green Giant)*, 1⅓ cups 4.0
florets *(Stilwell)*, 4 florets 4.0
chopped:
    10-oz. pkg. 13.6
    (Birds Eye), ⅓ cup 5.0
    (Green Giant), ¾ cup 4.0
    (Seabrook), ¾ cup, 3 oz. 4.0
cut:
    (Green Giant), 1 cup 4.0
    (Green Giant Harvest Fresh), ⅔ cup 4.0
    (Stilwell), ½ cup 4.0
stir-fry *(Birds Eye)*, 1 cup 4.0
in butter sauce, spears *(Green Giant)*, 4 oz. 7.0
in cheese sauce:
    (Birds Eye), ½ cup 7.0
    (Freezer Queen Family Side Dish), ⅔ cup. 6.0
    (Green Giant), ⅔ cup 9.0
Broccoli, cheese breaded, frozen *(Giorgio)*, 10 pieces 23.0
Broccoli combinations (see also "Vegetables, mixed"),
    frozen:
carrots and cauliflower *(Green Giant American*
    Mixtures), ¾ cup 5.0
carrots and water chestnuts *(Green Giant American*
    Mixtures), ¾ cup 6.0
cauliflower *(Birds Eye)*, ½ cup 4.0
cauliflower *(Stilwell)*, ½ cup 4.0
cauliflower and carrots:
    (Birds Eye), ½ cup 5.0
    (Green Giant Harvest Fresh), 1 cup 5.0
    in cheese sauce *(Birds Eye)*, ½ cup 7.0
    in cheese sauce *(Green Giant)*, ⅔ cup 11.0
    corn and peas, in butter sauce *(Green Giant)*, ¾ cup 8.0
cauliflower, peas, peppers *(Green Giant American*
    Mixtures), ¾ cup. 5.0
corn and red peppers *(Birds Eye)*, ½ cup 12.0
green beans, onions, and red peppers *(Birds Eye)*, ½ cup . . . 6.0
pasta, cauliflower, and carrots, in cheese sauce
    (Freezer Queen Family Side Dish), ⅔ cup. 10.0
pasta, peas, corn, and peppers, in butter sauce *(Green*
    Giant), ¾ cup 11.0
stir-fry *(Birds Eye)*, 1 cup 5.0

Broccoli rabe *(Frieda's Rapini)*, ¾ cup, 3 oz. 3.0
Broccoli stir-fry entree mix, see "Entree mix, frozen"
Broccoli-cheddar pocket, frozen
   (Ken & Robert's Veggie Pockets), 1 piece 38.0
Broccoli-cheese in pastry *(Pepperidge Farm)*, 1 piece 24.0
Broiling sauce, see "Grilling sauce"
Broth, see "Bouillon" and "Soup"
Broth concentrate, 2 tsp.:
beef flavor *(Knorr)* 1.0
chicken flavor *(Knorr)* . . . . <1.0
vegetable flavor *(Knorr)* 4.0
Brown gravy, ¼ cup:
with onions *(Franco-American)* 4.0
savory *(Heinz)* 2.0
mix*:
   (Durkee/French's) 3.0
   (Knorr Classic) 3.0
   (Loma Linda Gravy Quik) 4.0
   (Pillsbury) 3.0
   (Tone's Cook Up) 2.0
   (Weight Watchers) 0
   herb *(Durkee/French's)* 3.0
Brown gravy sauce *(La Choy)*, ¼ cup 66.0
Brownie, 1 piece, except as noted:
(Hostess Light), 1.4-oz. piece 29.0
(Oreo) 25.0
chocolate:
   (Awrey's Decadent) 30.0
   (Little Debbie Low Fat) 39.0
   Bavarian *(Awrey's)* 29.0
   peanut *(Awrey's Sensation)* 27.0
fudge:
   (Entenmann's Fat Free), ¹⁄₁₀ strip 27.0
   (Little Debbie) 46.0
   (Snack Well's) 26.0
   without nuts *(Awrey's)* 30.0
fudge nut:
   (Awrey's) 23.0
   (Drake's Reduced Fat) 33.0
   chewy *(Awrey's)* 28.0
fudge walnut *(Tastykake)* 52.0
mini *(Hostess Bites)*, 5 pieces 35.0

Brownie, frozen, 1 piece:
à la mode *(Weight Watchers)* 34.0
frosted *(Weight Watchers)* 22.0
peanut butter fudge *(Weight Watchers)* 21.0
Brownie mix:
(Arrowhead Mills), 1 piece* 27.0
(Arrowhead Mills Fat Free), 1 piece* 28.0
(Arrowhead Mills Wheat Free), 1 piece* 26.0
(Betty Crocker), ¹/₂₀ pkg. or 1 piece* 27.0
(Sweet Rewards Reduced Fat), ¹/₂₀ pkg. or 1 piece* 27.0
blonde, with white chocolate chunks *(Duncan Hines),*
  ¹/₂₀ pkg. or 1 piece* 25.0
caramel *(Betty Crocker),* ¹/₁₈ pkg. or 1 piece* 27.0
cheesecake swirl *(Pillsbury* Thick 'n Fudgy), ¹/₁₆ pkg.
  or 1 piece* 21.0
chocolate *(Pillsbury* Deluxe), ¹/₂₀ pkg. or 1 piece* 28.0
chocolate, dark, with *Hershey's* syrup *(Betty Crocker),*
  ¹/₁₈ pkg. or 1 piece* 28.0
chocolate, double *(Pillsbury* Thick 'n Fudgy),
  ¹/₁₆ pkg. or 1 piece* 23.0
chocolate, German *(Betty Crocker),* ¹/₁₈ pkg. 32.0
chocolate, German *(Betty Crocker),* 1 piece* 33.0
chocolate chip *(Betty Crocker),* ¹/₁₈ pkg. or 1 piece* 26.0
chocolate chunk *(Betty Crocker),* ¹/₂₀ pkg. or 1 piece* 24.0
cookies and cream:
  (Betty Crocker), ¹/₁₈ pkg. or 1 piece* 27.0
  no-cholesterol recipe *(Betty Crocker),* 1 piece* 28.0
dark 'n chunky *(Duncan Hines),* ¹/₂₀ pkg. or 1 piece* 26.0
devil's food *(SnackWell's),* 1 piece* 28.0
frosted *(Betty Crocker),* ¹/₂₀ pkg. 30.0
frosted *(Betty Crocker),* 1 piece* 31.0
fudge:
  (Betty Crocker), ¹/₁₂ pkg. or 1 piece* 29.0
  (Betty Crocker Family Size), ¹/₁₈ pkg. or 1 piece* 28.0
  (Betty Crocker Light), 1 piece* 26.0
  (Martha White Chewy Family Size), ¹/₂₀ pkg. or 1 piece* 25.0
  (Martha White Chewy Snack Size), ¹/₁₀ pkg. or 1 piece* 24.0
  (Martha White Moist 'n Fudgy), ¹/₂₀ pkg. or 1 piece* ... 24.0
  (Mother's Best Chewy), ¹/₁₀ pkg. or 1 piece* 24.0
  (Pillsbury Deluxe 15 oz.), ¹/₁₆ pkg. or 1 piece* 22.0
  (Pillsbury Deluxe 21.5 oz.), ¹/₂₀ pkg. or 1 piece* 25.0
  (Robin Hood/Gold Medal Pouch), ¹/₁₀ pkg. or 1 piece* .. 24.0

(SnackWell's), 1 piece* 29.0
(Sweet Rewards Low Fat), 1/18 pkg. 27.0
chewy *(Duncan Hines)*, 1/12 pkg. or 1 piece* 25.0
dark *(Duncan Hines)*, 1/18 pkg. or 1 piece* 25.0
dark chocolate *(Betty Crocker)*, 1/18 pkg. or 1 piece* . . . 27.0
double *(Duncan Hines)*, 1/20 pkg. 28.0
double *(Duncan Hines)*, 1 piece* 29.0
hot *(Betty Crocker)*, 1/18 pkg. or 1 piece* 25.0
hot *(Pillsbury* Deluxe), 1/24 pkg. or 1 piece* 24.0
milk chocolate chunk *(Duncan Hines)*, 1/20 pkg. or 1 piece* 26.0
Mississippi mud *(Duncan Hines)*, 1/20 pkg. or 1 piece* . . . 27.0
peanut butter candies with *Reese's Pieces (Betty Crocker)*,
  1/18 pkg. or 1 piece* 27.0
raspberry dark chocolate *(Duncan Hines)*, 1/20 pkg.
  or 1 piece* 23.0
walnut:
  (Betty Crocker), 1/18 pkg. or 1 piece* 24.0
  (Duncan Hines), 1/20 pkg. or 1 piece* 24.0
  (Martha White Deluxe Family Size), 1/20 pkg. or 1 piece* 23.0
  (Pillsbury Thick 'n Fudgy), 1/12 pkg. or 1 piece* 24.0
white chocolate swirl *(Betty Crocker)*, 1/18 pkg. 27.0
white chocolate swirl *(Betty Crocker)*, 1 piece* 28.0
Browning sauce *(Gravy Master)*, 1/4 tsp. 2.0
Brussels sprouts, fresh:
raw:
  (Dole), 1 cup 4.0
  untrimmed, 1 lb. 36.6
  1 sprout, approx. .7 oz. 1.7
  1/2 cup 3.9
boiled, drained, 1 sprout, .7 oz. 1.8
boiled, drained, 1/2 cup 6.8
Brussels sprouts, frozen:
(Birds Eye), 11 sprouts 7.0
(Stilwell), 6 sprouts 5.0
10-oz. pkg. 22.4
boiled, drained, 1/2 cup 6.5
baby, in butter sauce *(Green Giant)*, 2/3 cup 9.0
Buckwheat:
whole-grain, 1 oz. 20.3
whole-grain, 1 cup 121.6
Buckwheat flour:
(Arrowhead Mills), 1/4 cup 25.0

Buckwheat flour *(cont.)*
1 oz. 20.0
1 cup 84.7
Buckwheat groats:
brown *(Arrowhead Mills)*, ¼ cup 30.0
roasted, dry, 1 oz. 21.2
roasted, cooked, 1 cup 39.5
Bulgur, dry:
uncooked:
   (Arrowhead Mills), ¼ cup 33.0
   1 oz. 21.5
   1 cup 106.2
cooked, 1 cup 33.8
Bulgur pilaf mix *(Casbah)*, 1 oz. 20.0
Bulgur salad, see "Tabouli"
Bun, see "Roll"
Bun, sweet (see also "Danish"), 1 piece:
apple *(Entenmann's* Fat Free) 33.0
cheese:
   blueberry *(Entenmann's* Fat Free) 31.0
   pineapple *(Entenmann's* Fat Free) 30.0
   raspberry *(Entenmann's* Fat Free) 36.0
cinnamon *(Entenmann's)* 31.0
cinnamon raisin *(Entenmann's* Fat Free) 36.0
cinnamon roll:
   (Awrey's Homestyle) 46.0
   (Hostess) 34.0
   (Weight Watchers) 33.0
honey:
   (Grandma's) 48.0
   (Little Debbie), 3 oz. 39.0
   (Morton), 2.3 oz. 35.0
   (Morton Mini), 1.3 oz. 19.0
   glazed *(Entenmann's* Donut Dippers) 19.0
   glazed *(Hostess)* 34.0
   glazed or iced *(Tastykake)* 47.0
   iced *(Hostess)* 49.0
honey, frozen *(Rich's)* 32.0
pecan roll *(Little Debbie Spinwheels)* 32.0
Bun, sweet, frozen or refrigerated, 1 piece:
apple cinnamon, iced *(Pillsbury)* 23.0
caramel *(Pillsbury)* 24.0

cinnamon:
    (Pepperidge Farm) 33.0
    (Sara Lee Deluxe) 41.0
    iced *(Pillsbury)* 23.0
    iced *(Schwan's)* 43.0
    raisin, iced *(Pillsbury)* 26.0
orange, iced *(Pillsbury)* 25.0
Burbot, without added ingredients 0
Burdock root:
raw:
    untrimmed, 1 lb. 59.0
    trimmed, 1 medium, 7.3 oz. 13.6
    pieces, ½ cup 10.3
    Japanese *(Frieda's* Gobo Root), ¾ cup, 3 oz. 15.0
boiled, drained, 1″ pieces, ½ cup 13.2
Burger, see "Beef, frozen," "Beef sandwich," and specific
    restaurant listings
Burger King, 1 serving:
breakfast items:
    biscuit with bacon, egg, cheese 39.0
    biscuit with sausage 41.0
    Croissan'wich, sausage, egg, cheese 25.0
    French toast sticks 60.0
    hash browns 25.0
    A.M. Express jam, grape 7.0
    A.M. Express jam, strawberry 8.0
sandwiches:
    BK Big Fish 56.0
    BK Broiler chicken 41.0
    cheeseburger, regular, double, or double with bacon . . . 28.0
    chicken sandwich 54.0
    Double Whopper, regular 45.0
    Double Whopper, with cheese 46.0
    hamburger 28.0
    Whopper 45.0
    Whopper, with cheese 46.0
    Whopper Jr., regular or with cheese 29.0
Chicken Tenders, 8 pieces 19.0
dipping sauces, 1 oz., except as noted:
    A.M. Express 21.0
    barbecue 9.0
    Bull's Eye, ½ oz. 5.0

Burger King,* dipping sauces *(cont.)
  honey 23.0
  ranch 2.0
  sweet and sour 11.0
fries, regular or coated, medium 43.0
onion rings 41.0
salad, without dressing:
  chicken, broiled or garden 7.0
  side 4.0
salad dressings, 1.1 oz.:
  blue cheese 1.0
  French 11.0
  Italian, light 3.0
  ranch 2.0
  Thousand Island 7.0
shakes, medium:
  chocolate 54.0
  chocolate with syrup 84.0
  strawberry with syrup 83.0
  vanilla 53.0
Dutch apple pie 39.0
Burrito, frozen:
bean, black *(Amy's),* 6 oz. 54.0
bean and cheese *(Old El Paso),* 5 oz. 44.0
bean and cheese *(Tina's),* 5 oz. 52.0
bean and rice *(Amy's),* 6 oz. 44.0
bean, rice, and cheese *(Amy's),* 6 oz. 43.0
beef:
  (Hormel Quick Meal), 4 oz. 37.0
  (Tina's Red Hot), 5 oz. 49.0
  nacho *(Patio Britos),* 10 pieces, 6 oz. 48.0
beef and bean:
  (Patio Britos), 10 pieces, 6 oz. 51.0
  (Schwan's), 4.3 oz. 27.0
  hot *(Old El Paso),* 5 oz. 45.0
  medium *(Old El Paso),* 5 oz. 46.0
  mild *(Old El Paso),* 5 oz. 48.0
  steak *(Don Miguel),* 7 oz. 55.0
cheese *(Hormel Quick Meal),* 4 oz. 41.0
cheese, nacho *(Patio Britos),* 10 pieces, 6 oz. . 52.0
chicken:
  (Don Miguel), 7 oz. 54.0

and cheese, spicy *(Patio Britos)*, 10 pieces, 6 oz. 52.0
con queso *(Healthy Choice)*, 10.55 oz. 66.0
chili, red *(Hormel Quick Meal)*, 4 oz. 37.0
pizza, 3.5 oz.:
    cheese *(Old El Paso)* 27.0
    pepperoni *(Old El Paso)* 31.0
    sausage *(Old El Paso)* 32.0
Burrito, breakfast, frozen, 1 pkg.:
(Schwan's Bright Starts) 26.0
black bean *(Amy's)*, 6 oz. 38.0
egg, scrambled *(Swanson Great Starts Original)* 25.0
egg, scrambled, and bacon *(Swanson Great Starts)* 27.0
ham and cheese *(Swanson Great Starts)* 30.0
hot and spicy *(Swanson Great Starts)* 30.0
sausage *(Swanson Great Starts)* 24.0
Burrito dinner, frozen, beef or chicken
    (Chi-Chi's Burro), 15 oz. 73.0
Burrito entree, see "Burrito"
Burrito mix *(Old El Paso Dinner)*, 1 piece* 37.0
Burrito sauce *(Hunt's Manwich)*, ¼ cup 5.0
Burrito seasoning mix:
(Durkee Pouch), ¹⁄₁₀ pkg. 5.0
(Lawry's), 1 tbsp. 6.0
(Old El Paso), 2 tsp. 0
Butter (see also "Margarine"):
1 stick or 4 oz. 0
clarified *(Purity Farms Ghee)*, 1 tsp. 0
whipped, ½ cup or 1 stick . . . . <.1
whipped, 1 tbsp. . . . . <.1
Butter beans, see "Lima beans"
Butter salt *(Durkee)*, ½ tsp. 0
Butterbur:
fresh:
    raw, untrimmed, 1 lb. 14.4
    raw, 1 stalk, .2 oz. 2
    boiled, drained, 4 oz. 2.4
canned, chopped, ½ cup 2
Butterfish, without added ingredients 0
Buttermilk, see "Milk"
Buttercup squash *(Frieda's)*, ¾ cup, 3 oz. 7.0
Butternut, dried:
in shell, 1 lb. 14.8

Butternut *(cont.)*
shelled, 1 oz. 3.4
Butternut squash:
fresh:
    raw *(Frieda's)*, ¾ cup, 3 oz. 10.0
    raw, untrimmed, 1 lb. 44.6
    raw, cubed, ½ cup 8.1
    baked, cubed, ½ cup 10.7
frozen, 12-oz. pkg. 49.0
frozen, boiled, drained, mashed, ½ cup 12.1
Butterscotch, see "Candy"
Butterscotch chips, baking *(Nestlé Morsels)*, 1 tbsp. 10.0
Butterscotch topping, 2 tbsp.:
(Kraft) 28.0
(Mrs. Richardson's) 30.0
(Smucker's Special Recipe) 30.0
(Smucker's Sundae) 27.0
caramel *(Smucker's Fat Free)* 31.0
caramel fudge *(Mrs. Richardson's)* 30.0

C

Cabbage:
raw:
    (Dole), ¹⁄₁₂ medium head 6.0
    untrimmed, 1 lb. 19.5
    1 head, 5¾″-diam., approx. 2.5 lb. 49.3
    shredded, ½ cup 1.9
boiled, drained, 4 oz. 5.4
boiled, drained, shredded, ½ cup 3.4
Cabbage, Chinese:
raw, shredded *(Dole)*, ½ cup 1.0
bok choy:
    raw *(Frieda's)*, 1 cup, 3 oz. 2.0
    raw, untrimmed, 1 lb. 8.7
    raw, shredded, ½ cup 8
    boiled, drained, shredded, ½ cup 1.5
pe-tsai:
    raw, untrimmed, 1 lb. 13.6
    raw, shredded, ½ cup 1.2
    boiled, drained, shredded, ½ cup 1.4
Cabbage, mustard *(Frieda's* Gai Choy), 1 cup, 3 oz. 4.0
Cabbage, napa, raw:
(Frieda's), 1 cup, 3 oz. 3.0
shredded *(Dole)*, 3 oz. 1.0
Cabbage, pickled, spicy, see "Kimchee"
Cabbage, red:
raw, untrimmed, 1 lb. 22.2
raw, shredded, ½ cup 2.1
boiled, drained, shredded, ½ cup 3.5
shredded *(Dole)*, 3 oz. 5.0
Cabbage, red, sweet and sour, canned or in jars:
(Greenwood), ½ cup 24.0
(S&W), 2 tbsp. 3.0
(Seneca), ½ cup 19.0
Cabbage, savoy:
raw, untrimmed, 1 lb. 22.1

Cabbage, savoy *(cont.)*
raw, shredded, ½ cup 2.1
boiled, drained, shredded, ½ cup 4.0
Cabbage entree, stuffed, frozen, with potatoes
   (Lean Cuisine), 9.5 oz. 24.0
Cabbage salad, see "Coleslaw"
Cacciatore entree, see "Chicken entree" and
   "Entree mix, frozen"
Cactus, leaves or pads *(Frieda's),* ¾ cup, 3 oz. 4.0
Cactus, marinated *(Goya* Napolitos), 2–3 pieces 3.0
Cactus pear, see "Prickly pear"
Caesar salad, see "Salad, complete"
Caesar salad mix *(Just Add Lettuce),* ⅙ pkg.* 6.0
Cajun seasoning, all varieties, ¼ tsp. 0
Cake:
apple-spice crumb *(Entenmann's* Fat Free), ⅛ cake 30.0
banana:
   (Awrey's Sheet), 1/24 cake 40.0
   (Entenmann's Fat Free), ⅛ cake 34.0
   chocolate chip *(Awrey's* Marquise), 1/16 cake 40.0
   crunch *(Entenmann's),* ⅛ cake 32.0
   crunch *(Entenmann's* Fat Free), ⅛ cake 33.0
Black Forest torte *(Awrey's),* 1/12 cake 38.0
blueberry crunch *(Entenmann's* Fat Free), ⅛ cake 32.0
Boston creme *(Awrey's),* 1/16 cake 30.0
butter *(Entenmann's),* ⅙ loaf 31.0
butter, French crumb *(Entenmann's),* ⅛ cake 29.0
carrot:
   (Entenmann's), ⅛ cake 35.0
   (Entenmann's Fat Free), ⅛ cake 40.0
   cream cheese iced *(Awrey's),* 1/16 cake 44.0
   supreme *(Awrey's* Sheet), 1/24 cake 47.0
cherries cordial *(Awrey's* Marquise), 1/16 cake 30.0
chocolate:
   crunch *(Entenmann's* Fat Free), ⅛ cake 32.0
   fudge *(Entenmann's),* ⅙ cake 47.0
   fudge iced *(Entenmann's* Fat Free), ⅙ cake 51.0
   German *(Awrey's* Sheet), 1/24 cake 41.0
   German, layer *(Awrey's),* 1/16 cake 46.0
   loaf *(Entenmann's* Fat Free), ⅛ cake 30.0
   mocha iced *(Entenmann's* Fat Free), ⅙ cake 46.0
   peanut *(Awrey's* Marquise), 1/16 cake 38.0

tropical *(Awrey's* Marquise), 1/16 cake 34.0
white iced, layer *(Awrey's)*, 1/16 cake 34.0
chocolate, double:
    (Awrey's Sheet), 1/24 cake 48.0
    (Awrey's Torte), 1/12 cake 52.0
    3 layer *(Awrey's)*, 1/16 cake 48.0
    2 layer *(Awrey's)*, 1/16 cake 38.0
coconut buttercream *(Awrey's* Sheet), 1/24 cake 43.0
coconut buttercream, layer *(Awrey's)*, 1/16 cake 41.0
coffee:
    (Awrey's Long John), 1/12 cake 21.0
    cheese *(Entenmann's)*, 1/9 cake 24.0
    cheese, crumb *(Entenmann's)*, 1/8 cake 25.0
    cinnamon apple *(Entenmann's* Fat Free), 1/9 cake 29.0
    crumb *(Entenmann's)*, 1/10 cake 33.0
crunch, Louisiana *(Entenmann's)*, 1/9 cake 45.0
crunch, Louisiana *(Entenmann's* Fat Free), 1/6 cake 51.0
Danish cake:
    apple cinnamon *(Entenmann's* Fat Free), 1/8 cake 33.0
    Black Forest *(Entenmann's* Fat Free), 1/9 cake 32.0
    raspberry cheese *(Entenmann's* Fat Free), 1/9 cake 32.0
Danish ring, cinnamon filbert *(Entenmann's)*, 1/6 ring 27.0
Danish ring, pecan or walnut *(Entenmann's)*, 1/8 cake 23.0
Danish twist, 1/8 cake:
    apricot *(Entenmann's* Fat Free) 34.0
    cinnamon apple *(Entenmann's* Fat Free) 35.0
    lemon *(Entenmann's* Fat Free) 31.0
    raspberry *(Entenmann's)* 28.0
    raspberry *(Entenmann's* Fat Free) 33.0
devil's food, marshmallow iced *(Entenmann's)*, 1/6 cake 45.0
espresso, French *(Awrey's* Marquise), 1/16 cake 30.0
fruit *(Hostess)*, 1/12 cake 84.0
golden:
    crumb, French *(Entenmann's* Fat Free), 1/8 cake 35.0
    fudge, thick *(Entenmann's)*, 1/6 cake 48.0
    fudge iced *(Entenmann's* Fat Free), 1/6 cake 52.0
golden loaf *(Entenmann's* Fat Free), 1/8 cake 28.0
golden loaf, chocolatey chip *(Entenmann's* Fat Free), 1/8 cake 31.0
lemon layer *(Awrey's)*, 1/16 cake 38.0
marble loaf *(Entenmann's)*, 1/8 cake 25.0
marble loaf *(Entenmann's* Fat Free), 1/8 cake 29.0
Neapolitan *(Awrey's)*, 1/12 cake 41.0

Cake *(cont.)*

orange, frosty *(Awrey's* Sheet), ¹/₂₄ cake 43.0
orange, layer *(Awrey's)*, ¹/₁₆ cake 41.0
peach, Georgia *(Awrey's* Marquise), ¹/₁₆ cake 34.0
pound, golden *(Awrey's)*, ¹/₆ cake 37.0
raisin loaf *(Entenmann's)*, ¹/₈ cake 32.0
raisin loaf *(Entenmann's* Fat Free), ¹/₈ cake 33.0
raspberry and creme *(Awrey's* Marquise), ¹/₁₆ cake 34.0
raspberry nut *(Awrey's* Marquise), ¹/₁₆ cake 38.0
sour cream chip-nut loaf *(Entenmann's)*, ¹/₈ cake 28.0
sponge, uniced *(Awrey's)*, ¹/₂₄ cake 28.0
strawberry supreme *(Awrey's* Marquise), ¹/₁₆ cake 36.0
strawberry supreme, torte *(Awrey's)*, ¹/₁₂ cake 37.0
yellow, lemon iced, 2 layer *(Awrey's)*, ¹/₁₆ cake 34.0
yellow, white iced *(Awrey's* Sheet), ¹/₂₄ cake 42.0

Cake, frozen:

Boston creme *(Mrs. Smith's)*, ¹/₈ cake 29.0
Boston creme *(Pepperidge Farm)*, ¹/₈ cake 42.0
carrot *(Oregon Farms)*, ¹/₆ cake 38.0
carrot *(Pepperidge Farm* Deluxe), ¹/₈ cake 39.0
cheesecake:
    (Sara Lee Original Cream), ¹/₄ cake 49.0
    chocolate, triple *(Weight Watchers)*, 3.15-oz. cake 32.0
    French *(Sara Lee)*, ¹/₅ cake 41.0
    French style *(Weight Watchers)*, 3.9-oz. cake 28.0
    New York style *(Weight Watchers)*, 2.5-oz. cake 21.0
    strawberry *(Amy's)*, 4 oz. 38.0
    strawberry, French *(Sara Lee)*, ¹/₆ cake 43.0
chocolate:
    double, layer *(Sara Lee)*, ¹/₈ cake 37.0
    fudge *(Amy's)*, 3.25 oz. 60.0
    fudge, layer *(Pepperidge Farm)*, ¹/₆ cake 38.0
    fudge stripe, layer *(Pepperidge Farm)*, ¹/₆ cake 38.0
    German *(Sara Lee)*, ¹/₈ cake 34.0
    German, layer *(Pepperidge Farm)*, ¹/₆ cake 37.0
    mousse *(Pepperidge Farm)*, ¹/₈ cake 35.0
    mousse *(Sara Lee)*, ¹/₅ cake 37.0
    raspberry royale *(Weight Watchers)*, 3.5 oz. 39.0
coconut *(Sara Lee)*, ¹/₈ cake 34.0
coconut layer *(Pepperidge Farm)*, ¹/₆ cake 41.0
coffee cake:
    (Sara Lee), ¹/₈ cake 32.0

(Sara Lee Reduced Fat), 1/6 cake 28.0
raspberry *(Sara Lee)*, 1/6 cake 27.0
devil's food *(Oregon Farms* Divine), 1/6 cake 43.0
devil's food, layer *(Pepperidge Farm)*, 1/6 cake 40.0
fudge, double *(Weight Watchers)*, 2.75-oz. cake 36.0
golden layer *(Pepperidge Farm)*, 1/6 cake 40.0
golden layer, fudge *(Sara Lee)*, 1/8 cake 34.0
lemon mousse *(Pepperidge Farm)*, 1/8 cake 34.0
pineapple cream *(Pepperidge Farm)*, 1/9 cake 38.0
pound:
   (Goya), 1/4 cake 37.0
   (Sara Lee Reduced Fat), 1/4 cake 42.0
   butter *(Pepperidge Farm)*, 1/5 cake 39.0
   butter *(Sara Lee)*, 1/4 cake 38.0
   chocolate swirl *(Sara Lee)*, 1/4 cake 42.0
   strawberry swirl *(Sara Lee)*, 1/4 cake 44.0
strawberry cream *(Pepperidge Farm)*, 1/9 cake 38.0
strawberry stripe layer *(Pepperidge Farm)*, 1/6 cake 47.0
vanilla layer *(Pepperidge Farm)*, 1/6 cake 31.0
Cake, mix:
angel food:
   (Duncan Hines), 1/12 cake* 30.0
   (Gold Medal), 1/4 pkg. 37.0
   (Pillsbury Moist Supreme), 1/12 cake* 31.0
   (SuperMoist), 1/12 cake* 30.0
   chocolate swirl *(SuperMoist)*, 1/12 cake* 34.0
   confetti *(SuperMoist)*, 1/12 cake* 34.0
   lemon custard *(SuperMoist)*, 1/12 cake* 33.0
   strawberry *(Duncan Hines)*, 1/12 cake* 30.0
   white *(SuperMoist)*, 1/12 cake* 31.0
banana *(Duncan Hines* Supreme), 1/12 pkg. or 1/12 cake* . . . 36.0
banana *(Pillsbury Moist Supreme)*, 1/12 pkg. 35.0
banana *(Pillsbury Moist Supreme)*, 1/12 cake* 36.0
butter pecan *(SuperMoist)*, 1/12 pkg. or 1/12 cake* 34.0
butter recipe:
   (Pillsbury Moist Supreme), 1/12 pkg. 35.0
   (Pillsbury Moist Supreme), 1/12 cake* 36.0
   chocolate *(Pillsbury Moist Supreme)*, 1/12 pkg.
     or 1/12 cake* 33.0
   chocolate *(SuperMoist)*, 1/12 pkg. or 1/12 cake* 34.0
   fudge *(Duncan Hines)*, 1/10 pkg. or 1/10 cake* 40.0
   golden *(Duncan Hines)*, 1/10 pkg. or 1/10 cake* 42.0

Cake, mix, butter recipe *(cont.)*

yellow *(SuperMoist)*, 1/12 pkg. or 1/12 cake* 37.0

butterscotch *(Duncan Hines)*, 1/12 pkg. or 1/12 cake* 36.0

caramel *(Duncan Hines)*, 1/12 pkg. or 1/12 cake* 36.0

carrot *(Pillsbury Moist Supreme)*, 1/12 pkg. or 1/12 cake* 35.0

carrot *(SuperMoist)*, 1/10 pkg. or 1/10 cake* 41.0

cheesecake, 1/6 cake*:

(Jell-O Homestyle) 49.0

(Jell-O Real) 46.0

blueberry *(Jell-O)* 49.0

cherry *(Jell-O)* 51.0

strawberry *(Jell-O)* 52.0

chip, cherry *(SuperMoist)*, 1/10 pkg. or 1/10 cake* 40.0

chip, rainbow *(SuperMoist)*, 1/12 pkg. or 1/12 cake* 34.0

chocolate:

(Pillsbury Moist Supreme), 1/12 pkg. or 1/12 cake* 35.0

caramel nut *(Pillsbury Bundt)*, 1/16 pkg. or 1/16 cake* . . . 28.0

caramel nut *(Pillsbury Streusel Swirl)*, 1/16 pkg.

or 1/16 cake* 37.0

chip *(SuperMoist)*, 1/12 pkg. 34.0

chip *(SuperMoist)*, 1/12 cake* 35.0

dark *(Pillsbury Moist Supreme)*, 1/12 pkg. or 1/12 cake* . . 35.0

fudge *(SuperMoist)*, 1/12 pkg. or 1/12 cake* 34.0

German *(Pillsbury Moist Supreme)*, 1/12 pkg. or 1/12 cake* 34.0

German *(SuperMoist)*, 1/12 pkg. or 1/12 cake* 34.0

milk *(SuperMoist)*, 1/12 pkg. or 1/12 cake* 33.0

mocha *(Duncan Hines)*, 1/12 pkg. or 1/12 cake* 34.0

swirl, double *(SuperMoist)*, 1/12 pkg. or 1/12 cake* 35.0

Swiss *(Duncan Hines)*, 1/12 pkg. or 1/12 cake* 34.0

coffee *(Aunt Jemima* Easy Mix), 1/3 cup mix 12.0

date nut roll *(Dromedary)*, 1/3 pkg. 31.0

devil's food:

(Duncan Hines), 1/12 pkg. or 1/12 cake* 34.0

(Pillsbury Moist Supreme), 1/12 pkg. or 1/12 cake* 33.0

(Robin Hood Pouch), 1/5 pkg. or 1/5 cake* 36.0

(SnackWell's), 1/6 pkg. or 1/6 cake* 38.0

(SuperMoist), 1/12 pkg. 34.0

(SuperMoist), 1/12 cake* 33.0

(SuperMoist Light), 1/10 pkg. 42.0

(SuperMoist Light), 1/10 cake* 43.0

(Sweet Rewards Reduced Fat)*, 1/12 pkg. or 1/12 cake* . . . 20.0

fudge:

    dark, dutch *(Duncan Hines)*, 1/12 pkg. or 1/12 cake* 34.0

    hot *(Pillsbury Bundt)*, 1/16 pkg. or 1/16 cake* 39.0

    swirl *(Pillsbury Moist Supreme)*, 1/12 pkg. or 1/12 cake* . . 37.0

gingerbread, see "Bread mix, sweet"

lemon:

    (Duncan Hines Supreme), 1/12 pkg. or 1/12 cake* 36.0

    (Pillsbury Moist Supreme), 1/10 pkg. or 1/10 cake* 42.0

    (SuperMoist), 1/12 pkg. 35.0

    (SuperMoist), 1/12 cake* 36.0

lime, key *(Duncan Hines)*, 1/12 pkg. or 1/12 cake* 36.0

marble, fudge *(Duncan Hines)*, 1/12 pkg. or 1/12 cake* 36.0

marble, fudge *(SuperMoist)*, 1/12 pkg. or 1/12 cake* 36.0

orange *(Duncan Hines Supreme)*, 1/12 pkg. or 1/12 cake* 36.0

peanut butter chocolate swirl *(SuperMoist)*, 1/12 pkg.

    or 1/12 cake* 34.0

(Pillsbury Moist Supreme Funfetti), 1/12 pkg. or 1/12 cake* . . . 36.0

pineapple *(Duncan Hines Supreme)*, 1/12 pkg. or 1/12 cake* . . 36.0

pound, 1/8 pkg., except as noted:

    (Betty Crocker) 40.0

    (Dromedary) 38.0

    (Martha White), 1/4 pkg. or 1/4 cake* 44.0

raspberry *(Duncan Hines)*, 1/12 pkg. or 1/12 cake* 36.0

spice:

    (Duncan Hines), 1/12 pkg. or 1/12 cake* 36.0

    (SuperMoist), 1/12 pkg. 34.0

    (SuperMoist), 1/12 cake* 35.0

strawberry:

    (Duncan Hines Supreme), 1/12 pkg. or 1/12 cake* 36.0

    (Pillsbury Moist Supreme), 1/12 pkg. or 1/12 cake* 36.0

    cream cheese *(Pillsbury Bundt)*, 1/16 pkg. or 1/16 cake* . . 34.0

    swirl *(SuperMoist)*, 1/10 pkg. or 1/10 cake* 42.0

swirl, party *(SuperMoist)*, 1/12 pkg. or 1/12 cake* 35.0

vanilla, French:

    (Duncan Hines), 1/12 pkg. or 1/12 cake* 36.0

    (Pillsbury Moist Supreme), 1/10 pkg. or 1/10 cake* 42.0

    (SuperMoist), 1/12 pkg. or 1/12 cake* 35.0

vanilla, golden *(SuperMoist)*, 1/12 pkg. or 1/12 cake* 35.0

vanilla, wild cherry *(Duncan Hines)*, 1/12 pkg. or 1/12 cake* . . 36.0

white:

    (Duncan Hines), 1/12 pkg. or 1/12 cake* 35.0

    (Pillsbury Moist Supreme/Plus), 1/10 pkg. or 1/10 cake* . . 41.0

Cake, mix, white *(cont.)*

    (SnackWell's), ¹⁄₆ pkg. or ¹⁄₆ cake* 39.0

    (SuperMoist), ¹⁄₁₂ pkg. or ¹⁄₁₂ cake* 35.0

    (SuperMoist Light), ¹⁄₁₀ pkg. or ¹⁄₁₀ cake* 43.0

    (Sweet Rewards Reduced Fat), ¹⁄₁₂ pkg. or ¹⁄₁₂ cake* . . . 35.0

    Olympic party *(SuperMoist)*, ¹⁄₁₂ pkg. or ¹⁄₁₂ cake* 33.0

    sour cream *(SuperMoist)*, ¹⁄₁₀ pkg. or ¹⁄₁₀ cake* 39.0

white chocolate swirl *(SuperMoist)*, ¹⁄₁₂ pkg. 35.0

white chocolate swirl *(SuperMoist)*, ¹⁄₁₂ cake* 36.0

white 'n fudge swirl *(Pillsbury Moist Supreme)*, ¹⁄₁₂ pkg.

    or ¹⁄₁₂ cake* 37.0

yellow:

    (Duncan Hines), ¹⁄₁₂ pkg. or ¹⁄₁₂ cake* 36.0

    (Pillsbury Moist Supreme), ¹⁄₁₂ pkg. or ¹⁄₁₂ cake* 35.0

    (Robin Hood Pouch), ¹⁄₅ pkg. or ¹⁄₅ cake* 37.0

    (SnackWell's), ¹⁄₆ pkg. or ¹⁄₆ cake* 39.0

    (SuperMoist), ¹⁄₁₂ pkg. or ¹⁄₁₂ cake* 34.0

    (SuperMoist Light), ¹⁄₁₀ pkg. or ¹⁄₁₀ cake* 43.0

    (Sweet Rewards Reduced Fat), ¹⁄₁₂ pkg. or ¹⁄₁₂ cake* . . . 36.0

Cake, snack (see also specific listings),

    1 piece, except as noted:

(Tastykake Koffee Kake), 2.5 oz. 43.0

(Tastykake Kreme Krimpies), 2 pieces 37.0

all varieties *(Health Valley* Healthy Tarts) 35.0

apple, date, or raisin *(Health Valley* Bakes) . . . . •. 18.0

apple bar *(Health Valley)* 35.0

apple filled *(Tastykake Krimpets* Low Fat), 2 pieces 36.0

apricot bar *(Health Valley)* 35.0

banana:

    (Little Debbie Twins) 39.0

    (SnackWell's) 27.0

    (Tastykake Creamies) 27.0

Boston creme *(Drake's)* 25.0

brownie, fudge filled *(Health Valley)* 26.0

butterscotch iced *(Tastykake Krimpets)*, 2 pieces 26.0

cheesecake *(Boar's Head* New York), 4 oz. 40.0

cheesecake bar, all varieties *(Health Valley)* 34.0

chocolate:

    (Devil Dogs), 1.6 oz. 28.0

    (Ding Dongs), 2 pieces 45.0

    (Funny Bones), 2 pieces 42.0

    (Ho-Hos), 3 pieces 50.0

    (Hostess Choco-Diles) 34.0
    (Hostess Choco Licious), 2 pieces 60.0
    (Ring Dings), 2 pieces 42.0
    (Suzy Q's), 2 pieces 70.0
    (Tastykake Creamies) 26.0
    (Tastykake Juniors), 3.3 oz. 57.0
    (Tastykake Kandy Kakes), 3 pieces 35.0
    (Yodels), 2 pieces 35.0
chocolate chip *(Chips Ahoy)* 25.0
chocolate chip *(Little Debbie)* 37.0
coconut covered:
    (Sno Balls), 2 pieces 62.0
    (Tastykake Juniors), 3.3 oz. 59.0
    (Tastykake Kandy Kakes), 3 pieces 34.0
coffee cake:
    (Drake's) 18.0
    (Drake's Low Fat) 20.0
    (Little Debbie) 39.0
crumb *(Hostess)*, 3 pieces 56.0
crumb *(Hostess Light)*, 3 pieces 58.0
cupcake, 2 pieces, except as noted:
    (Tastykake Kreme Kup) 31.0
    (Yankee Doodles) 32.0
    apple filled *(Tastykake Koffee Kake Low Fat)* 33.0
    buttercreme, iced *(Tastykake)* 42.0
    buttercreme, iced, mini *(Tastykake)* 18.0
    chocolate *(Hostess)* 60.0
    chocolate *(Hostess Light)* 56.0
    chocolate *(Tastykake)* 39.0
    chocolate *(Tastykake)*, 3 pieces 58.0
    chocolate, creme *(Tastykake Low Fat)* 42.0
    chocolate iced, creme *(Tastykake)* 41.0
    chocolate iced, creme, mini *(Tastykake)* 18.0
    chocolate iced, creme, vanilla, mini *(Tastykake)* 17.0
    creme *(Tastykake Koffee Kake)* 35.0
    creme, mini *(Tastykake Koffee Kake)* 16.0
    lemon filled *(Tastykake Koffee Kake Low Fat)* 34.0
    orange *(Hostess)* 55.0
    raspberry filled *(Tastykake Koffee Kake Low Fat)* 34.0
    vanilla, creme *(Tastykake Low Fat)* 44.0
date bar *(Health Valley)* 34.0
devil's food *(Little Debbie Devil Cremes)* 56.0

Cake, snack *(cont.)*

frosty *(Tastykake Kandy Kakes)*, 3 pieces	38.0
fudge, frosted *(Little Debbie)*	14.0
fudge, rounds *(Little Debbie)*	12.0
golden *(SnackWell's)*.	27.0

golden, creme-filled:

(Hostess Dessert Cup)	18.0
(Little Debbie Golden Cremes)	42.0
(Sunny Doodles), 2 pieces	33.0
(Sunny Doodles Reduced Fat), 2 pieces	33.0
(Twinkies), 1.4 oz.	51.0
(Twinkies Light), 1.4 oz.	53.0
jelly filled *(Tastykake Krimpets)*, 2 pieces	38.0
jelly filled *(Tastykake Krimpets* Low Fat), 2 pieces	40.0
lemon filled *(Tastykake Krimpets* Low Fat), 2 pieces	38.0
peanut butter *(Tastykake Kandy Kakes)*, 3 pieces	32.0
pound *(Awrey's)*.	31.0
pound *(Tastykake)*	46.0
raisin bar *(Health Valley* Fat Free)	35.0
sprinkled *(Tastykake* Creamies)	25.0

stick, dunking:

(Little Debbie)	30.0
(Tastykake Stix)	45.0
twin sticks *(Awrey's)*, 2.75 oz.	32.0
strawberry, iced *(Tastykake Krimpets)*, 2 pieces	39.0
strawberry shortcake *(Little Debbie)*.	49.0
Swiss roll *(Little Debbie)*	48.0
vanilla *(Little Debbie)*	53.0
vanilla *(Tastykake* Creamies)	26.0
zebra *(Little Debbie)*	53.0

Cake, snack, mix (see also specific listings):

(Betty Crocker Easy Layer Bar), 1/16 pkg.	20.0
(Betty Crocker Easy Layer Bar), 1 bar*	21.0
apple cinnamon *(Sweet Rewards)*, 1/8 pkg. or 1/8 cake*	39.0
apple streusel bar *(Pillsbury)*, 1/24 pkg.	22.0
apple streusel bar *(Pillsbury)*, 1 bar*	23.0
banana *(Sweet Rewards)*, 1/8 pkg. or 1/8 cake*	39.0
Boston cream pie *(Betty Crocker)*, 1/10 pkg.	27.0
Boston cream pie *(Betty Crocker)*, 1/10 pie*	28.0
caramel oatmeal bar *(Betty Crocker)*, 1/20 pkg. or 1 bar* . . .	24.0
cheesecake bar, strawberry swirl *(Betty Crocker)*, 1/24 pkg. . .	22.0
cheesecake bar, strawberry swirl *(Betty Crocker)*, 1 bar* . . .	23.0

chocolate *(Sweet Rewards)*, 1/8 pkg. or 1/8 cake* 38.0
chocolate bar:
    chip *(Pillsbury Chips Ahoy!)*, 1/20 pkg. or 1 bar* 25.0
    chunk *(Betty Crocker)*, 1/32 pkg. or 1 bar* 17.0
    peanut butter *(Betty Crocker)*, 1/12 pkg. or 1 bar* 25.0
chocolate cookie bar *(Pillsbury Oreo)*, 1/18 pkg. or 1 bar* . . 26.0
chocolate pudding *(Betty Crocker)*, 1/8 pkg. or 1/8 cake* 33.0
cookie bar:
    (Betty Crocker Hershey), 1/16 pkg. or 1 bar* 21.0
    (Betty Crocker M&M's), 1/20 pkg. 25.0
    (Betty Crocker M&M's), 1 bar* 24.0
    (Pillsbury M&M's), 1/18 pkg. or 1 bar* 27.0
    double decker *(Duncan Hines)*, 1/30 pkg. or 1 bar* 18.0
    milk chocolate chunk *(Duncan Hines)*, 1/27 pkg. or 1 bar* 18.0
cupcake, dirt *(Duncan Hines)*, 1/6 pkg. or 2 pieces* 35.0
cupcake, polka dot angel food *(Duncan Hines)*, 1/8 pkg.
    or 3 pieces* 35.0
date bar *(Betty Crocker)*, 1/12 pkg.* 23.0
fudge swirl cookie *(Pillsbury)*, 1/20 pkg. or 1 bar* 25.0
gingerbread *(Betty Crocker)*, 1/8 pkg. or 1/8 cake* 38.0
lemon:
    (Sweet Rewards), 1/8 pkg. or 1/8 cake* 39.0
    bar *(Betty Crocker Sunkist)*, 1/16 pkg. or 1 bar* 24.0
    chiffon *(Betty Crocker)*, 1/16 pkg. or 1/16 cake* 26.0
    pudding *(Betty Crocker)*, 1/8 pkg. or 1/8 cake* 33.0
lemon cheesecake bar *(Pillsbury)*, 1/24 pkg. or 1 bar* 22.0
peanut butter bar *(Pillsbury Nutter Butter)*, 1/18 pkg.
    or 1 bar* 26.0
pineapple upside-down cake *(Betty Crocker)*, 1/6 pkg.
    or 1/6 cake* 63.0
pound cake *(Betty Crocker)*, 1/8 pkg. 40.0
pound cake *(Betty Crocker)*, 1/8 cake* 41.0
raspberry bar *(Betty Crocker)*, 1/20 pkg. or 1 bar* 26.0
S'mores bar *(Betty Crocker)*, 1/24 pkg. or 1 bar* 26.0
Cake decoration (see also "Frosting"), 1 tsp., except as
    noted:
(Dec-A-Cake Dec-A-Cone) 3.0
confetti or nonpareils *(Dec-A-Cake)* 3.0
hearts, bats, or pumpkins *(Dec-A-Cake)* 4.0
party imperials or fruit cocktail *(Dec-A-Cake)*, 9 pieces 4.0
rainbow *(Dec-A-Cake)* 4.0

Cake decoration *(cont.)*
sprinkles:
    (Hershey's Cookies n' Mint), 2 tbsp. 11.0
    chocolate, milk *(Hershey's)*, 2 tbsp. 22.0
    fun *(Dec-A-Cake)* 4.0
    holiday *(Dec-A-Cake)* 3.0
    peanut butter *(Reese's)*, 2 tbsp. 17.0
sugar crystals *(Dec-A-Cake)* 3.0
trims, chocolate *(Dec-A-Cake)*. 2.0
trims, chocolate mint *(Dec-A-Cake)* 3.0
Calves' liver, see "Liver"
Calzone, refrigerated, 6-oz. piece:
cheese *(Stefano's)* 43.0
pepperoni *(Stefano's)* 46.0
spinach *(Stefano's)* 46.0
Canary beans, dry *(Goya)*, ¼ cup 35.0
Candy:
(Baby Ruth), 2.1-oz. bar 38.0
(Baby Ruth Fun Size), 2 bars 27.0
(Bar None), 1.65-oz. bar 25.0
(Buncha Crunch), 1.4 oz. 26.0
butter rum *(Lifesavers)*, 2 pieces 5.0
butter rum *(Pearson Nips)*, 2 pieces 12.0
buttercrunch/almond *(Almond Roca)*, 4 pieces 25.0
(Butterfinger), 2.1-oz. bar 41.0
(Butterfinger Fun Size), 2 bars 30.0
(Butterfinger BB's), 1.7-oz. bag 34.0
butterscotch *(Brach's Disks)*, 3 pieces 17.0
butterscotch *(Hershey's Tastetations)*, 3 pieces 11.0
candy corn *(Heide/Heide Indian)*, 1 oz. 27.0
caramel:
    (Kraft), 5 pieces 32.0
    (Pearson Nips), 2 pieces 12.0
    hard *(Hershey's Tastetations)*, 3 pieces 12.0
caramel, chocolate coated:
    (Milk Duds), 1.85-oz. box 38.0
    (Pom Poms), 1.58-oz. box 35.0
    (Rolo), 1.9 oz. 35.0
caramel, with cookies:
    (Twix), 1-oz. piece 19.0
    (Twix King Size), .8-oz. bar 16.0
    (Twix Miniatures), 3 pieces 19.0

(Twix Singles), 2 bars, 2 oz. 37.0
(Twix Fun Size), .6-oz. piece 10.0
cherry, chocolate coated *(Perugina),* 1.21 oz. 26.0
chocolate:
 (Cella's Dark/Milk), 2 pieces, 1 oz. 18.0
 hard *(Hershey's Tastetations),* 3 pieces 12.0
 with hazelnuts *(Ferraro Rocher),* 3 pieces 17.0
 milk, see "chocolate, milk," below
 parfait *(Pearson Nips),* 2 pieces 11.0
chocolate, candy coated:
 (M&M's), 1.5 oz. 30.0
 (M&M's King Size), ½ bag, 1.6 oz. 34.0
 (M&M's Singles), 1.68-oz. bag. 32.0
 (M&M's Fun Size), .75-oz. bag. 15.0
 with almonds *(M&M's),* 1.5 oz. 25.0
 with almonds *(M&M's* Singles), 1.3-oz. bag 21.0
 mini *(M&M's),* 3 boxes, 1.5 oz. 29.0
 mini *(M&M's* Tube), 1.25-oz. tube 24.0
 peanut butter *(M&M's),* 1.5 oz. 24.0
 peanut butter *(M&M's* Singles), 1.6-oz. bag 27.0
 peanut butter *(M&M's Fun Size),* .75-oz. bag 12.0
 with peanuts *(M&M's),* 1.5 oz. 26.0
 with peanuts *(M&M's* King Size), ½ bag, 1.6 oz. 28.0
 with peanuts *(M&M's* Singles), 1.74-oz. bag 30.0
 with peanuts *(M&M's Fun Size),* .75-oz. bag 13.0
chocolate, dark:
 (Dove), ¼ of 6-oz. bar 26.0
 (Dove Mini), 7 pieces, 1.5 oz. 26.0
 (Dove Singles), 1.3-oz. bar 22.0
 (Ghirardelli), 1.5 oz. 26.0
 (Ghirardelli), 1.25-oz. bar 22.0
 (Hershey's Special Dark), 1.45-oz. bar 25.0
 with almonds *(Ghirardelli),* 1.5-oz. bar 23.0
 bittersweet *(Toblerone),* ⅓ of 3.5-oz. bar 21.0
 with raspberries *(Ghirardelli),* 4 pieces 26.0
chocolate, milk:
 (Dove), ¼ of 6-oz. bar 25.0
 (Dove Doves), .8-oz. piece 14.0
 (Dove Mini), 7 pieces, 1.5 oz. 25.0
 (Dove Single), 1.3-oz. bar 22.0
 (Ghirardelli), 1.25 oz. 22.0
 (Ghirardelli), 1.25-oz. bar 25.0

Candy, chocolate, milk *(cont.)*

(Hershey's), 1.55-oz. bar	25.0
(Hershey's Nuggets), 4 pieces	23.0
(Hershey's Kisses), 8 pieces	23.0
(Hershey's Hugs), 8 pieces	23.0
(Hershey's Miniatures), 5 pieces	25.0
(Nestlé), 1.45-oz. bar	23.0
(Symphony), 1.5-oz. bar	22.0
with almonds *(Cadbury)*, 9 blocks	21.0
with almonds *(Ghirardelli)*, 1.25-oz. bar	19.0
with almonds *(Ghirardelli)*, 1.5 oz.	22.0
with almonds *(Ghirardelli)*, 2.1-oz. bar	32.0
with almonds *(Hershey's)*, 1.45-oz. bar	20.0
with almonds *(Hershey's Golden)*, 2.8-oz. bar	36.0
with almonds *(Hershey's Golden Solitaire)*, 2.8-oz. bag	37.0
with almonds *(Hershey's Nuggets)*, 4 pieces	19.0
with almonds *(Hershey's Hugs)*, 9 pieces	22.0
with almonds *(Hershey's Kisses)*, 8 pieces	19.0
with almonds and toffee *(Symphony)*, 1.5-oz. bar	20.0
with caramel *(Caramello)*, 1.6-oz. bar	29.0
cookies and cream *(Ghirardelli)*, 1.3 oz.	22.0
cookies and cream *(Hershey's Nuggets)*, 4 pieces	22.0
with crisps *(Cadbury Krisp)*, 9 blocks	25.0
with crisps *(Crunch)*, 1.55-oz. bar	28.0
with crisps *(Crunch Fun Size)*, 4 bars	25.0
with crisps *(Ghirardelli)*, 1.25-oz. bar	22.0
with crisps *(Ghirardelli)*, 2.1-oz. bar	37.0
with crisps *(Ghirardelli)*, 2.5-oz. bar	44.0
with crisps *(Krackel)*, 1.4-oz. bar	25.0
with fruit and nuts *(Chunky)*, 1.4-oz. bar	22.0
with hazelnuts *(Mon Cheri)*, 3 pieces	20.0
with honey and nougat *(Toblerone)*, ⅓ of 3.5-oz. bar	20.0
with macadamias *(Ghirardelli)*, 1.25-oz. bar	19.0
with macadamias *(Hershey's Golden)*, 2.4-oz. bar	35.0
with peanuts *(Mr. Goodbar)*, 1.75-oz. bar	25.0
with pecans *(Ghirardelli)*, 4 pieces, 1.5 oz.	22.0
thins *(Lindt Swiss)*, 15 pieces, 1.5 oz.	22.0
with toffee *(Ghirardelli)*, 4 pieces, 1.5 oz.	26.0
wafers *(Ghirardelli)*, 11 pieces, 1.5 oz.	29.0
chocolate, white, and cookie *(Hershey's Cookies 'n' Creme)*, 1.5-oz. bar	24.0

chocolate, white, with crisps:
  (*Nestlé White Crunch*), 1.4-oz. bar 23.0
  (*Nestlé White Crunch* Giant), ⅓ of 4.5-oz. bar 24.0
chocolate, white, raspberry cream (*Ghirardelli*), 4 pieces,
  ⅓ oz. 21.0
chocolate mint:
  (*Cadbury* Mint), 5 blocks 27.0
  (*Ghirardelli*), 1½ oz. 26.0
  (*Ghirardelli*), 2.1-oz. bar 37.0
  (*Pearson Nips*), 2 pieces 11.0
  candy coated (*M&M's*), 1.5 oz. 30.0
  cookies and (*Hershey's*), 1.55-oz. bar 27.0
  cookies and (*Hershey's* Nuggets), 4 pieces 24.0
  wafers (*Ghirardelli*), 11 pieces, 1.5 oz. 27.0
coconut, chocolate coated (*Mounds*), 1.9-oz. bar 31.0
coconut, chocolate coated, with almonds
  (*Almond Joy*), 1.76-oz. bar 29.0
coffee (*Pearson Nips*), 2 pieces 12.0
coffee beans, espresso, chocolate covered, milk chocolate
  or hazelnut flavor (*Snap!*), 1.5-oz. pkg. 23.0
creme egg (*Milky Way*), 1.2-oz. piece 18.0
creme egg (*Snickers*), 1.2-oz. piece 19.0
fruit flavor:
  (*Frooties*), 12 pieces, 1.3 oz. 31.0
  (*Skittles*), 1.5 oz. 39.0
  (*Skittles* Singles), 2.2-oz. bag 54.0
  (*Skittles Fun Size*), 3 bags, 1.6 oz. 41.0
  chews, all flavors (*Starburst*), 8 pieces, 1.4 oz. 33.0
  chews, all flavors (*Starburst* Singles), 2.1-oz. pack 48.0
  tropical or wild berry (*Skittles*), 1.5 oz. 37.0
  tropical or wild berry (*Skittles* Singles), 2.2-oz. bag . . . 56.0
  tropical or wild berry (*Skittles Fun Size*), 2 bags, 1.4 oz. 36.0
  twists (*Starburst*), 4 pieces, 1.5 oz. 34.0
  twists (*Starburst* Singles), 2-oz. bag 35.0
fruit flavor, gummed:
  (*Amazin' Fruit*), 1.9 oz. 41.0
  (*Brach's Fruit Bunch*), 3 pieces, 1.6 oz. 37.0
  (*Gummi Savers*), 1.5 oz.
  original or tropical (*Dots*), 12 pieces, 1.5 oz. 37.0
  original or tropical (*Dots*), 2.25-oz. box 56.0
fudge (*Kraft Fudgies*), 5 pieces, 1.4 oz. 32.0
gum, chewing, all flavors, 1 piece 2.0

Candy *(cont.)*

gum, bubble, 1 piece:

(Blow Pop Ball) 11.0

(Bubble Yum) 6.0

(Bubble Yum Sugarless) 3.0

(Care*Free) 2.0

stick (Care*Free) 2.0

hard, all flavors:

(Brach's Sparklers), 3 pieces, .6 oz. 17.0

(Charms), 2 pieces, .2 oz. 6.0

(Farley's Clearly Fruit), 3 pieces, .6 oz. 17.0

(Lifesavers), 2 pieces 5.0

(Pez), .3-oz. roll 9.0

(Pez Sugar Free), .3-oz. roll 8.0

(Tootsie Pop Drops), 1 piece, .2 oz. 5.0

hard, chocolate dipped (Bodgon's Reception Sticks), 1 piece . 3.0

honey (Bit-O-Honey), 1.7-oz. bar 41.0

jelled:

(Chuckles Rings), 4 pieces, 1.6 oz. 37.0

(Jujubes), 58 pieces, 1.4 oz. 32.0

(Jujyfruits), 15 pieces, 1.4 oz. 33.0

spearmint leaves (Brach's), 5 pieces 34.0

jelly beans, assorted flavors:

(Jelly Belly), 1 oz. 26.0

(Jelly Belly), 35 pieces, 1.4 oz. 37.0

(Smucker's), 24 pieces, 1.4 oz. 37.0

(Starburst), 1.5 oz. 38.0

(Starburst Singles), 1.25-oz. bag 32.0

egg (Starburst), 2-oz. egg 51.0

licorice:

(Crows), 12 pieces, 1.5 oz. 37.0

(Nibs), 22 pieces 31.0

(Pearson Nips), 2 pieces 12.0

(Twizzlers), 4 pieces 33.0

bridge mix (Goelitz), 2 tbsp., 1.4 oz. 37.0

cherry (Nibs), 22 pieces 31.0

cherry (Twizzler Pull-n-Peel), 1.3-oz. piece 23.0

chocolate (Twizzlers), 5 pieces 33.0

strawberry (Twizzlers), 4 pieces 33.0

licorice, candy coated (Good & Fruity), 1.8-oz. box 35.0

licorice, candy coated (Good & Plenty), 1.4 oz. 33.0

lollipop, all flavors, 1 pop, except as noted:
   (Astro Pops), 1 oz. 27.0
   (Blow Pop), .65 oz. 17.0
   (Blow Pop), .9 oz. 24.0
   (Blow Pop), 1.35 oz. 36.0
   (Blow Pop Junior)*, .5 oz. 13.0
   (Caramel Apple), .5 oz. 13.0
   (Caramel Apple), .6 oz. 17.0
   (Charms), .5 oz. 14.0
   (Charms Sweet/Sour)*, .6 oz. 18.0
   (Dum-Dums), .6 oz. 18.0
   (Fiesta), .7 oz. 19.0
   (Lifesavers), .4 oz. 11.0
   (Mutant Fruitant), .6 oz. 16.0
   (Save-A-Sucker/Suck An Egg), 1 oz. 27.0
   (Save-A-Sucker), 2 oz. 54.0
   (Sugar Daddy), 1.7 oz. 43.0
   (Sugar Daddy Junior)*, 3 pops, 1.3 oz. 34.0
   (Tootsie Pop), .6 oz. 16.0
   (Tootsie Pop), .45 oz 12.0
   (Tootsie Roll Candy Cane)*, .7 oz. 19.0
   (Tootsie Roll Candy Cane)*, .5 oz. 13.0
   (Zip-A-Dee-Doo-Da), 3 pops, .5 oz. 15.0
malted milk balls *(Whoppers)*, 1.4 oz. 30.0
(Mars), 1.76-oz. bar 31.0
(Mars Fun Size), 2 bars 24.0
marshmallow:
   (Funmallows), 4 pieces 26.0
   (Kraft Jet-Puffed)*, 5 pieces, 1.2 oz. 27.0
   mini *(Funmallows)*, ½ cup 25.0
   mini *(Kraft)*, ½ cup 25.0
   peanut *(Spangler)*, 6 pieces 41.0
(Mexican Midgee), 12 pieces, 1.3 oz. 30.0
(Milky Way Original Miniatures)*, 5 pieces, 1.5 oz. 30.0
(Milky Way Original Singles)*, 2-oz. bar 41.0
(Milky Way Original *Fun Size)*, 2 bars, 1.4 oz. 28.0
(Milky Way Dark Miniatures)*, 5 pieces, 1.45 oz. 30.0
(Milky Way Dark Singles)*, 1.76-oz. bar 36.0
(Milky Way Dark *Fun Size)*, 2 bars, 1.4 oz. 28.0
(Milky Way Lite Miniatures)*, 5 pieces, 1.4 oz. 29.0
(Milky Way Lite Singles)*, 1.57-oz. bar 34.0

Candy *(cont.)*
mint:
    (Lifesavers Cryst-O-Mint), 2 pieces 5.0
    (Pez Peppermint), 3 pieces 2.0
    all flavors *(Breath Savers)*, 1 piece 2.0
    all flavors *(Lifesavers)*, 3 pieces 5.0
    butter *(Kraft)*, 7 pieces 14.0
    chocolate coated *(After Eight)*, 5 pieces 32.0
    chocolate coated *(Junior* Mints), 1.6-oz. box 38.0
    chocolate coated *(Junior* Mints), 16 pieces 34.0
    chocolate coated *(Junior* Mints Mini), 3 boxes, 1.5 oz. . . . 36.0
    chocolate coated *(Pearson)*, 5 pieces 31.0
    chocolate coated *(York* Peppermint Pattie), 1.5-oz. piece 33.0
    chocolate coated *(York* Peppermint Pattie Mini),
      3 pieces, 1.4 oz. 33.0
    party *(Kraft)*, 7 pieces 14.0
(Nestlé Turtles), 2 pieces 20.0
nonpareils *(Ghirardelli)*, 1.4 oz. 29.0
nonpareils *(Sno-Caps)*, 2.3 oz. 48.0
nougat *(Brach's)*, 4 pieces 38.0
nougat *(Charleston Chew* Vanilla), 5 pieces, 1.2 oz. 26.0
nougat bar, chocolate covered:
    chocolate or vanilla *(Charleston Chew)*, 1.9-oz. bar 40.0
    chocolate *(Charleston Chew)*, .35-oz. bar 7.0
    chocolate *(Charleston Chew)*, 2.5-oz. bar 53.0
    strawberry *(Charleston Chew)*, 1.9-oz. bar 42.0
    strawberry *(Charleston Chew)*, 2.5-oz. bar 56.0
    vanilla *(Charleston Chew)*, .35-oz. bar 8.0
    vanilla *(Charleston Chew)*, 2.5-oz. bar 53.0
(Oh Henry!), 1.8-oz. bar 32.0
(100 Grand), 1.5-oz. bar 30.0
(Pay Day), 1.85-oz. bar 30.0
peanut *(Planters)*, 1.6-oz. bar 22.0
peanut, chocolate coated *(Goobers)*, 1.38 oz. 19.0
peanut brittle *(Kraft)*, 1.3 oz. 29.0
peanut butter, chocolate:
    (5th Avenue), 2-oz. bar 38.0
    with cookie *(Twix)*, .9-oz. bar 13.0
    with cookie *(Twix* Singles), 2 bars, 1.7 oz. 26.0
    cup *(Reese's)*, 2 pieces, 1.6-oz. pkg. 25.0
    cup *(Reese's* Crunchy Cookie), 2 pieces, 1.44-oz. pkg. . . . 23.0
peanut butter parfait *(Pearson Nips)*, 2 pieces 11.0

popcorn, caramel, see "Popcorn, popped"
pretzel, chocolate covered *(Price's)*, 2 pieces 23.0
pretzel, frosted *(Price's)*, 2 pieces 25.0
raisins, chocolate coated *(Raisinets)*, 1.58 oz. 31.0
raisins, yogurt coated:
    strawberry or vanilla *(Del Monte)*, .9-oz. bag 20.0
    vanilla *(Del Monte)*, 1-oz. bag 22.0
    vanilla *(Del Monte)*, 3 tbsp. 23.0
rock *(Brach's)*, 1 oz. 27.0
(Snickers King Size), 1/3 bar 21.0
(Snickers Miniatures), 4 pieces, 1.26 oz. 22.0
(Snickers Singles), 2.07-oz. bar 35.0
(Snickers Fun Size), 2 bars, 1.4 oz. 24.0
(Snickers Munch), 1.4-oz. bar 17.0
(Sugar Babies), 30 pieces 39.0
(Sugar Babies Christmas Pouch), 18 pieces, 9.3 oz. 47.0
(Sugar Babies Pouch), 1.7-oz. bag 43.0
(Sugar Daddy Chewz), 5 pieces, 1.5 oz. 33.0
(Sugar Daddy Nuggets), 5 pieces, 1.5 oz. 37.0
(3 Musketeers), 2.13-oz. bar 46.0
(3 Musketeers Miniatures), 7 bars 32.0
(3 Musketeers Fun Size), 2 bars 26.0
toffee:
    (Brach's Treasures), 3 pieces 15.0
    bar *(Heath)*, 1.4 oz. 25.0
    bar *(Skor)*, 1.4 oz. 23.0
(Tootsie Flavor Roll Twisties), 6 pieces, 1.4 oz. 35.0
(Tootsie Roll Midges), 6 pieces, 1.4 oz. 33.0
(Tootsie Roll Snack Bar), 2 pieces, 1 oz. 23.0
wafer, chocolate coated *(Kit Kat)*, 1½-oz. bar 26.0
(Whatchamacallit), 1.7-oz. bar 29.0
Cane syrup, 1 tbsp. 13.4
Cannellini beans, see "Kidney beans"
Cannelloni dinner, frozen *(Amy's)*, 10 oz. 32.0
Cannelloni entree, frozen, cheese *(Lean Cuisine)*, 9 1/8 oz. . . 29.0
Cantaloupe:
(Dole), 1/4 fruit 11.0
untrimmed, 1 lb. 19.3
½ of 5"-diam. melon 22.3
pulp, cubed, ½ cup 6.7
Cantaloupe cocktail *(Snapple)*, 8 fl. oz. 32.0
Caperberries, in jars *(Haddon House)*, 2 tbsp. 1.0

Capers:
(B&G), 1 tbsp. 1.0
(Crosse & Blackwell), 1 tbsp. 1.0
(Krinos), 1 tsp. 0
(Progresso), 1 tsp. 0
with pimientos *(Goya)*, ¼ cup 0
Capon, without added ingredients 0
Caponata, see "Artichoke appetizer" and "Eggplant
    appetizer"
Cappacola, see "Ham lunch meat"
Cappuccino, iced:
(Jamaican Gold), 11 oz. 29.0
coffee *(Maxwell House)*, 8 fl. oz. 24.0
mocha or vanilla *(Maxwell House)*, 8 fl. oz. 27.0
Cappuccino bar, frozen *(Frozfruit)*, 1 bar 18.0
Cappuccino mix, see "Coffee, flavored, mix"
Carambola:
fresh:
    (Frieda's), 5 oz. 11.0
    untrimmed, 1 lb. 33.7
    1 medium, 4.7 oz. 9.9
dried *(Frieda's* Starfruit)*, ⅓ cup, 1.4 oz. 29.0
dried *(Sonoma)*, 1.4 oz. 34.0
Caramel custard, see "Pudding mix"
Caramel dip, 2 tbsp.:
(Marie's) 24.0
(Marie's Low Fat)* 29.0
(Smucker's Fruit Fat Free)* 30.0
Caramel topping, 2 tbsp.:
(Kraft) 28.0
(Mrs. Richardson's Fat Free)* 32.0
(Smucker's Sundae)* 27.0
hot *(Smucker's)* 29.0
Caraway seed:
(McCormick), ¼ tsp. 3
1 tbsp. 3.3
1 tsp. 1.1
Carbonara sauce mix *(Knorr)*, 2 tbsp. 5.0
Cardamom:
(McCormick), ¼ tsp. 4
ground:
    (Tone's), 1 tsp. 1.3

1 tbsp. 4.0
1 tsp. 1.4
seed *(Spice Islands)*, 1 tsp. 1.3
Cardoon:
raw, untrimmed, 1 lb. 10.9
raw, shredded, ½ cup 4.4
boiled, drained, 4 oz. 6.0
Carissa:
untrimmed, 1 lb. 53.2
1 medium, .8 oz. 2.7
sliced, ½ cup 10.2
Carl's Jr., 1 serving:
breakfast items:
    bacon, 2 strips 0
    burrito, breakfast 29.0
    English muffin, with margarine 30.0
    French toast dips, without syrup 40.0
    quesadilla, breakfast 27.0
    sausage, 1 patty 0
    scrambled eggs 1.0
    Sunrise Sandwich 31.0
    table syrup, 1 oz. 22.0
chicken stars, 6 pieces 11.0
sauces:
    barbecue sauce 11.0
    honey sauce 23.0
    mustard sauce 10.0
    salsa 2.0
    sweet n' sour sauce 11.0
sandwiches:
    Big Burger 46.0
    Carl's Catch Fish Sandwich 54.0
    chicken, barbequed 34.0
    chicken, ranch 56.0
    chicken, Santa Fe 36.0
    chicken bacon Swiss 57.0
    chicken club 37.0
    double cheeseburger, ⅓ lb. 37.0
    Double Western Bacon Cheeseburger 58.0
    Famous Big Star hamburger 42.0
    hamburger 23.0
    Hot & Crispy sandwich 35.0

Carl's Jr., sandwiches (cont.)
 Super Star hamburger 41.0
 Western Bacon Cheeseburger. 59.0
"Great Stuff" potatoes:
 bacon and cheese 76.0
 broccoli and cheese 76.0
 potato, plain 68.0
 sour cream and chive 70.0
Entree Salads-To-Go:
 chicken 11.0
 garden 4.0
salad dressings, 2 oz.:
 blue cheese 1.0
 French, fat free 18.0
 house 3.0
 Italian, fat free 4.0
 Thousand Island 7.0
side dishes:
 CrissCut Fries, large 55.0
 fries, regular 44.0
 hash brown nuggets 27.0
 onion rings 63.0
 zucchini 38.0
bakery products:
 blueberry muffin 49.0
 bran muffin 61.0
 cheese Danish 49.0
 cheesecake, strawberry swirl 31.0
 chocolate cake 49.0
 chocolate chip cookie 49.0
 cinnamon roll 68.0
shake, small:
 chocolate 74.0
 strawberry 77.0
 vanilla 54.0
Carnival squash *(Frieda's)*, ¾ cup, 3 oz. 7.0
Carob drink mix, powder, 3 tsp. 11.2
Carob flour, 1 cup 91.6
Carp, without added ingredients 0
Carrot, fresh:
raw:
 (Dole), 7″ long, 1¼″ diam. 9.0

untrimmed, 1 lb. 41.0
whole, 7½" long, 2.8 oz. 7.3
shredded, ½ cup 5.6
shredded *(Dole)*, 3 oz. 9.0
baby, 1 medium, 2¾" long 8
mini *(Frieda's)*, 1 oz. 2.7
mini, peeled *(Dole)*, 3 oz. 9.0
boiled, drained, 1 medium, 1.6 oz. 4.8
boiled, drained, sliced, ½ cup 8.2
Carrot, canned, ½ cup, except as noted:
all varieties *(S&W)* 6.0
all varieties *(Seneca)* 6.0
baby, whole *(LeSueur)* 8.0
whole or sliced *(Stokely)*, 4.5 oz. 5.0
sliced:
   (Allens/Crest Top) 8.0
   (Del Monte) 8.0
   (Goya) 6.0
   (Green Giant) 6.0
   (Stokely No Salt) 5.0
   with liquid 6.2
   drained 4.0
Carrot, frozen:
boiled, drained, sliced, ½ cup 6.0
baby, whole:
   (Birds Eye), ½ cup 9.0
   (Schwan's), 13 pieces 7.0
   (Stilwell), ⅔ cup 6.0
baby, cut *(Green Giant)*, ¾ cup 7.0
baby, cut *(Green Giant Harvest Fresh)*, ⅔ cup 5.0
crinkle *(Stilwell)*, ⅔ cup 6.0
green beans and cauliflower *(Green Giant American*
   Mixtures), ¾ cup 5.0
Carvel:
ice cream, soft serve, ½ cup:
   chocolate 21.0
   chocolate, no fat 19.0
   vanilla 21.0
   vanilla, no fat 24.0
sherbet, all flavors, ½ cup 33.0
yogurt, soft serve, vanilla, no sugar, ½ cup 12.0

Carvel (cont.)
novelties, 1 piece:
Brown Bonnet cone 43.0
Chipsters 50.0
Flying Saucer 33.0
ice cream cupcake 27.0
Casaba:
untrimmed, 1 lb. 16.9
1/10 of 73/4" melon 10.2
pulp, cubed, 1/2 cup 5.3
Cashew:
(Frito-Lay), 1.5 oz. 9.0
whole *(Paradise/White Swan),* 1/4 cup, 1.2 oz. 8.0
dry-roasted, 1 oz., 14 large or 18 medium 9.3
dry-roasted, whole or halves, 1 cup 44.8
honey-roasted:
(Planters), 1 oz. 11.0
(Planters), 2-oz. pkg. 23.0
and peanuts *(Planters),* 1 oz. 10.0
oil-roasted:
(Master Choice), 1 oz. 8.0
(Planters), 1-oz. pkg. 8.0
(Planters), 1.5-oz. pkg. 12.0
(Planters Fancy), 1 oz. 8.0
(Planters Fancy), 2-oz. pkg. 16.0
(Planters Halves), 1 oz. 8.0
(Planters Halves Lightly Salted), 1 oz. 9.0
(Planters Munch 'N Go Singles), 2-oz. pkg. 16.0
1 oz., 14 large or 18 medium 8.1
whole or halves, 1 cup 37.1
Cashew butter:
(Roaster Fresh), 1 oz. 9.0
1 oz. 7.8
Catfish, without added ingredients 0
Catfish entree, frozen, breaded *(Schwan's),* 4 oz. 15.0
Catjang:
raw, 1 oz. 16.9
boiled, 1/2 cup 17.5
Catsup, see "Ketchup"
Cauliflower, fresh:
raw:
(Dole), 1/6 medium head 5.0

untrimmed, 1 lb. 8.7
3 florets, approx. 5 oz. 2.9
1″ pieces, ½ cup 2.6
boiled, drained, 1″ pieces, ½ cup 2.6
green:
    raw *(Dole)*, ⅕ head 7.0
    raw, ⅕ head 5.7
    raw, 1″ pieces, ½ cup 3.0
    boiled, drained, 1″ pieces, ½ cup 3.9
Cauliflower, frozen:
(Stilwell), 1 cup 3.0
boiled, drained, 1″ pieces, ½ cup 3.4
florets *(Green Giant),* 1 cup 4.0
in cheese sauce *(Green Giant),* ½ cup 8.0
Cauliflower, pickled, sweet *(Vlasic),* 1 oz. 9.0
Cauliflower combinations, frozen:
broccoli, see "Broccoli combinations"
carrots, sugar snap peas, and sweet peas *(Green Giant
    American Mixtures),* ¾ cup 7.0
Cavatelli, frozen *(Celentano),* 3.2 oz. 79.0
Caviar (see also "Roe"), 1 tbsp.:
black or red 6
carp roe *(Krinos* Tarama) 0
lumpfish, black or red *(Romanoff)* 0
salmon, red *(Romanoff)* 0
whitefish, black *(Romanoff)* 1.0
Caviar spread *(Krinos* Taramosalata), 1 tbsp. 0
Cayenne, see "Pepper"
Ceci, see "Chickpeas"
Celeriac:
raw:
    (Frieda's Celery Root), ¾ cup, 3 oz. 8.0
    untrimmed, 1 lb. 35.9
    trimmed, ½ cup 10.4
boiled, drained, 4 oz. 7.2
Celery:
raw:
    (Dole), 2 medium stalks, 3.9 oz. 5.0
    untrimmed, 1 lb. 14.7
    7½″ stalk, 1.6 oz. 1.5
    diced, ½ cup 2.2
boiled, drained, diced, ½ cup 3.0

Celery, Chinese *(Frieda's* Kun Choy), 1 cup, 3 oz. 3.0
Celery, dried:
flakes or seed *(Tone's)*, 1 tsp. .9
seed, 1 tbsp. 2.7
seed, 1 tsp. 8
Celery root or knob, see "Celeriac"
Celery salt *(Tone's)*, 1 tsp. .6
Celery seed, see "Celery, dried"
Cellophane noodle, see "Noodle, Chinese"
Celtus:
untrimmed, 1 lb. 12.4
trimmed, 1 oz. 1.0
1 leaf, approx. .4 oz. 3
Cereal, ready-to-eat (see also specific grains):
amaranth flakes *(Arrowhead Mills)*, 1 cup 21.0
bran (see also "oat bran," below):
   (Kellogg's All-Bran/Kellogg's All-Bran Extra Fiber), ½ cup 22.0
   (Kellogg's Bran Buds), ⅓ cup 24.0
   (Kellogg's Frosted Bran), ¾ cup 26.0
   (Kellogg's Fruitful Bran), 1¼ cups 44.0
   (Nabisco 100% Bran), ⅓ cup 23.0
   (Post Bran'nola), ½ cup 43.0
   flakes *(Arrowhead Mills)*, 1 cup 22.0
   flakes *(Kellogg's Complete)*, ¾ cup 25.0
   flakes *(New Morning* Multi-Bran), 1 cup 21.0
   flakes *(Post)*, ⅔ cup 22.0
   raisin *(Kellogg's)*, 1 cup 43.0
   raisin *(Malt-O-Meal)*, 1 cup 43.0
   raisin *(New Morning* Multi-Bran), 1 cup 22.0
   raisin *(Post)*, 1 cup 46.0
   raisin *(Post Bran'nola)*, ½ cup 44.0
   with raisins *(Total* Raisin Bran), 1 cup 43.0
   with raisins and nuts *(Raisin Nut Bran)*, ¾ cup 41.0
corn:
   (Arrowhead Mills Maple Corns), 1 cup 43.0
   (Barbara's Frosted Funnies), 1 cup 27.0
   (Barbara's Puffins), ¾ cup 23.0
   (Berry Colossal Crunch), ¾ cup 25.0
   (Cap'N Crunch), ¾ cup 23.0
   (Cap'N Crunch with Cranberries), ¾ cup 22.0
   (Cap'N Crunch Peanut Butter Crunch), ¾ cup 22.0
   (Cocoa Comets), ¾ cup 27.0

(Colossal Crunch), ¾ cup 26.0
(Corn Burst), 1 cup 27.0
(Kellogg's Corn Pops), 1 cup 27.0
(Nut & Honey Crunch), 1¼ cups 45.0
(Perky's Nutty Rice), ¾ cup 50.0
(Post Toasties), 1 cup 24.0
almond raisin *(New Morning Crunchy)*, ¾ cup 22.0
bran *(Quaker* Crunchy), ¾ cup 23.0
chocolate flavor *(Coco-Roos)*, ¾ cup 27.0
chocolate flavor *(Cocoa Puffs)*, 1 cup 27.0
flakes *(Arrowhead Mills)*, 1 cup 30.0
flakes *(Barbara's)*, 1 cup 26.0
flakes *(Country* Corn Flakes), 1 cup 26.0
flakes *(Kellogg's Corn Flakes)*, 1 cup 26.0
flakes *(Kellogg's Frosted Flakes)*, ¾ cup 28.0
flakes *(Malt-O-Meal* Frosted), ¾ cup 27.0
flakes *(New Morning)*, 1 cup 26.0
flakes *(Total* Corn Flakes), 1⅓ cups 25.0
flakes, frosted *(Quaker By the Bag)*, ¾ cup 28.0
flakes, honey frosted *(New Morning)*, ⅔ cup 25.0
honey roasted pecan *(Kellogg's Temptations)*, 1 cup . . . 24.0
with marshmallow bits *(Count Chocula)*, 1 cup 26.0
with marshmallow bits *(Frankenberry)*, 1 cup 27.0
puffed *(Arrowhead Mills)*, 1 cup 16.0
puffed *(Body Buddies)*, 1 cup 26.0
puffed, honey *(Health Valley)*, 1 cup 20.0
Quakes (Quaker By the Bag), ¾ cup 25.0
corn and oat, cinnamon *(Kellogg's* Mini Buns), ¾ cup 27.0
corn and oat, vanilla almond *(Kellogg's Temptations)*, ¾ cup 24.0
corn and rice *(Kellogg's Crispix)*, 1 cup 26.0
corn and rice *(Kellogg's Double Dip Crunch)*, ¾ cup 27.0
granola:
   (C.W. Post Hearty), ⅔ cup 45.0
   (Heartland), ½ cup 41.0
   (Heartland Lowfat), ½ cup 40.0
   (Kellogg's Lowfat), ½ cup 43.0
   (New Morning Oatiola), ¾ cup 42.0
   almond *(Sun Country)*, ½ cup 38.0
   blueberries, milk *(Mountain House)*, ⅓ cup 18.0
   carob cashew *(Roman Meal)*, ½ cup 37.0
   figs and filberts *(Roman Meal)*, ½ cup 39.0
   honey nut *(Roman Meal)*, ½ cup 37.0

Cereal, ready-to-eat, granola *(cont.)*

    low fat, with fruit *(Nature Valley)*, ⅔ cup 44.0

    raisin *(Heartland)*, ½ cup 42.0

    raisin *(Kellogg's* Low Fat), ⅔ cup 43.0

    raisin and date *(Sun Country)*, ½ cup 43.0

    raisin nut *(Roman Meal)*, ½ cup 37.0

kamut, 1 cup:

    (New Morning Kamutios) 23.0

    flakes *(Arrowhead Mills)* 25.0

    puffed *(Arrowhead Mills)*. 19.0

millet, puffed *(Arrowhead Mills)*, 1 cup 19.0

mixed/multi grain:

    (Apple Jacks), 1 cup 27.0

    (Arrowhead Mills Crispy Puffs), 1 cup 16.0

    (Barbara's Shredded Spoonfuls), ¾ cup 23.0

    (Barbara's High 5), ¾ cup. 23.0

    (Basic 4), 1 cup 42.0

    (Berry Berry Kix), ¾ cup 26.0

    (Cinnamon Toast Crunch), ¾ cup 24.0

    (Fiber One), ½ cup 24.0

    (Froot Loops), 1 cup 26.0

    (Fruiteo's), 1 cup 25.0

    (Golden Grahams), ¾ cup 25.0

    (Grape-Nuts), ½ cup 47.0

    (Grape-Nuts Flakes), ¾ cup. 24.0

    (Just Right Crunchy Nuggets), 1 cup 46.0

    (Kaboom), 1¼ cups 24.0

    (Kellogg's Mueslix Crispy), ⅔ cup 42.0

    (Kellogg's Mueslix Golden Crunch), ¾ cup 40.0

    (Kix), 1⅓ cups 26.0

    (Multi•Grain Cheerios), 1 cup 24.0

    (Product 19), 1 cup 25.0

    (Quaker Life), ¾ cup 25.0

    (Quaker Life Cinnamon), ¾ cup 26.0

    (Quaker 100% Natural), ½ cup 31.0

    (Quaker 100% Natural Low Fat), ½ cup. 44.0

    (Quaker 100% Natural With Raisins), ½ cup 34.0

    (Team Flakes), 1¼ cups 49.0

    (Tootie Fruities), 1 cup 26.0

    (Total Whole Grain), ¾ cup 24.0

    (Trix), 1 cup 26.0

    all varieties *(Granola O's)*, ¾ cup 26.0

all varieties *(Health Valley* Honey Clusters & Flakes),
  ¾ cup 31.0
brown sugar cinnamon *(Pop-Tarts Crunch)*, ¾ cup 26.0
cocoa *(Startoons)*, 1 cup 26.0
dates, raisins, walnuts *(Fruit & Fibre)*, 1 cup 46.0
flakes *(Arrowhead Mills)*, 1 cup 29.0
flakes *(Healthy Choice)*, 1 cup 25.0
fruit-nut *(Just Right)*, 1 cup 46.0
granola, see "granola," above
honey *(Startoons)*, 1 cup 26.0
with marshmallow bits *(S'Mores)*, ¾ cup 26.0
peaches, raisins, almonds *(Fruit & Fibre)*, 1 cup 46.0
pecan *(Great Grains)*, ⅔ cup 38.0
raisins, dates, pecans *(Great Grains)*, ⅔ cup 39.0
raisins, oats, almonds *(Healthy Choice)*, 1 cup 45.0
squares *(Healthy Choice)*, 1¼ cups 45.0
strawberry *(Pop-Tarts Crunch)*, ¾ cup 27.0
oat:
  (Alpha-Bits), 1 cup 27.0
  (Apple Cinnamon Cheerios), ¾ cup 25.0
  (Arrowhead Mills Nature O's), 1 cup 24.0
  (Barbara's Breakfast O's), 1 cup 22.0
  (Cheerios), 1 cup 23.0
  (Frosted Cheerios), 1 cup 23.0
  (Honey Bunches of Oats), ¾ cup 25.0
  (Honey Nut Cheerios), 1 cup 24.0
  (Kellogg's Nut & Honey Crunch O's), ¾ cup 24.0
  (New Morning Oatios Original), 1 cup 21.0
  (Toasty O's), 1 cup 22.0
  (Toasty O's Frosted), 1 cup 25.0
  almonds *(General Mills* Oatmeal Crisp Almond), 1 cup . . 42.0
  almonds *(Honey Bunches of Oats)*, ¾ cup 24.0
  apple cinnamon *(General Mills* Oatmeal Crisp), 1 cup . . . 46.0
  apple cinnamon *(New Morning Oatios)*, 1 cup 18.0
  apple cinnamon *(Toasty O's)*, ¾ cup 25.0
  blueberry *(New Morning Oatiola)*, 1 cup 41.0
  cinnamon raisin *(Nature Valley* 100% Natural Oat
    Cinnamon & Raisin), ¾ cup 38.0
  cocoa *(New Morning Oatios)*, 1 cup 37.0
  fruit and nut *(Nature Valley* 100% Natural Oat Fruit &
    Nut), ⅔ cup 34.0

Cereal, ready-to-eat, oat *(cont.)*

and honey *(Nature Valley 100% Natural Oat Toasted
   Oats & Honey)*, ¾ cup 36.0
honey and nut *(Toasty O's)*, 1 cup 24.0
honey almond *(New Morning Oatios)*, 1 cup 22.0
honey graham *(Quaker Oh!s)*, ¾ cup 23.0
honey nut *(Quaker By the Bag)*, 1 cup 24.0
marshmallow *(Alpha-Bits)*, 1 cup 25.0
marshmallow *(Lucky Charms)*, 1 cup 25.0
marshmallow *(Mateys)*, 1 cup 25.0
with raisins *(General Mills Oatmeal Crisp Raisin)*, 1 cup   44.0
oat bran:
   (Common Sense), ¾ cup 23.0
   (Cracklin' Oat Bran), ¾ cup 40.0
   (New Morning Ultimate Oat Bran), 1 cup 20.0
   (Quaker), 1¼ cups 41.0
   flakes *(Arrowhead Mills)*, 1 cup 22.0
oatmeal:
   (Quaker Squares), 1 cup 43.0
   (Quaker Toasted), 1 cup 39.0
   cinnamon *(Quaker Squares)*, 1 cup 47.0
   honey nut *(Quaker Toasted)*, 1 cup 39.0
rice:
   (Apple Cinnamon Rice Krispies), ¾ cup 27.0
   (Cocoa Krispies), ¾ cup 27.0
   (Frosted Krispies), ¾ cup 27.0
   (Fruity Marshmallow Krispies), ¾ cup 27.0
   (Perky's Nutty Rice), ¾ cup 46.0
   (Rice Krispies), 1¼ cups 26.0
   (Rice Krispies Treats), ¾ cup 25.0
   (Special K), 1 cup 21.0
   crispy *(Malt-O-Meal)*, 1 cup 26.0
   puffed *(Arrowhead Mills)*, 1 cup 19.0
   puffed *(Malt-O-Meal)*, 1 cup 13.0
   puffed *(Quaker)*, 1 cup 12.0
rice, brown, crisp, 1 cup:
   (Barbara's) 25.0
   (Health Valley) 30.0
   (New Morning) 23.0
   frosted *(New Morning)* 45.0
rice and corn, almond raisin *(Nutri-Grain)*, 1¼ cups 44.0
rice and rye *(Kellogg's Apple Raisin Crisp)*, 1 cup 46.0

spelt flakes *(Arrowhead Mills)*, 1 cup 22.0
wheat:
    (Clusters), 1 cup 44.0
    (Golden Puffs), 3/4 cup 26.0
    (Honey Frosted Wheaties), 3/4 cup 27.0
    (Kellogg's Apple Cinnamon/Blueberry Squares), 3/4 cup . . 44.0
    (Kellogg's Frosted Mini-Wheats), 1 cup 45.0
    (Kellogg's Raisin Squares), 3/4 cup 44.0
    (Kellogg's Smacks), 3/4 cup 26.0
    (Kellogg's Strawberry Squares), 3/4 cup 44.0
    (Nabisco Frosted Wheat Bites), 1 cup 44.0
    (Nutri-Grain Golden), 3/4 cup 24.0
    (Wheaties), 1 cup 24.0
    blueberry or strawberry *(Nabisco Wheat Bites)*, 3/4 cup . . 41.0
    honey grahams *(New Morning)*, 2 pieces 24.0
    puffed *(Arrowhead Mills)*, 1 cup 20.0
    puffed *(Malt-O-Meal)*, 1 cup 11.0
    puffed *(Quaker)*, 1 cup 11.0
    raisin *(Nutri-Grain Golden)*, 1 1/4 cups 45.0
    with raisins *(Crispy Wheaties 'n Raisins)*, 1 cup 44.0
    raspberry *(Nabisco Wheat Bites)*, 3/4 cup 40.0
wheat, shredded:
    (Barbara's), 2 pieces 31.0
    (Nabisco), 2 pieces 38.0
    (Nabisco Shredded Wheat 'n Bran), 1 1/4 cups 47.0
    (Nabisco Spoon Size), 1 cup 41.0
    (Quaker), 3 pieces 50.0
wheat and barley *(Perky's Nutty Wheat & Barley)*, 3/4 cup . . 47.0
Cereal, cooking/hot (see also specific grains), uncooked,
    1 pkt., except as noted:
barley *(Arrowhead Mills Bits O Barley)*, 1/3 cup 35.0
barley, banana nut *(Fantastic Cup)*, 1.6 oz. 39.0
farina, see "wheat," below
mixed/multi grain:
    (Mothers), 1/2 cup 28.0
    (Pritikin) 34.0
    (Quaker), 1/2 cup 29.0
    (Roman Meal) 25.0
    (Roman Meal Instant) 21.0
    3 grain, maple raisin *(Fantastic Cup)*, 1.8 oz. 42.0
    3 grain, strawberry banana *(Fantastic Cup)*, 1.7 oz. 40.0
    4 grain, with flax *(Arrowhead Mills)*, 1/4 cup 28.0

Cereal, cooking/hot, mixed/multi grain *(cont.)*

7 grain *(Arrowhead Mills)*, ⅓ cup 25.0
7 grain *(Arrowhead Mills* Wheat Free), ¼ cup 25.0
apple cinnamon *(Roman Meal/Roman Meal* Instant) 24.0
raisin date-nut *(Roman Meal)* 26.0
raisin date-nut *(Roman Meal* Instant) 25.0

oat bran:

(Mothers), ½ cup 24.0
(Quaker), ½ cup 25.0
mango *(Fantastic* Cup), 1.8 oz. 39.0

oat flakes, raisin and spice *(H-O* Instant) 32.0

oatmeal, instant:

(Arrowhead Mills) 19.0
(H-O), ½ cup 27.0
(Maypo), ⅓ cup 27.0
(Mothers), ½ cup 23.0
(Quaker) 19.0
(Quaker Microwave) 19.0
(Roman Meal Premium) 40.0
apple cinnamon *(Fantastic* Cup), 1.7 oz. 37.0
with apples and cinnamon *(Quaker)* 27.0
apple spice *(Quaker* Microwave) 35.0
bananas and cream *(Quaker)* 26.0
blueberries and cream *(Quaker)* 26.0
brown sugar cinnamon *(Quaker* Microwave) 31.0
cinnamon double raisin *(Quaker* Microwave) 35.0
cinnamon raisin almond *(Arrowhead Mills)* 24.0
cinnamon spice *(Quaker)* 36.0
cinnamon toast *(Quaker)* 27.0
chocolate chip cookie *(Quaker Kids' Choice)* 32.0
cookies 'n cream *(Quaker Kids' Choice)* 31.0
cranberry orange *(Fantastic* Cup), 1.7 oz. 38.0
fruity marshmallow *(Quaker Kids' Choice)* 31.0
honey bran *(Quaker* Microwave) 30.0
maple *(Maypo)*, ½ cup 36.0
maple, apple, spice *(Arrowhead Mills)* 25.0
maple brown sugar *(Quaker)* 33.0
oatmeal raisin cookie *(Quaker Kids' Choice)* 32.0
peaches and cream *(Quaker)* 26.0
raisin, date, walnut *(Quaker)* 27.0
raisin spice *(Quaker)* 33.0
raspberry *(Quaker Kids' Choice)* 29.0

S'mores *(Quaker Kids' Choice)* 32.0
strawberries and cream *(Quaker)* 26.0
strawberries'n stuff *(Quaker Kids' Choice)* 30.0
strawberry-banana *(Quaker Kids' Choice)* 31.0
oats *(H-O* Quick), ½ cup 27.0
oats *(H-O* Quick Oats'n Fiber) 17.0
oats, rolled:
    (H-O Instant) 18.0
    (H-O Sweet & Mellow Instant) 30.0
    (Mothers), ½ cup 27.0
    (Quaker Quick/Old Fashioned), ½ cup 27.0
    almond raisin *(H-O* Explo Instant) 32.0
    apple and cinnamon *(H-O* Instant) 26.0
    apple maple spice *(H-O* Explo Instant) 33.0
    apricot honey *(H-O* Explo Instant) 33.0
    banana creme *(H-O* Explo Instant) 32.0
    maple and brown sugar *(H-O* Instant) 32.0
oats, toasted *(H-O* Old Fashioned), ⅓ cup 28.0
rice:
    (Arrowhead Mills Rice & Shine), ¼ cup 32.0
    almond, sweet *(Lundberg* Hot 'n Creamy), ⅓ cup 40.0
    amber grain *(Lundberg* Hot 'n Creamy), ⅓ cup 44.0
    cinnamon raisin *(Lundberg* Hot 'n Creamy), ⅓ cup 42.0
    purely organic *(Lundberg* Hot 'n Creamy), ⅓ cup 43.0
rye, cream of *(Roman Meal)* 25.0
rye, cream of *(Roman Meal* Instant) 20.0
wheat:
    (Arrowhead Mills Bear Mush), ¼ cup 33.0
    (Malt-O-Meal Quick), 3 tbsp. 26.0
    (Mothers), ½ cup 30.0
    (Wheat Hearts), ¼ cup 26.0
    (Wheatena), ⅓ cup 32.0
    all varieties *(Malt-O-Meal)*, 3 tbsp. 28.0
    cracked *(Arrowhead Mills)*, ¼ cup 29.0
    farina *(H-O)*, 3 tbsp. 26.0
    whole *(Mothers/Quaker)*, ½ cup 30.0
    n'berries *(Fantastic* Cup), 1.7 oz. 40.0
    and oat, peachberry *(Fantastic* Cup), 1.8 oz. 42.0
Cereal bar, see "Granola and cereal bar"
Cereal beverage, see "Coffee substitute"
Charcoal seasoning *(Durkee)*, ¼ tsp. 0

Chayote:

raw:

    (Frieda's), ²/₃ cup 5.0

    untrimmed, 1 lb. 24.3

    1 medium, 7.2 oz. 11.0

    1″ pieces, ½ cup 3.6

boiled, drained, 1″ pieces, ½ cup 4.1

Cheese (see also "Cheese food" and "Cheese product"):

American, processed:

    (Boar's Head Loaf), 1 oz. 1.0

    (Borden), ²/₃-oz. slice 1.0

    (Borden), ³/₄-oz. slice 1.0

    (Borden Loaf), 1 oz. 1.0

    (Harvest Moon), ²/₃-oz. slice 0

    (Kraft Deluxe Loaf), 1 oz. . . . . <1.0

    (Kraft Deluxe Slice), ²/₃-oz. slice . . . . <1.0

    (Kraft Deluxe Slice), ³/₄-oz. slice . . . . <1.0

    (Kraft Deluxe Slice), 1-oz. slice . . . . <1.0

    (Old English Loaf), 1 oz. . . . . <1.0

    (Old English Slice), 1-oz. slice . . . . <1.0

    (Schwan's), ²/₃-oz. slice . . . . <1.0

    sharp *(Borden)*, 1 oz. 1.0

(Bel Paese):

    medallions, ³/₄ oz. 1.5

    flavored varieties, 1 oz. 1.0

    with basil and sun-dried tomatoes, 1 oz. 7

blue *(Kraft)*, 1 oz. . . . . <1.0

blue, crumbled *(Sargento)*, ¼ cup 1.0

brick *(Kraft)*, 1 oz. 0

Brie, 1 oz. 1

butterkase, plain or smoked *(Boar's Head)*, 1 oz. 0

cheddar, 1 oz., except as noted:

    (Alpine Lace Reduced Fat) 1.0

    (Boar's Head Double Glouster) 0

    (Dorman) 1.0

    (Dorman Reduced Fat) 0

    (Heluva Good Low Sodium) 0

    (Kraft Cracker Barrel/Kraft Cracker Barrel ¹/₃ *Less Fat)* . . <1.0

    (Land O Lakes) . . . . <1.0

    (Land O Lakes Cheddarella) 0

    mild *(Heluva Good Reduced Fat)* 1.0

    mild *(Kraft* ¹/₃ *Less Fat)* 0

mild, light, snack *(MooTown Snackers)*, .8-oz. piece ...<1.0
mild or sharp *(MooTown Snackers)*, .8-oz. piece 1.0
mild or sharp *(Weight Watchers* Natural) 1.0
mild, sharp, or extra sharp *(Heluva* Good) 1.0
sharp *(Boar's Head* Slicing) ....<1.0
sharp *(Kraft* Less Fat).......................<1.0
sharp *(Sargento* Sliced) 1.0
nacho, with peppers *(Kraft)* 0
cheddar, shredded, ¼ cup, except as noted:
  (Kraft) ....<1.0
  fat free *(Kraft Healthy Favorites)* 1.0
  fine *(Kraft)* ....<1.0
  mild *(Heluva* Good) 1.0
  mild *(Kraft* ⅓ Less Fat) ....<1.0
  mild *(Sargento Preferred Light)* ....<1.0
  mild or sharp *(Sargento)* 1.0
  sharp *(Kraft Cracker Barrel* ⅓ Less Fat) ....<1.0
  sharp, New York State *(Heluva* Good), 1 oz. 1.0
Cheshire, 1 oz. 1.4
Colby, 1 oz., except as noted:
  (Alpine Lace Reduced Fat) 1.0
  (Dorman Sandwich), 1.1-oz. slice 1.0
  (Kraft) ....<1.0
  (Kraft ⅓ Less Fat) 0
  (Sargento Sliced) 0
  mild *(Heluva* Good Longhorn) 0
Colby Jack:
  (Heluva Good), 1 oz. 0
  shredded *(Heluva* Good), ¼ cup 1.0
  shredded *(Sargento)*, ¼ cup ....<1.0
  snack *(MooTown Snackers)*, .8-oz. piece ....<1.0
Colby Monterey Jack *(Kraft)*, 1 oz. 0
Colby Monterey Jack, shredded *(Kraft)*, ¼ cup ....<1.0
cottage, ½ cup, except as noted:
  4% *(Breakstone's)* 4.0
  4% *(Friendship* California Style) 4.0
  4% *(Sealtest)* 4.0
  4%, large curd *(Knudsen)* 4.0
  4%, small curd *(Knudsen)*...................3.0
  2% *(Breakstone's)* 4.0
  2% *(Knudsen)*.........................3.0
  2% *(Sealtest)* 4.0

Cheese, cottage *(cont.)*

2% *(Weight Watchers)* 4.0
1% *(Friendship/Friendship* Low Sodium) 4.0
1% *(Light n' Lively)* 4.0
1% *(Weight Watchers)* 4.0
dry curd *(Breakstone's),* 1/4 cup 0
garden salad, 1% *(Light n' Lively)* 5.0
peach, 1.5% *(Knudsen),* 4 oz. 12.0
peach and pineapple, 1% *(Light n' Lively)* 14.0
pineapple, 4% *(Friendship)* 16.0
pineapple *(Friendship* Lowfat) 17.0
pot style, 2% *(Friendship)* 3.0
tropical fruit *(Knudsen),* 4 oz. 15.0

cottage, nonfat, 1/2 cup:
(Friendship) 5.0
(Knudsen Free) 4.0
(Light n' Lively Free) 3.0
peach *(Friendship)* 15.0

cream cheese, 1 oz., except as noted:
(Boar's Head) 2.0
(Philadelphia Brand) ....<1.0
(Western Creamy), 2 tbsp., 1.1 oz. 1.0
(Western Creamy Light), 2 tbsp., 1.1 oz. 0
with chive or pimiento *(Philadelphia Brand)* ....<1.0
fat free *(Philadelphia Brand)* 2.0
reduced fat *(Friendship)* 0

cream cheese, soft, 2 tbsp.:
plain *(Friendship)* 2.0
plain *(Philadelphia Brand)* 1.0
plain *(Philadelphia Brand* Fat Free/Light) 2.0
with chives and onion *(Philadelphia Brand)* 2.0
with herb and garlic *(Philadelphia Brand)* 2.0
with olive and pimiento *(Philadelphia Brand)* 2.0
with pineapple *(Philadelphia Brand)* 4.0
with smoked salmon *(Philadelphia Brand)* 1.0
with strawberries *(Philadelphia Brand)* 5.0

cream cheese, whipped, 3 tbsp.:
plain *(Breakstone's Temp-Tee)* 1.0
plain *(Philadelphia Brand)* 1.0
with smoked salmon *(Philadelphia Brand)* 1.0

curd, extra sharp *(Heluva Good),* 1 oz. 1.0
Edam *(Boar's Head),* 1 oz. 0

Edam *(Dorman* Sliced), 1 oz. 0
farmer:
    (Friendship/Friendship No Salt), 1 oz., approx. 2 tbsp. 0
    (Kraft), 1 oz. . . . . <1.0
    (Western Creamy), 2.3 oz. 2.0
    dry *(Western Creamy* Fat Free), 2 oz. 1.0
    hoop *(Friendship),* 1 oz., approx. 2 tbsp. 0
feta, 1 oz.:
    (Alpine Lace Reduced Fat) 1.0
    (Classika Portions) 2.0
    (Krinos Imported) 0
fontina *(Classica),* 1 oz. . . . . <1.0
goat, 1 oz.:
    hard type 6
    semisoft type 7
    soft type 3
Gorgonzola *(Galbani* Dolcelatte), 1 oz. . . . . <1.0
Gouda, 1 oz.:
    (Boar's Head) 0
    (Dorman Sliced) 0
    (Kraft) . . . . <1.0
Gruyère, 1 oz. 1
Havarti, 1 oz.:
    (Boar's Head) 0
    (Dorman Sliced) 0
    (Kraft Casino) 0
hot pepper *(Alpine Lace),* 1 oz. 2.0
Italian:
    (Classica Italiana), 1 oz. 1.0
    blend, shredded *(Heluva* Good), ¼ cup 0
    style, grated *(Kraft* ⅓ Less Fat), 2 tsp. 1.0
    style, shredded *(Sargento Recipe Blend),* ¼ cup 0
Jarlsberg *(Sargento),* 1.2-oz. slice 1.0
(Laughing Cow Original Wedge), 1 oz. 1.0
(Laughing Cow Babybel 7 oz.), 1 oz. 0
(Laughing Cow Babybel Mini), ¾-oz. piece 0
Limburger *(Kraft Mohawk Valley),* 1 oz. 0
mascarpone *(Classica* Domestic), 1 oz. 1.0
mascarpone *(Galbani* Imported), 1 oz. 1.0
Mexican, 4, shredded *(Sargento Recipe Blend),* ¼ cup . . . . <1.0
Monterey Jack:
    (Boar's Head), 1 oz. 0

Cheese, Monterey Jack *(cont.)*

(*Dorman/Dorman* Reduced Fat), 1 oz. 0
(*Dorman*), 1.2-oz. slice 1.0
(*Dorman* Reduced Fat), 1.5-oz. slice 1.0
(*Heluva* Good/*Heluva* Good Jalapeño), 1 oz. 0
(*Kraft/Kraft* ⅓ Less Fat), 1 oz. 0
(*Land O Lakes*), 1 oz. . . . . <1.0
(*Sargento* Sliced), 1 oz. 0
shredded *(Dorman)*, ⅓ cup, 1 oz. 0
shredded *(Heluva* Good), ¼ cup 1.0
shredded *(Kraft)*, ¼ cup . . . . <1.0
shredded *(Sargento)*, ¼ cup 0
jalapeño *(Boar's Head)*, 1 oz. 0
jalapeño *(Kraft)*, 1 oz. . . . . <1.0
peppers *(Kraft* ⅓ Less Fat), 1 oz. . . . . <1.0
mozzarella (see also "string," below), 1 oz., except as
noted:
(*Boar's Head*) . . . . <1.0
(*Polly-O* Fat Free) . . . . <1.0
(*Polly-O* Fior Di Latte) 0
(*Polly-O* Lite) . . . . <1.0
whole milk *(Heluva* Good) 2.0
whole milk *(Polly-O)* . . . . <1.0
part skim *(Alpine Lace* Reduced Fat) 1.0
part skim *(Dorman)* 1.0
part skim *(Heluva* Good) . . . . <1.0
part skim *(Kraft)* . . . . <1.0
part skim *(Polly-O)*, ¼ cup . . . . <1.0
sliced *(Sargento)*, 1.6-oz. slice 2.0
sliced *(Sargento Preferred Light)*, 1.6 oz. 0
mozzarella, shredded, ¼ cup:
(*Heluva* Good) 1.0
(*Sargento*) 1.0
(*Sargento Preferred Light*) . . . . <1.0
whole milk *(Kraft)* . . . . <1.0
whole milk *(Polly-O)* . . . . <1.0
part skim *(Kraft)* . . . . <1.0
part skim *(Kraft* ⅓ Less Fat) . . . . <1.0
part skim *(Polly-O)* 1.0
part skim, fine *(Kraft)* . . . . <1.0
fat free *(Kraft Healthy Favorites)* 2.0
fat free *(Polly-O)* 1.0

light *(Polly-O* Lite) 1.0
Muenster:
    (Alpine Lace Reduced Sodium), 1 oz. 1.0
    (Boar's Head/Boar's Head Low Sodium), 1 oz. 0
    (Dorman), 1-oz. slice 0
    (Dorman), 1.5-oz. slice 1.0
    (Dorman Reduced Fat/Reduced Sodium), 1.5 oz. 0
    (Heluva Good), 1 oz. 0
    (Kraft), 1 oz. 0
    (Sargento Sliced), 1 oz. . . . . <1.0
Neufchâtel *(Philadelphia Brand),* 1 oz. . . . . <1.0
Parmesan:
    grated, 1 tbsp. 2
    shredded, 1 tbsp. 0
    shredded *(Sargento),* ¼ cup 1.0
Parmesan-Romano, grated, 1 tbsp. 0
Parmesan-Romano, shredded *(Sargento),* ¼ cup 1.0
pimiento, processed *(Kraft* Deluxe), 1 oz. . . . . <1.0
pizza, shredded, ¼ cup:
    (Heluva Good) 1.0
    (Sargento) 0
    (Sargento Pizza Double Cheese) 1.0
    all varieties *(Kraft)* . . . . <1.0
Port du Salut, 1 oz. 2
provolone, 1 oz., except as noted:
    (Alpine Lace Reduced Fat) 1.0
    (Boar's Head) 1.0
    (Dorman) 1.0
    (Dorman Reduced Fat), 1.5 oz. 1.0
    (Sargento Sliced) 0
    smoke flavor *(Kraft)* . . . . <1.0
ricotta, ¼ cup:
    (Breakstone's) 3.0
    (Polly-O Light) 3.0
    (Sargento Light/Old Fashioned) 3.0
    whole milk 1.9
    whole milk *(Polly-O)* 2.0
    part skim *(Polly-O)* 2.0
    part skim *(Sargento)* 2.0
    fat free *(Polly-O)* 2.0
Romano, grated or shredded, 1 tbsp. 0
Romano-Parmesan, grated *(Polly-O),* 2 tsp. 0

Cheese *(cont.)*

Roquefort, 1 oz. 6

string:

(Polly-O), 1 oz. . . . . <1.0

(Polly-O Light Mozzarella), 1 oz. . . . . <1.0

part skim (Heluva Good Mozzarella), 1 oz. . . . . <1.0

snack (Handi-Snacks/Kraft), 1 piece . . . . <1.0

snack (MooTown Snackers), .8-oz. piece . . . . <1.0

snack (Polly-O), ¾ oz. . . . . <1.0

snack, light (MooTown Snackers), .8-oz. piece . . . . . . <1.0

Swiss, 1 oz., except as noted:

(Alpine Lace Reduced Fat) 1.0

(Boar's Head Domestic) . . . . <1.0

(Boar's Head Gold Label Imported/No Salt) . . . . <1.0

(Borden) 1.0

(Dorman), 1.2-oz. slice 1.0

(Dorman Low Sodium), 1.2-oz. slice 0

(Dorman Reduced Fat), 1.2-oz. slice 1.0

(Dorman Sandwich) 1.0

(Dorman Very Low Sodium) 0

(Kraft) 0

(Sargento Sliced), ¾-oz. slice 0

(Sargento Preferred Light Sliced) . . . . <1.0

(Sargento Wafer Thin Sliced), 2 slices 0

baby (Boar's Head) . . . . <1.0

baby (Kraft Cracker Barrel) 0

processed (Kraft Deluxe), ¾-oz. slice 0

processed (Kraft Deluxe), 1-oz. slice . . . . <1.0

Swiss, shredded (Kraft), ¼ cup . . . . <1.0

Swiss, shredded (Sargento), ¼ cup 0

taco, shredded, ¼ cup:

(Heluva Good) 1.0

(Sargento) 1.0

(Sargento Preferred Light) . . . . <1.0

cheddar and Monterey Jack (Kraft) . . . . <1.0

nacho and taco (Sargento) 1.0

(Tal-Fino Taleggio), 1 oz. 2.0

white or yellow (Weight Watchers Natural), 1 oz. 1.0

"Cheese," substitute and nondairy:

(Sandwich-Mate), .7-oz. slice 1.0

all varieties, 1 oz., except as noted:

(AlmondRella) 3.0

    (Smart Beat), ⅔ oz. 3.0
    (TofuRella) 2.0
    (VeganRella) 7.0
    (Zero-FatRella) 3.0
American flavor:
    (Borden), 1 slice 1.0
    (Cheeztwo/Sandwich-Mate), 1 slice 1.0
    (Golden Image), ¾ oz. 1.0
    (Lunchwagon), ⅔ oz. . . . . <1.0
    (Lunchwagon), ¾ oz. 1.0
    (Smart Beat Fat Free), ⅔ oz. 3.0
    (Weight Watchers Reduced Sodium Slices), .75-oz. slice . 3.0
    shredded *(Harvest Moon)*, ¼ cup 3.0
cheddar flavor:
    (Borden), 1 oz. 2.0
    (Borden Taco Mate/Fortified), 1 oz. 3.0
    (Weight Watchers Fat Free Slices), .75-oz. slice 3.0
    shredded *(Harvest Moon)*, ¼ cup 3.0
    shredded *(Sargento)*, ¼ cup 2.0
cream cheese, all varieties *(Tofutti Better Than Cream*
    Cheese), 1 oz. 1.0
Italian topping, grated *(Weight Watchers)*, 1 tbsp. 2.0
Jamaican Jack style *(HempRella)*, 1 oz. 1.0
Monterey Jack *(Borden)*, 1 oz. 1.0
mozzarella, shredded:
    (Borden), 1 oz. 1.0
    (Harvest Moon), ¼ cup 1.0
    (Sargento), ¼ cup . . . . <1.0
    imitation *(Borden)*, 1 oz. 2.0
Swiss *(Borden)*, 1 slice 1.0
Swiss *(Weight Watchers* Fat Free Slices), .75-oz. slice 2.0
white or yellow *(Weight Watchers* Fat Free Slices), .75-oz.
    slice 3.0
Cheese dip, 2 tbsp.:
(Chi-Chi's Fiesta) 3.0
and bacon *(Nalley)* 3.0
blue *(Kraft* Premium) 2.0
cheddar:
    jalapeño *(Heluva* Good Light) 4.0
    mild *(Frito-Lay)* 4.0
    mild *(Old Dutch)* 3.0
chili *(Fritos)* 3.0

Cheese dip *(cont.)*
hot *(Price's* Fiesta) 2.0
nacho:
   (Knudsen Premium) 3.0
   (Kraft Premium) 2.0
   (Nalley) 3.0
   (Old Dutch) 3.0
Parmesan garlic *(Marie's)* 2.0
salsa:
   (Heluva Good Cheese 'N Salsa) 3.0
   (Old El Paso/Old El Paso Low Fat) 3.0
   (Tostitos Con Queso/Con Queso Low Fat) 5.0
Cheese entree mix, see "Entree mix, frozen"
Cheese food (see also "Cheese" and "Cheese spread"):
American:
   (Borden), .7-oz. slice 2.0
   (Heluva Good), 1 oz. 2.0
   (Kraft Singles), ⅔-oz. slice 2.0
   (Kraft Singles), ¾-oz. slice 2.0
   (Kraft Singles), 1.2-oz. slice 3.0
   grated *(Kraft),* 1 tbsp. 1.0
cheddar:
   sharp *(Kaukauna* Premium Blend), 1 oz. 2.0
   sharp *(Kaukauna Lite 50),* 1 oz. 5.0
   sharp *(Kraft Cracker Barrel),* 2 tbsp. 4.0
   sharp or extra sharp *(Kaukauna),* 1 oz. 3.0
   extra sharp *(Kraft Cracker Barrel),* 2 tbsp. 3.0
with garlic *(Kraft),* 1 oz. 2.0
with jalapeños:
   (Kraft), 1 oz. 2.0
   (Kraft Mexican Singles), ¾-oz. slice 2.0
   shredded, hot or mild *(Velveeta* Mexican), ¼ cup 3.0
Monterey *(Kraft* Singles), ¾-oz. slice 2.0
with pimiento *(Kraft* Singles), ⅔-oz. slice 1.0
with pimiento *(Kraft* Singles), ¾-oz. slice 2.0
port wine:
   (Kaukauna), 1 oz. 4.0
   (Kaukauna Premium Blend), 1 oz. 2.0
   (Kaukauna Lite), 1 oz. 5.0
   (Wispride Cup), 2 tbsp. 2.0
   (Wispride Light Cup), 2 tbsp. 5.0
sharp *(Kraft* Singles), ¾-oz. slice . . . . <1.0

shredded *(Velveeta)*, ¼ cup 3.0
smoke flavor *(Kaukauna Smokey)*, 1 oz. 3.0
smoke flavor *(Kaukauna Lite 50 Smokey)*, 1 oz. 5.0
Swiss:
    (Borden), 1 slice 1.0
    (Kraft Singles), ¾-oz. slice 1.0
    almond *(Kaukauna)*, 1 oz. 3.0
    almond *(Kaukauna Lite 50)*, 1 oz. 5.0
Cheese nuggets, breaded, frozen *(Schwan's)*, ¼ cup 7.0
Cheese pastry, see "Danish"
Cheese product (see also "Cheese food"):
(Cheez Whiz Light), 2 tbsp. 6.0
(Kraft Free Singles), ⅔-oz. slice 3.0
(Kraft Free Singles), ¾-oz. slice 3.0
(Velveeta Light), 1 oz. 3.0
all varieties *(Borden Fat Free)*, 1 slice 2.0
all varieties *(Lite-Line)*, .7-oz. slice 1.0
American flavor:
    (Alpine Lace), 1 oz. 2.0
    (Alpine Lace Nonfat), 1 oz. 2.0
    (Alpine Lace Nonfat), ¾-oz. slice 1.0
    (Borden Fat Free/Light), ¾-oz. slice 1.0
    (Borden Lowfat), 1 slice 1.0
    (Harvest Moon), ⅔ oz. 1.0
    (Kraft Deluxe 25% Less Fat), ¾-oz. slice 1.0
    (Kraft Singles Less Fat), ¾-oz. slice 2.0
    (Light n' Lively 50% Less Fat), ¾-oz. slice 2.0
cheddar flavor:
    (Alpine Lace Nonfat), 1 oz. 2.0
    all varieties *(Spreadery)*, 2 tbsp. 3.0
    sharp *(Kraft Singles ⅓ Less Fat)*, ¾-oz. slice 2.0
    sharp *(Kraft Free Singles)*, ¾-oz.slice 3.0
mozzarella *(Alpine Lace Nonfat)*, 1 oz. 2.0
Neufchâtel, garlic herb or ranch *(Spreadery)*, 2 tbsp. 1.0
Neufchâtel, vegetable *(Spreadery)*, 2 tbsp. 2.0
pimiento *(Spreadery)*, 2 tbsp. 3.0
Swiss flavor *(Kraft Singles Less Fat)*, ¾-oz. slice 2.0
Swiss flavor *(Kraft Free Singles)*, ¾-oz. slice 3.0
Cheese sandwich, frozen, grilled *(Swanson Fun Feast)*,
  1 pkg. 56.0
Cheese sauce, 2 tbsp., except as noted:
(Cheez Whiz Squeezable) 4.0

Cheese sauce *(cont.)*
(Cheez Whiz Zap-A-Park Original/Salsa) 3.0
(Franco-American), ¼ cup 4.0
all varieties *(Kaukauna Micro Melt)* 2.0
nacho *(Kaukauna)* 4.0
Cheese sauce mix:
(Durkee), ¼ pkg. 4.0
(French's), ¼ pkg. 4.0
four *(Knorr),* ⅓ pkg. 4.0
nacho *(Durkee),* ⅕ pkg. 2.0
Cheese spread (see also "Cheese" and "Cheese product"):
(Cheez Whiz), 2 tbsp. 2.0
(Squeez-A-Snak), 2 tbsp. . . . . <1.0
(Velveeta), 1 oz. 3.0
(Velveeta Italiana), 1 oz. 2.0
all varieties *(Heluva* Good), 2 tbsp. 3.0
American:
    (Borden), 1 oz. 3.0
    (Easy Cheese), 2 tbsp. 2.0
    (Harvest Moon), ⅔ oz. 2.0
    (Harvest Moon), ¾ oz. 2.0
    (The Big!), 1 slice 2.0
with bacon *(Kraft),* 2 tbsp. . . . . <1.0
blue cheese *(Kraft Roka),* 2 tbsp. 2.0
cheddar, regular, bacon or sharp *(Easy Cheese),* 2 tbsp. 3.0
with jalapeños:
    (Cheez Whiz), 2 tbsp. 2.0
    (Kraft), 1 oz. 2.0
    hot *(Velveeta* Mexican), 1 oz. 2.0
    mild *(Velveeta* Mexican), 1 oz. 3.0
Limburger *(Mohawk Valley),* 2 tbsp. 0
nacho *(Easy Cheese),* 2 tbsp. 3.0
nacho *(The Big!),* 1 slice 2.0
Neufchâtel, all varieties *(Kaukauna),* 1 oz. 1.0
olive and pimiento *(Kraft),* 2 tbsp. 3.0
pimiento, 2 tbsp.:
    (Kraft) 3.0
    (Price's) 2.0
    (Price's Light) 3.0
pineapple *(Kraft),* 2 tbsp. 4.0
salsa, hot or mild *(Cheez Whiz),* 2 tbsp. 2.0
sharp *(Old English),* 2 tbsp. <1.0

slices:
    (Velveeta), ¾ oz. 2.0
    (Velveeta), ⁴/₅ oz. 2.0
    (Velveeta), 1.2 oz. 3.0
Cheese sticks:
cornmeal coated *(Goya Surullitos)*, 7 pieces 48.0
mozzarella, breaded, frozen *(Giorgio)*, 2 pieces 9.0
mozzarella, breaded, frozen *(Schwan's)*, 2 pieces, 1 oz. 6.0
Cheese-ham roll, mozzarella and prosciutto
    (Volpi Rotola), 2 oz. . . . . <1.0
Cheese-nut log, sharp *(Wispride)*, 2 tbsp. 4.0
Cheeseburger, see "Beef sandwich"
Cheesecake, see "Cake, frozen," "Cake, mix," and "Cake,
    snack"
Cherimoya (see also "Custard apple"):
(Frieda's), 5 oz. 34.0
untrimmed, 1 lb. 70.8
1 medium, 1.9 lb. 131.3
Cherries jubilee *(Lucky Leaf/Musselman's)*, ¼ cup 20.0
Cherry, fresh:
(Dole), 21 cherries, 5 oz. 23.0
sour, red:
    with pits, 1 lb. 49.7
    with pits, ½ cup 6.3
    with pits, 1 oz. 3.5
    pitted, ½ cup 9.4
sweet:
    with pits, 1 lb. 67.6
    with pits, ½ cup 12.0
    10 medium, 2.6 oz. 11.3
Cherry, candied, green or red:
(Paradise/White Swan), .2-oz. piece 4.0
(S&W Glace), 5 pieces 20.0
and pineapple mix *(Paradise/White Swan)*, 2 tbsp., 1.3 oz. 29.0
Cherry, canned, ½ cup:
Royal Anne *(Comstock)* 26.0
sour, pitted:
    red, in water *(Comstock)* 11.0
    red, in water *(Lucky Leaf/Musselman's)* 13.0
    red, in heavy syrup *(Comstock)* 36.0
    in heavy syrup 29.8

Cherry, canned *(cont.)*
sweet:
    pitted, dark *(S&W)* 34.0
    pitted, dark, in heavy syrup *(Comstock)* 26.0
    pitted, dark, in heavy syrup *(Del Monte)* 24.0
    pitted, dark, in heavy syrup *(Oregon* Bing) 26.0
    pitted, light *(S&W* Royal Anne) 33.0
    pitted, in heavy syrup 27.4
    unpitted, dark, in heavy syrup *(Oregon)* 24.0
Cherry, dried, pitted:
(Sonoma), ¼ cup 34.0
bing *(Frieda's),* ¼ cup, 1.4 oz. 26.0
tart *(Frieda's),* ⅓ cup, 1.4 oz. 33.0
Cherry, frozen:
dark, sweet *(Big Valley),* ¾ cup 20.0
dark, sweet *(Schwan's),* ⅔ cup 31.0
sour, red, unsweetened, 4 oz. 12.5
sweet, sweetened, 4 oz. 25.4
tart, red *(Stilwell),* 1 cup 14.0
Cherry, maraschino, green or red:
(Haddon House), 1 piece 2.0
(S&W), 1 piece 3.0
with liquid, 1 oz. 8.3
Cherry drink, 8 fl. oz., except as noted:
(After the Fall Very Cherry) 26.0
(Farmer's Market) 31.0
apple *(Schwan's Vita Sun)* 25.0
wild *(Capri Sun),* 6.75 fl. oz. 30.0
Cherry drink mix* *(Kool Aid),* 8 fl. oz. 25.0
Cherry dumpling, frozen *(Pepperidge Farm),* 1 piece 47.0
Cherry glacé, see "Cherry, candied"
Cherry juice, 8 fl. oz., except as noted:
(Juicy Juice) 32.0
(Minute Maid Box), 8.45 fl. oz. 33.0
black *(Heinke's)* 43.0
black *(R.W. Knudsen)* 43.0
Cherry juice blend, 8 fl. oz.:
(Apple & Eve Nothin' But Juice) 29.0
(Dole Mountain) 30.0
(Veryfine Juice-Ups) 33.0
black, concentrate* *(R.W. Knudsen)* 23.0

cider:
- (Heinke's) 28.0
- (R.W. Knudsen Aseptic) 31.0
- frozen* (R.W. Knudsen) 33.0

Cherry nectar (Santa Cruz), 8 fl. oz. 26.0
Cherry pocket pastry (Tastykake), 1 piece 45.0
Cherry syrup, 2 tbsp.:
- black (Fox's) 21.0
- black (Fox's No Cal) 0

Chervil, dried:
- (McCormick), ¼ tsp. 1
- 1 tbsp. 9
- 1 tsp. 3

Chestnut, Chinese:
- raw, in shell, 1 lb. .187.0
- dried, shelled, 1 oz. 22.7
- boiled or steamed, 1 oz. 9.6
- roasted, 1 oz. 14.9

Chestnut, European:
- raw, in shell, 1 lb. .152.8
- raw, shelled, with peel, 1 cup or 13 kernels 66.0
- dried, peeled, 1 oz. 22.3
- boiled or steamed, 1 oz. 7.9
- roasted:
  - in shell, 1 lb. .151.3
  - peeled, 1 oz. 15.0
  - peeled, 1 cup, approx. 17 kernels 75.7

Chestnut, Japanese:
- raw, in shell, 1 lb. .104.5
- boiled or steamed, 1 oz. 3.6
- dried, 1 oz. 23.1
- roasted, 1 oz. 12.8

Chia seeds, dried, 1 oz. 13.6
Chicken, without added ingredients 0
Chicken, canned, chunk, 2 oz., ¼ cup, except as noted:
- all varieties (Hormel) 0
- in broth (Swanson Mixin') 0
- in water (Swanson Premium), ¼ cup or 3 oz. . . . . <1.0
- white (Swanson), 3 oz. 0
- white, in water (Swanson Premium) . . . . <1.0

Chicken, ground, without added ingredients 0

Chicken, refrigerated or frozen (see also "Chicken entree, frozen"):

whole, cooked:

all cuts, unseasoned *(Perdue/Perdue Oven Stuffer)*, 3 oz. . . 0
all cuts, seasoned, roasted *(Perdue)*, 4 oz. 1.0
barbecued *(Empire* Kosher), 5 oz. edible 1.0
all cuts, unseasoned *(Perdue)*, 4 oz. 0
all cuts, unseasoned *(Tyson)*, 4 oz. 0
breast, raw, halves or quarters *(Tyson)*, 4 oz. 1.0
breast, raw, halves, skinless *(Tyson)*, 4 oz. 0
breast, raw, boneless:

all cuts *(Tyson)*, 4 oz. 0
filet *(Schwan's)*, 4 oz. 0
filet, breaded *(Schwan's)*, 5-oz. piece 15.0
breast, cooked, unseasoned, split, roasted *(Tyson)*, ½ breast . . 0
breast, breaded, cooked:

cutlet *(Perdue* Original), 3.5-oz. piece 14.0
cutlet, battered, breaded *(Empire* Kosher), 3.3-oz. piece   11.0
cutlet, Parmesan *(Perdue* Kit), 3-oz. piece 20.0
fried, battered and breaded *(Empire* Kosher), 3 oz. edible . 3.0
patties *(Perdue Individually Frozen)*, 3-oz. piece 11.0
tenderloin *(Perdue* Original/*Perdue Individually Frozen)*,
3 oz. 13.0
tenderloin *(Perdue Kick'n Chicken)*, 3-oz. piece 12.0
breast, seasoned, raw, 4 oz., except as noted:

barbecue *(Perdue)* 10.0
barbecue *(Perdue Individually Frozen)*, 5.7-oz. piece 7.0
Cajun *(Chicken By George)* 2.0
Caribbean grill *(Chicken By George)* 8.0
garlic and herb *(Chicken By George)* 3.0
Italian *(Perdue)* 4.0
Italian *(Perdue Individually Frozen)*, 5.7-oz. piece 2.0
Italian blue cheese *(Chicken By George)* 2.0
lemon herb *(Chicken By George)* 3.0
lemon oregano *(Chicken By George)* 3.0
lemon pepper *(Perdue)* 2.0
lemon pepper *(Perdue Individually Frozen)*, 5.7-oz. piece . 2.0
lemon pepper *(Schwan's)*, 4.5-oz. piece 6.0
mesquite barbecue *(Chicken By George)* 5.0
mustard dill *(Chicken By George)* 1.0
Oriental *(Perdue)* 5.0
teriyaki *(Chicken By George)* 6.0

teriyaki *(Perdue Individually Frozen)*, 5.7-oz. piece 4.0
teriyaki *(Schwan's)* 2.0
tomato herb with basil *(Chicken By George)* 5.0
breast, seasoned, cooked:
   barbecue *(Perdue)*, 3 oz. 10.0
   barbecue *(Perdue Individually Frozen)*, 4.3-oz. piece 4.0
   with barbecue sauce *(Perdue)*, ½ cup 19.0
   honey roasted, carved *(Perdue Short Cuts)*, ½ cup 4.0
   Italian *(Perdue)*, 3 oz. 2.0
   Italian *(Perdue Individually Frozen)*, 4.3-oz. piece 1.0
   Italian, carved *(Perdue Short Cuts)*, ½ cup 1.0
   lemon pepper *(Perdue)*, 3 oz. 2.0
   lemon pepper *(Perdue Individually Frozen)*, 4.3-oz. piece . 1.0
   lemon pepper, carved *(Perdue Short Cuts)*, ½ cup 2.0
   mesquite, carved *(Perdue Short Cuts)*, ½ cup 2.0
   Oriental *(Perdue)*, 3 oz. 3.0
   roasted, carved *(Perdue Short Cuts Original)*, ½ cup 2.0
   strips, fajita *(Schwan's)*, 3 oz. 1.0
   teriyaki *(Perdue Individually Frozen)*, 4.3-oz. piece 2.0
chunks, cooked *(Tyson Chick'n Chunks)*, 6 pieces, 3 oz. . . . 14.0
cutlet, see "breast," above
diced, cooked *(Schwan's)*, 3 oz. 0
drum and thigh, fried *(Empire Kosher)*, 3 oz. edible 7.0
drumstick, roasted *(Tyson)*, 3 pieces 1.0
half, roasted, without skin *(Tyson)*, 3 oz. 0
nuggets, breaded, cooked:
   (Empire Kosher), 5 pieces, 3 oz. 12.0
   (Perdue Original), 5 pieces, 3.4 oz. 14.0
   (Perdue Fun Shapes Chik-Tac-Toe), 5 pieces, 3 oz. 12.0
   (Schwan's), 6 pieces 11.0
   breast *(Perdue Individually Frozen)*, approx. 12, 3.4 oz. . 15.0
   and cheese *(Perdue)*, 5 pieces, 3.5 oz. 15.0
   dinosaur *(Perdue Fun Shapes)*, 3 nuggets, 3 oz. 12.0
   football, baseball, and basketball *(Perdue Fun Shapes)*,
      4 pieces, 3 oz. 14.0
   star and drumstick *(Perdue Fun Shapes)*, 4 pieces, 3 oz. 13.0
patties, breaded, cheddar *(Tyson Chick'n with Cheddar)*,
   1 piece 12.0
roundelet *(Tyson)*, 2.6-oz. piece 10.0
shredded, cooked, in barbecue sauce *(Lloyd's)*, ¼ cup 8.0
sticks *(Empire* Kosher Stix), 4 pieces, 3.1 oz. 6.0

Chicken, refrigerated or frozen *(cont.)*
thigh:
fajita, raw *(Perdue)*, 3.2-oz. piece 2.0
fajita, cooked *(Perdue)*, 2.4-oz. piece 1.0
honey mustard, raw *(Perdue)*, 3.2-oz. piece 5.0
honey mustard, cooked *(Perdue)*, 2.4-oz. piece 4.0
roasted *(Tyson)*, 3.6-oz. piece 1.0
wing, hot and spicy, cooked *(Perdue)*, 3 oz. 3.0
wing, hot and spicy, cooked *(Perdue Individually Frozen)*,
3 oz. 1.0
"Chicken," vegetarian:
canned:
diced *(Worthington Chik)*, ¼ cup 1.0
fried *(Worthington FriChik)*, 2 pieces 1.0
fried *(Worthington FriChik Low Fat)*, 2 pieces 2.0
fried, with gravy *(Loma Linda Chik'n)*, 2 pieces 3.0
sliced *(Worthington Chik)*, 3 slices 1.0
frozen:
(Worthington Chik-Stiks), 1 piece 3.0
fried *(Loma Linda Chik'n)*, 1 piece . . . . <1.0
nuggets *(Loma Linda)*, 5 pieces 13.0
nuggets *(Morningstar Farms)*, 4 pieces 17.0
patties *(Morningstar Farms Chik)*, 1 patty 13.0
patties *(Worthington Crispy Chik)*, 1 patty 15.0
roll *(Worthington Chic-Ketts)*, 2 slices, ⅜" 2.0
roll or sliced *(Worthington)*, 2 slices 1.0
mix *(Loma Linda Supreme)*, ⅓ cup 6.0
Chicken dinner, frozen:
barbecue:
mesquite *(The Budget Gourmet)*, 11 oz. 38.0
mesquite *(Healthy Choice)*, 10.5 oz. 44.0
with potato and vegetables *(Tyson)*, 1 pkg. 73.0
boneless *(Swanson Hungry Man)*, 1 pkg. 76.0
breaded, country *(Healthy Choice)*, 10¼ oz. 53.0
breast:
herb roasted *(Schwan's)*, 1 pkg. 40.0
herbed, with fettuccini *(The Budget Gourmet)*, 11 oz. . . . 32.0
honey mustard *(The Budget Gourmet)*, 11 oz. 45.0
roasted, with herb gravy *(The Budget Gourmet)*, 11 oz.   34.0
broccoli Alfredo *(Healthy Choice)*, 11.5 oz. 38.0
cacciatore *(Healthy Choice)*, 12.5 oz. 36.0
Cantonese *(Healthy Choice)*, 10¾ oz. 35.0

Dijon *(Healthy Choice)*, 11 oz. 33.0
fingers, and BBQ sauce *(Freezer Queen* Meal), 9 oz. 32.0
Francesca *(Healthy Choice)*, 12.5 oz. 46.0
fried:
    (Banquet Extra Helping), 18 oz. 72.0
    country, with gravy *(Marie Callender's)*, 14 oz. 67.0
    dark *(Swanson)*, 1 pkg. 50.0
    dark *(Swanson* Budget), 1 pkg. 46.0
    dark *(Swanson Hungry Man)*, 1 pkg. 76.0
    Southern *(Banquet* Extra Helping), 17.5 oz. 67.0
    white *(Banquet* Extra Helping), 18 oz. 72.0
    white *(Swanson)*, 1 pkg. 54.0
    white, mostly *(Swanson Hungry Man)*, 1 pkg. 77.0
ginger, Hunan *(Healthy Choice)*, 12.6 oz. 59.0
grilled:
    patties *(Swanson Hungry Man)*, 1 pkg. 67.0
    Southwestern *(Healthy Choice)*, 10.2 oz. 23.0
    white, in garlic sauce *(Swanson)*, 1 pkg. 35.0
herb, country *(Healthy Choice)*, 12.15 oz. 49.0
nuggets *(Freezer Queen* Meal), 6 oz. 34.0
nuggets *(Swanson)*, 1 pkg. 48.0
parmigiana:
    (Banquet Extra Helping), 19 oz. 64.0
    (The Budget Gourmet), 11 oz. 34.0
    (Healthy Choice), 11.5 oz. 47.0
    (Marie Callender's), 16 oz. 63.0
    (Swanson), 1 pkg. 43.0
    (Swanson Budget), 1 pkg. 33.0
pasta and *(Swanson* Budget), 1 pkg. 30.0
patty *(Freezer Queen* Meal), 7.5 oz. 29.0
picante *(Healthy Choice)*, 10.75 oz. 30.0
roasted:
    (Healthy Choice), 11 oz. 27.0
    herb *(Swanson)*, 1 pkg. 42.0
    herb, with mashed potatoes *(Marie Callender's)*, 14 oz. 32.0
sesame, Shanghai *(Healthy Choice)*, 12 oz. 47.0
sweet and sour *(Healthy Choice)*, 11 oz. 53.0
tenders, platter *(Swanson)*, 1 pkg. 39.0
teriyaki:
    (The Budget Gourmet), 11 oz. 48.0
    (Healthy Choice), 11 oz. 32.0
    (Schwan's), 10 oz. 66.0

Chicken entree, canned:

à la king *(Swanson* Main Dish), 1 cup 17.0
à la king *(Top Shelf)*, 10 oz. 47.0
breast, glazed *(Top Shelf)*, 10 oz. 17.0
cacciatore *(Top Shelf)*, 10 oz. 26.0
chow mein *(Chun King/La Choy* Bi-Pack), 1 cup 10.0
chow mein *(La Choy* Entree), 1 cup 6.0
and dumplings *(Dinty Moore* Cup), 7½ oz. 20.0
and dumplings *(Swanson* Main Dish), 1 cup 22.0
fiesta *(Top Shelf)*, 10 oz. 45.0
hot and spicy *(Chun King* Bi-Pack), 1 cup 11.0
with mashed potato *(Dinty Moore American Classics)*,
    10 oz. 25.0
and noodles *(Dinty Moore American Classics)*, 10 oz. 26.0
noodles and, see "Noodle entree"
Oriental, with noodles *(La Choy)*, 1 cup 18.0
and pasta *(Chef Boyardee* Bowl), 7½ oz. 21.0
salad *(Swanson* Lunch Kit), 1 cup 16.0
spicy *(La Choy* Szechwan Bi-Pack), 1 cup 11.0
stew:
    (Dinty Moore), 1 cup 16.0
    (Dinty Moore Cup), 7½ oz. 18.0
    (Swanson Main Dish), 1 cup 17.0
sweet and sour *(Chun King/La Choy* Bi-Pack), 1 cup 29.0
teriyaki *(La Choy* Bi-Pack), 1 cup 15.0
Chicken entree, freeze-dried, 1 cup:
à la king and noodles *(Mountain House)* 31.0
honey lime, with rice *(Mountain House)* 43.0
noodles and *(Mountain House)* 33.0
Polynesian with rice *(Mountain House)* 34.0
rice and *(Mountain House)* 44.0
stew *(Mountain House)* 24.0
teriyaki, with rice *(Mountain House)* 37.0
Chicken entree, frozen (see also "Chicken, refrigerated or
    frozen"):
à la king:
    (Banquet Toppers), 4.5-oz. bag 7.0
    (Freezer Queen Cook-in-Pouch), 4-oz. pkg. 7.0
    (Stouffer's), 9½ oz. 41.0
au gratin *(The Budget Gourmet* Light), 9.1 oz. 29.0
baked, with whipped potato and gravy *(Stouffer's*
    Homestyle), 8⅞ oz. 19.0

baked, with whipped potato and stuffing *(Lean Cuisine)*,
8.5 oz. 31.0
barbecue, with potato and vegetable *(Tyson)*, 8.9 oz. 38.0
barbecue style *(Banquet* Country), 9 oz. 36.0
with basil cream sauce *(Lean Cuisine Cafe Classics)*, 8.5 oz. 31.0
biryani *(Curry Classics)*, 10 oz. 58.0
and biscuits *(Freezer Queen* Family), 1 cup, 7.9 oz. 29.0
blackened, with rice and corn *(Tyson)*, 8.9 oz. 36.0
breaded cutlet, pasta marinara *(Celentano)*, 10 oz. 36.0
breast, with gravy *(Schwan's)*, 1 cup 8.0
breast, in wine sauce *(Lean Cuisine* Cafe Classics), 8⅛ oz. 25.0
breast, stuffed:
   asparagus and cheese *(Barber Foods)*, 6-oz. piece 19.0
   asparagus and cheese *(Schwan's)*, 6-oz. piece 15.0
   broccoli and cheese *(Barber Foods)*, 6-oz. piece 20.0
   broccoli and cheese *(Schwan's)*, 4-oz. piece 5.0
   broccoli, cheese, and ham *(Schwan's)*, 5-oz. piece 15.0
   Cordon Bleu *(Barber Foods)*, 6-oz. piece 14.0
   Cordon Bleu *(Schwan's)*, 5-oz. piece 15.0
   Kiev *(Barber Foods)*, 6-oz. piece 16.0
   Kiev *(Schwan's)*, 5-oz. piece 16.0
   skinless *(Barber Foods)*, 6-oz. piece 21.0
breast strips, breaded *(Schwan's)*, 3 strips, 4 oz. 21.0
breast tenderloin, breaded *(Schwan's)*, 2 pieces, 2.86 oz. . . 16.0
breast tenderloin, breaded, Southern *(Schwan's)*, 2 pieces,
3 oz. 17.0
breast tenders:
   (Banquet), 3 pieces, 3 oz. 16.0
   (Tyson), 5 pieces, 3 oz. 8.0
   Southern *(Banquet)*, 3 pieces, 3 oz. 16.0
and broccoli *(Healthy Choice Hearty Handfuls)*, 6.1 oz. 51.0
with broccoli and cheese *(Tyson)*, 8.9 oz. 19.0
cacciatore *(Tyson)*, 14.9 oz. 64.0
calypso *(Lean Cuisine* Cafe Classics), 8.5 oz. 42.0
carbonara *(Lean Cuisine* Cafe Classics), 9 oz. 33.0
casserole *(Schwan's)*, 1 cup 35.0
chow mein:
   (Banquet), 9 oz. 28.0
   (Chun King), 13 oz. 45.0
   (Lean Cuisine), 9 oz. 38.0
   (Smart Ones), 9 oz. 34.0
   (Stouffer's), 10⅝ oz. 40.0

Chicken entree, frozen *(cont.)*
chunks, breaded:
    (Country Skillet), 5 pieces, 3.3 oz. 18.0
    and cheddar *(Banquet),* 4 pieces, 2.9 oz. 13.0
    Southern *(Banquet),* 5 pieces, 3.1 oz. 16.0
    Southern *(Country Skillet),* 5 pieces, 3.3 oz. 16.0
creamed *(Stouffer's),* 6½ oz. 8.0
creamy, and broccoli *(Stouffer's),* 8⅞ oz. 26.0
croquettes:
    (Goya), 3 pieces 30.0
    (Tyson), 3.5 oz. 21.0
    gravy and *(Freezer Queen* Family), ⅙ of 28-oz. pkg. . . . 15.0
drumlets *(Swanson Fun Feast),* 1 pkg. 50.0
and dumplings *(Banquet* Family Size), 1 cup, 7 oz. 30.0
and dumplings *(Banquet* Homestyle), 10 oz. 35.0
enchilada, see "Enchilada entree"
escalloped, and noodles *(Stouffer's),* 10 oz. 32.0
escalloped, and noodles *(Stouffer's* 76 oz.), 8.4 oz. 23.0
fajita, see "Fajita entree"
fettuccine:
    (The Budget Gourmet), 10 oz. 33.0
    (Lean Cuisine), 9¼ oz. 38.0
    (Stouffer's Homestyle), 10.5 oz. 32.0
    (Weight Watchers), 10 oz. 39.0
    Alfredo *(Healthy Choice),* 8.5 oz. 35.0
fiesta *(Lean Cuisine),* 8.5 oz. 34.0
fiesta *(Smart Ones),* 8.5 oz. 38.0
Français *(Tyson),* 8.9 oz. 23.0
French recipe *(The Budget Gourmet* Light), 9 oz. 19.0
fricassee with rice *(Goya),* 1 pkg. 118.0
fried:
    (Banquet Country), 9 oz. 35.0
    (Kid Cuisine High Flying), 10.1 oz. 49.0
    (Morton), 9 oz. 30.0
    (Swanson Fun Feast Frazzlin'), 1 pkg. 50.0
    Southern *(Banquet* Country), 8¾ oz. 44.0
    with mashed potatoes and gravy *(Tyson),* 10.9 oz. 39.0
    with whipped potatoes *(Stouffer's* Homestyle), 7.5 oz. . . 33.0
    with whipped potatoes *(Swanson),* 1 pkg. 34.0
    white meat *(Banquet* Country), 8¾ oz. 33.0
fried, pieces, 3 oz., except as noted:
    (Banquet) 13.0

  (Country Skillet) 13.0
  breast *(Banquet)*, 5.5-oz. piece 18.0
  country *(Banquet)* 13.0
  drums and thighs *(Banquet)* 10.0
  hot 'n spicy *(Banquet)* 13.0
  skinless, plain or honey BBQ *(Banquet)* 7.0
  Southern *(Banquet)* 13.0
  wing, hot and spicy *(Banquet)*, 4 pieces, 4 oz. 5.0
garlic *(Healthy Choice Hearty Handfuls)*, 6.1 oz. 53.0
garlic, Milano *(Healthy Choice)*, 9.5 oz. 34.0
glazed:
  (Stouffer's 63 oz.), 4.2 oz. 5.0
  country *(Healthy Choice)*, 8.5 oz. 30.0
  with rice, broccoli, and carrots *(Tyson)*, 9.1 oz........ 30.0
  with vegetable rice *(Lean Cuisine)*, 8.5 oz. 25.0
grilled:
  (Healthy Choice Sonoma), 9 oz. 34.0
  angel-hair pasta *(Stouffer's)*, 10⅞ oz. 40.0
  with corn, beans *(Tyson)*, 8.9 oz. 29.0
  Italian, with linguine *(Tyson)*, 8.9 oz. 19.0
  with mashed potatoes *(Healthy Choice)*, 8 oz. 18.0
  salsa *(Lean Cuisine Cafe Classics)*, 8⅞ oz. 36.0
gumbo *(Goya Asopao de Pollo)*, 1 pkg. 25.0
honey mustard:
  (Healthy Choice), 9.5 oz. 40.0
  (Lean Cuisine Cafe Classics), 8 oz. 39.0
  (Smart Ones), 8.5 oz. 37.0
  with pasta and peas *(Tyson)*, 11.36 oz. 49.0
imperial *(Healthy Choice)*, 9 oz. 31.0
imperial, with rice *(Freezer Queen Homestyle)*, 9 oz. 48.0
Italian, with fettuccine *(Lean Cuisine)*, 9 oz. 31.0
Kiev *(Tyson)*, 9.1 oz. 36.0
lo mein *(Banquet)*, 10.5 oz. 43.0
mandarin:
  (The Budget Gourmet Light), 10 oz. 40.0
  (Healthy Choice), 10 oz. 44.0
  (Lean Cuisine Lunch Classics), 9 oz. 37.0
marinara rotini *(Lean Cuisine Lunch Classics)*, 9.5 oz. 40.0
Marsala:
  (The Budget Gourmet), 9 oz. 34.0
  with potato, carrots *(Tyson)*, 8.9 oz. 18.0
  and vegetables *(Healthy Choice)*, 11.5 oz. 32.0

Chicken entree, frozen *(cont.)*

Mediterranean *(Lean Cuisine* Cafe Classics), 10.5 oz. 32.0
mesquite *(Tyson),* 8.9 oz. 41.0
Mirabella *(Smart Ones),* 9.2 oz. 26.0
Monterey *(Stouffer's* Homestyle), 9⅜ oz. 35.0
and mushroom *(Healthy Choice Hearty Handfuls),* 6.1 oz. . . 49.0
with mushroom sauce *(Tyson),* 8.9 oz. 27.0
nibbles *(Swanson),* 1 pkg. 31.0
and noodles *(The Budget Gourmet),* 9 oz. 29.0
noodle casserole *(Swanson),* 1 pkg. 33.0
noodle casserole, with vegetables *(Swanson),* 1 pkg. 32.0
nuggets:
    (Banquet), 6 pieces, 3 oz. 12.0
    (Banquet), 6 pieces, 4.5 oz. 25.0
    (Banquet Homestyle), 6¾ oz. 38.0
    (Country Skillet), 10 pieces, 3.3 oz. 16.0
    (Freezer Queen Family), 6 pieces, 3 oz. 13.0
    (Kid Cuisine Cosmic), 9.1 oz. 54.0
    (Morton), 7 oz. 30.0
    (Schwan's), 6 nuggets, 3 oz. 11.0
    mozzarella *(Banquet),* 6 pieces, 2.9 oz. 18.0
    Southern *(Banquet),* 6 pieces, 4.5 oz. 22.0
à l'orange *(Lean Cuisine),* 9 oz. 40.0
orange glazed *(The Budget Gourmet* Light), 9 oz. 56.0
Oriental:
    (Banquet), 9 oz. 34.0
    (The Budget Gourmet Light), 9 oz. 48.0
    (Lean Cuisine), 9 oz. 31.0
Parmesan *(Lean Cuisine* Cafe Classics), 10⅞ oz. 25.0
parmigiana:
    (Banquet), 9.5 oz. 27.0
    (Banquet Family), 4.7-oz. piece 18.0
    (Stouffer's Homestyle), 12 oz. 54.0
    (Tyson), 13.8 oz. 55.0
    Italian style *(Banquet),* 4.6-oz. piece 17.0
patties, breaded:
    (Banquet), 2.3-oz. piece 10.0
    (Banquet Country), 10.2 oz. 31.0
    (Country Skillet), 2½-oz. piece 12.0
    (Morton), 6¾ oz. 24.0
    (Schwan's), 3-oz. piece 11.0
    breaded strips *(Swanson),* 1 pkg. 31.0

Southern *(Banquet)*, 2.3-oz. piece 10.0
Southern *(Country Skillet)*, 3.3-oz. piece 12.0
in peanut sauce *(Lean Cuisine)*, 9 oz. 33.0
penne pollo *(Weight Watchers)*, 10 oz. 40.0
piccata:
    (Lean Cuisine Cafe Classics), 9 oz. 41.0
    lemon herb *(Smart Ones)*, 8.5 oz. 34.0
    with potato, broccoli *(Tyson)*, 8.9 oz. 18.0
pie or potpie:
    (Banquet), 7-oz. pie 36.0
    (Banquet Family Size), 1 cup, 8 oz. 39.0
    (Empire Kosher) 41.0
    (Lean Cuisine), 9.5 oz. 39.0
    (Marie Callender's), 10-oz. pie 54.0
    (Marie Callender's), 1 cup, 8½ oz. 49.0
    (Stouffer's), 10-oz. pie 40.0
    (Stouffer's), about 1 cup, ½ of 16-oz. pie 40.0
    (Swanson), 1 pkg. 45.0
    (Swanson Deluxe), 1 pkg. 56.0
    (Swanson Hungry Man), 1 pkg. 64.0
    (Tyson), 8.9 oz. 50.0
    (Tyson All Meat), 8.9 oz. 49.0
    au gratin *(Marie Callender's)*, 10-oz. pie 53.0
    au gratin *(Marie Callender's)*, 1 cup, 8.5 oz. 46.0
    and broccoli *(Marie Callender's)*, 10-oz. pie 88.0
    and broccoli *(Marie Callender's)*, 1 cup, 8.5 oz. 61.0
    broccoli and cheese *(Tyson)*, 8.9-oz. pie 51.0
primavera, pasta *(Banquet)*, 10.5 oz. 40.0
primavera, pasta *(Tyson)*, 11.35 oz. 42.0
with rice *(Goya* Arroz con Pollo), 1 pkg. 79.0
and rice, stir-fry casserole *(Swanson)*, 1 pkg. 40.0
roasted:
    herb *(Lean Cuisine* Cafe Classics), 8 oz. 25.0
    herb *(Tyson)*, 11.35 oz. 39.0
    honey mustard *(Tyson)*, 11.35 oz. 19.0
sandwich, see "Chicken sandwich"
sesame *(Healthy Choice)*, 9.75 oz. 38.0
sliced, gravy and *(Freezer Queen* Cook-in-Pouch), 4-oz. pkg. . 4.0
sweet and sour *(The Budget Gourmet)*, 10 oz. 54.0
sweet and sour, with rice *(Freezer Queen* Homestyle), 9 oz. 46.0
tikka *(Curry Classics* Makhanwala), 10 oz. 15.0
and vegetables *(Lean Cuisine)*, 10.5 oz. 31.0

Chicken entree, frozen *(cont.)*
and vegetables, with linguine *(Freezer Queen* Deluxe Family),
　1 cup, 8.6 oz. 30.0
and vegetables, with noodles *(Freezer Queen* Homestyle),
　9 oz. 30.0
walnut, crunchy *(Chun King),* 13 oz. 56.0
wings:
　(Schwan's Hot Wings), 6 pieces, 3.3 oz. 1.0
　(Tyson Wings of Fire), 4 pieces, 3.4 oz. 1.0
　barbecue *(Schwan's),* 6 pieces, 3.3 oz. 2.0
　barbecue *(Tyson),* 4 pieces, 3.4 oz. 2.0
　breaded *(Schwan's* Drummies), 3 pieces, 2.75 oz. 11.0
Chicken entree mix, dry, except as noted:
Alfredo *(Dinner Sensations),* 1 cup dry or 1 cup* 29.0
stir-fried *(Skillet Chicken Helper),* ¼ cup or 1 cup* 30.0
sweet and sour *(Dinner Sensations),* ⅔ cup dry or 1 cup* 57.0
Chicken entree mix, frozen, see "Entree mix, frozen"
Chicken fat:
1 oz. 0
rendered *(Empire* Kosher), 1 tbsp. .... <1.0
"Chicken" fat, imitation *(Rokeach* Nyafat), 1 tbsp. 0
Chicken frankfurter:
(Empire Kosher), 2-oz. link 1.0
and turkey, see "Turkey frankfurter"
Chicken giblets, simmered:
4 oz. 1.1
chopped, 1 cup 1.4
Chicken gravy, ¼ cup:
(Franco-American) 3.0
(Heinz Home Style Classic/Fat Free) 3.0
all varieties *(Pepperidge Farm)* 3.0
giblet *(Franco-American)* 3.0
mix*:
　(Durkee) 4.0
　(French's) 4.0
　(McCormick) 4.0
　(Pillsbury with Water) 3.0
　(Pillsbury with Water, Skim Milk) 4.0
　(Weight Watchers) 1.0
　roasted *(Knorr)* 3.0
　vegetarian *(Loma Linda Gravy Quik)* 3.0
Chicken liver pâté, see "Pâté"

Chicken lunch meat, breast:
baked *(Louis Rich Carving Board)*, 2 slices, 1.6 oz. 2.0
grilled *(Louis Rich Carving Board)*, 2 slices, 1.6 oz. 2.0
honey flavored *(Tyson)*, 2 slices, 1.5 oz. 2.0
honey glazed *(Louis Rich Carving Board)*, 2 slices, 1.6 oz. . 2.0
honey glazed *(Oscar Mayer Deli-Thin)*, 4 slices, 1.8 oz. 2.0
mesquite *(Tyson)*, 2 slices, 1.5 oz. 1.0
oven roasted:
    (Boar's Head Golden), 2 oz. . . . . <1.0
    (Hebrew National), 2 oz. 0
    (Louis Rich Deluxe), 1-oz. slice 1.0
    (Louis Rich Deli-Thin), 4 slices, 1.8 oz. 1.0
    (Oscar Mayer Fat Free), 4 slices, 1.8 oz. 1.0
    (Tyson), 2 slices, 1.5 oz. 1.0
    white *(Louis Rich)*, 1-oz. slice 1.0
peppered *(Tyson)*, 2 slices, 1.5 oz. 1.0
smoked *(Boar's Head* Hickory), 2 oz. . . . . <1.0
smoked *(Tyson* Hickory), 2 slices, 1.5 oz. 1.0
Chicken pie, see "Chicken entree, frozen"
Chicken sandwich, frozen, 1 piece:
(Hormel Quick Meal) 42.0
(Kid Cuisine Super Charging), 9.4 oz. 71.0
(Schwan's), 3.3 oz. 25.0
broccoli supreme *(Lean Pockets)*, 4.5 oz. 34.0
broccoli and cheddar *(Croissant Pockets)*, 4.5 oz. 37.0
broccoli and cheddar *(Schwan's)*, 4.4 oz. 33.0
and cheddar with broccoli *(Hot Pockets)*, 4.5 oz. 37.0
fajita *(Lean Pockets)*, 4.5 oz. 36.0
fajita *(Totino's* Big & Hearty), 4.8 oz. 35.0
grilled *(Hormel Quick Meal)* 36.0
grilled *(Tyson* Microwave), 3.45 oz. 25.0
Parmesan *(Lean Pockets)*, 4.5 oz. 40.0
pastry *(Mrs. Paterson's Aussie Pie)* 45.0
Chicken sauce (see also specific listings):
barbecue flavor *(Hunt's Chicken Sensations)*, 1 tbsp. 3.0
cacciatore *(Ragú Chicken Tonight)*, ½ cup 14.0
Caesar *(Lawry's)*, 2 tbsp. 5.0
country French *(Ragú Chicken Tonight)*, ½ cup 6.0
creamy, with mushrooms *(Ragú Chicken Tonight)*, ½ cup . . . 5.0
creamy, primavera *(Ragú Chicken Tonight)*, ½ cup 7.0
herbed, with wine *(Ragú Chicken Tonight)*, ½ cup 6.0
Italian garlic *(Hunt's Chicken Sensations)*, 1 tbsp. 1.0

Chicken sauce *(cont.)*
lemon herb *(Hunt's Chicken Sensations)*, 1 tbsp. 2.0
sherried *(Lawry's)*, 1 tbsp. 5.0
Southwestern *(Hunt's Chicken Sensations)*, 1 tbsp. 1.0
sweet and sour *(Ragú Chicken Tonight)*, ½ cup 30.0
Thai, satay *(Lawry's)*, 1 tbsp. 4.0
wing:
    (Stubb's Legendary Original/Inferno), 1 tbsp. 2.0
    Buffalo style *(World Harbors Hot Zings)*, 2 tbsp. 7.0
    hot *(Nance's)*, 2 tbsp. 3.0
    mild *(Nance's)*, 2 tbsp. 4.0
Chicken sauce mix, teriyaki *(McCormick)*, 1⅔ tbsp., ¼ pkg. . 7.0
Chicken sausage, cooked:
all varieties *(Gerhard's Sausage)*, 2.5 oz. 4.0
apple and herb *(McKenzie)*, 2.4-oz. link 5.0
and apricot *(Bilinski)*, 3.3-oz. link 8.0
and broccoli *(Bilinski)*, 3.3-oz. link 1.0
Italian, with pepper and onion *(Bilinski)*, 3.3-oz. link 1.0
and jalapeño *(Bilinski)*, 3.3-oz. link 1.0
and pesto *(Bilinski)*, 3.3-oz. link 0
pomodoro *(McKenzie)*, 2.4-oz. link 3.0
smoked, with apple and onion *(McKenzie)*, 2.4-oz. link 6.0
and spinach *(Bilinski)*, 3.3-oz. link 2.0
and sun-dried tomato with basil *(Bilinski)*, 3.3-oz. link 5.0
Thai brand *(McKenzie)*, 2.4-oz. link 2.0
Chicken seasoning and coating mix:
(Durkee/French's Roasting Bag), ⅙ pkg. 4.0
(McCormick Bag 'n Season), 1 tbsp. 4.0
(Shake'n Bake Original Recipe), ⅛ pkg. 7.0
barbecue *(Durkee Roasting Bag)*, ⅙ pkg. 8.0
barbecue glaze *(Shake'n Bake)*, ⅛ pkg. 9.0
Buffalo wing, all varieties *(Durkee)*, ⅛ pkg. 3.0
cacciatore *(Durkee Easy)*, ¹⁄₁₀ pkg. 3.0
coq au vin *(Knorr Recipe)*, 1 tbsp. 5.0
country *(Durkee Roasting Bag)*, ⅙ pkg. 3.0
Dijon, country *(Lawry's Chicken Saute)*, 2 tbsp. 7.0
Dijonne *(Knorr Recipe)*, ⅙ pkg. 5.0
extra crispy *(Oven Fry)*, ⅛ pkg. 10.0
garlic Italian *(Lawry's Chicken Saute)*, 2 tbsp. 3.0
homestyle flour *(Oven Fry)*, ⅛ pkg. 7.0
hot, spicy *(McCormick Bag 'n Season)*, 1 tbsp. 5.0
hot and spicy *(Shake'n Bake)*, ⅛ pkg. 7.0

lemon herb *(Lawry's Chicken Saute)*, 2 tbsp. 4.0
Mexican salsa *(Durkee Easy)*, ¹⁄₁₀ pkg. 3.0
mushroom *(Durkee Easy)*, ¹⁄₈ pkg. 3.0
Southwest, marinade *(Lawry's)*, 1 tsp. 1.0
stir-fry *(McCormick)*, 2 tsp., ¹⁄₆ pkg. 4.0
sweet and sour *(Durkee Easy)*, ¹⁄₉ pkg. 5.0
teriyaki *(Lawry's Chicken Saute)*, 2 tbsp. 9.0
Chicken spread:
chunky *(Underwood)*, ¼ cup 2.0
chunky, with crackers *(Red Devil* Snackers), 1 pkg. 20.0
salad *(Libby's Spreadables)*, ⅓ cup 7.0
Chicken wing sauce, see "Chicken sauce"
Chick-fil-A, 1 serving:
chicken dishes:
   chargrilled, 2.8 oz. 0
   Chick-fil-A Nuggets, 8-pack 12.0
   Chick-n-Strips, 4 pieces 10.0
   Chick-n-Strips salad 21.0
   salad, chargrilled garden 10.0
   salad plate 40.0
chicken sandwiches:
   regular 29.0
   chargrilled 36.0
   chargrilled, deluxe 38.0
   chargrilled club, without dressing 38.0
   Chick-n-Q 36.0
   deluxe 31.0
   salad, whole wheat 42.0
side dishes, small:
   carrot raisin salad 28.0
   chicken soup, 1 cup 14.0
   coleslaw 11.0
   tossed salad 13.0
   Waffle fries, salted or unsalted 49.0
desserts:
   brownie, fudge nut 41.0
   cheesecake 7.0
   cheesecake, with blueberry 9.0
   cheesecake, with strawberry 8.0
   Icedream, small cone 16.0
   Icedream, small cup 50.0
   lemon pie 19.0

Chickpea flour *(Arrowhead Mills)*, 2 oz. 35.0
Chickpeas:
dry:
    (Arrowhead Mills), ¼ cup 29.0
    ½ cup 60.7
    boiled, ½ cup 22.5
canned, ½ cup:
    (Allens/East Texas Fair) 19.0
    (Eden Organic/Organic Jars) 19.0
    (Goya) 20.0
    (Green Giant/Joan of Arc) 18.0
    (Old El Paso Garbanzo) 16.0
    (Progresso) 20.0
    (Progresso Garbanzo) 18.0
    (Seneca Garbanzo) 19.0
    (Stokely) 17.0
    with liquid 27.1
Chicory, witloof:
(Frieda's Belgian Endive), 2 cups, 3 oz. 3.0
untrimmed, 1 lb. 12.9
5–7"-long head, 2.1 oz. 2.1
½ cup 1.8
Chicory greens:
untrimmed, 1 lb. 17.5
trimmed, 1 oz. 1.3
chopped, ½ cup 4.2
Chicory root:
untrimmed, 1 lb. 65.1
1 medium, 2.6 oz. 10.5
1" pieces, ½ cup 7.0
Chili, canned (see also "Chili base"), 1 cup, except as
  noted:
with beans:
    (Broadcast) 20.0
    (Chi-Chi's San Antonio) 23.0
    (Gebhardt) 32.0
    (Hormel) 30.0
    (Hormel), 7½-oz. can 23.0
    (Hormel Micro Cup), 1 cont. 23.0
    (Hormel Micro Cup), 10.5-oz. cont. 41.0
    (Just Rite) 30.0
    (Libby's) 29.0

(Libby's Diner), 7¾ oz. 23.0
(Nalley Microwave)*, 7½ oz. 28.0
(Nalley Real Hearty) 27.0
(Nalley Thick) 32.0
(Old El Paso) 15.0
(Open Range) 25.0
(Van Camp's) 28.0
(Wolf) 30.0
with beef and hot dogs *(Nalley* Chili Dog) 27.0
cheddar *(Nalley)* 28.0
cheddar *(Nalley* Microwave)*, 7½ oz. 22.0
chunky *(Hormel)* 30.0
hot *(Hormel)* 30.0
hot *(Hormel/Hormel* Micro Cup)*, 7½ oz. 23.0
hot *(Nalley* Microwave)*, 7½ oz. 26.0
jalapeño *(Wolf)* 30.0
jalapeño hot *(Nalley)* 30.0
without beans:
    (Gebhardt) 11.0
    (Hormel) 16.0
    (Hormel), 7½-oz. can 13.0
    (Hormel Micro Cup)*, 1 cont. 15.0
    (Libby's) 16.0
    (Nalley Big Chunk) 13.0
    (Open Range) 19.0
    (Wolf) 20.0
    hot *(Hormel)* 16.0
    jalapeño *(Wolf)* 20.0
    onion *(Nalley* Walla Walla) 20.0
with franks, see "Beans and franks"
with macaroni *(Hormel* Chili Mac), 7.5-oz. can 17.0
with macaroni *(Hormel* Chili Mac Micro Cup), 1 cont. 17.0
turkey, with beans *(Hormel)* 26.0
turkey, without beans *(Hormel)* 17.0
vegetarian:
    (Hormel) 38.0
    (Natural Touch) 21.0
    (Worthington/Worthington Low Fat) 21.0
    all varieties *(Health Valley* Nonfat)*, ½ cup 15.0
Chili, freeze-dried:
with beef and beans *(Mountain House)*, 1 cup 27.0
with beef and macaroni *(Mountain House)*, 1 cup 30.0

Chili, freeze-dried *(cont.)*
meatless *(AlpineAire* Mountain), 1½ cups 54.0
Chili, frozen:
with beans *(Stouffer's),* 8¾ oz. 29.0
with corn bread *(Marie Callender's* Dinner), 16 oz. 45.0
three bean *(Lean Cuisine),* 10 oz. 23.0
vegetarian *(Tabatchnik* Side Dish), 7.5 oz. 28.0
Chili base, canned, ½ cup:
(Hunt's Homestyle Fixings) 18.5
(S&W Chili Makin's) 20.0
(Stubb's Legendary Chili Fixin's) 9.0
black bean *(S&W* Chili Makin's) 19.0
homestyle *(S&W* Chili Makin's) 19.0
Santa Fe *(S&W* Chili Makin's) 18.0
Chili beans (see also "Mexican beans"), canned, ½ cup:
(Gebhardt) 30.0
(Hunt's) 17.0
(S&W) 23.0
(Stokely) 21.0
(Sun-Vista) 24.0
(Van Camp's Mexican Style) 21.0
hot *(S&W* Chipotle) 21.0
with jalapeños and red peppers *(Eden* Organic) 21.0
spicy *(Green Giant/Joan of Arc)* 20.0
zesty *(Campbell's)* 21.0
Chili dip, green *(La Victoria),* 2 tbsp. 2.0
Chili dip mix, caliente *(Knorr),* ½ tsp. 1.0
Chili dinner or entree, see "Chili, frozen"
Chili mix:
all varieties *(Health Valley* Chili in a Cup), ⅓ cup 21.0
4 bean *(Knorr* Cup), 1 pkg. 53.0
3 bean *(Spice Islands* Quick Meal), 1 pkg. 34.0
vegetarian *(Spice Islands* Quick Meal), 1 pkg. 32.0
Chili pepper, see "Pepper, chili"
Chili powder:
(Gebhardt Eagle), ¼ tsp. 0
(Tone's), ¼ tsp. 0
1 tbsp. 4.1
1 tsp. 1.4
Chili sauce (see also "Pepper sauce" and "Szechwan
  sauce"):
(Del Monte), 1 tbsp. 5.0

(Hunt's), 2 tbsp. 8.0
(Las Palmas), 1/4 cup 2.0
(Nance's), 2 tbsp. 5.0
(S&W Steakhouse), 1 tbsp. 4.0
hot dog:
    (Gebhardt), 1/4 cup 6.0
    (Just Rite), 2 oz. 5.0
    (Open Range), 1/4 cup 6.0
    (Wolf), 1 tbsp. 2.0
    with beef *(Stenger)*, 1/4 cup 7.0
Chili seasoning mix:
(Adolph's Meal Makers), 1 tbsp. 9.0
(Durkee), 1/5 pkg. 7.0
(Durkee Pot-O), 1/8 pkg. 7.0
(Gebhardt Chili Quik), 2 tbsp. 8.0
(Lawry's), 1 tbsp. 5.0
(Lawry's Tex-Mex), 2 tbsp. 8.0
(McCormick), approximately 4 tsp. 5.0
(Mick Fowler's 2-Alarm Family), 2 tbsp. 9.0
(Mick Fowler's 2-Alarm Kit), 3 tbsp. 10.0
(Old El Paso), 1 tbsp. 0
mild *(Durkee)*, 1/5 pkg. 5.0
Texas red *(Durkee)*, 1/3 pkg. 2.0
Chimichanga, frozen:
beef *(Old El Paso)*, 4.3-oz. piece 37.0
beef steak and bean *(Don Miguel)*, 7 oz. 55.0
chicken *(Don Miguel)*, 7 oz. 54.0
chicken *(Old El Paso)*, 4.3-oz. piece 39.0
Chimichanga dinner, frozen:
beef *(Chi-Chi's)*, 15 oz. 70.0
chicken *(Chi-Chi's)*, 15 oz. 74.0
Chimichanga entree, frozen *(Banquet)*, 9.5 oz. 56.0
Chitterlings, pork 0
Chives:
fresh, 1 oz. 1.2
fresh, chopped, 1 tbsp. 1
freeze-dried:
    (McCormick), 1/4 tsp. 0
    (Tone's), 1/4 tsp. 0
    1/4 cup 5
    1 tbsp. 1
Chives, Chinese *(Frieda's Gil Choy)*, 1 tbsp. 0

Chocolate, see "Candy"
Chocolate, baking (see also specific listings):
(Choco Bake), ½ oz. 5.0
bars:
  (Hershey's), ½ of 1-oz. bar 4.0
  bittersweet *(Ghirardelli)*, 3 squares, 1.5 oz. 24.0
  bittersweet *(Hershey's)*, ½ oz. 8.0
  milk *(Ghirardelli)*, 3 squares, 1.5 oz. 25.0
  milk *(Ghirardelli)*, 1 oz. 17.0
  semisweet *(Baker's)*, 1 oz. 17.0
  semisweet *(Ghirardelli)*, 3 squares, 1.5 oz. 25.0
  semisweet *(Hershey's)*, ½ oz. 9.0
  semisweet *(Nestlé)*, ½ oz. 9.0
  sweet *(Baker's German)*, ½ oz. 8.0
  sweet, dark *(Ghirardelli)*, 3 squares, 1.5 oz. 26.0
  unsweetened *(Baker's)*, 1 oz. 9.0
  unsweetened *(Ghirardelli)*, 3 squares, 1.5 oz. 12.0
  unsweetened *(Nestlé)*, ½ oz. 5.0
  white *(Baker's)*, 1 oz. 17.0
  white *(Ghirardelli)*, 3 squares, 1.5 oz. 25.0
  white *(Nestlé)*, ½ oz. 8.0
bits, holiday *(Hershey's)*, 1 tbsp. 11.0
chips or morsels, ½ oz. or 1 tbsp.:
  (Ghirardelli Flickettes) 10.0
  milk *(Baker's)* 9.0
  milk *(Ghirardelli)* 10.0
  milk *(Hershey's)* 10.0
  milk *(M&M's)* 10.0
  milk *(Nestlé)* 10.0
  mint *(Nestlé)* 9.0
  semisweet *(Ghirardelli)* 10.0
  semisweet *(Hershey's/Hershey's Reduced Fat)* 10.0
  white *(Ghirardelli)* 10.0
  white *(Hershey's Bake Shoppe)* 9.0
chunks *(Hershey's Semisweet)*, 6 chunks 9.0
kiss *(Hershey's Mini)*, 11 pieces 9.0
semisweet, ½ oz.:
  (Baker's Real) 9.0
  (M&M's) 9.0
  (Nestlé) 9.0
  flavor *(Baker's)* 10.0
  mint *(Nestlé)* 9.0

Chocolate drink:
bottled *(Yoo-Hoo)*, 9 fl. oz. 33.0
canned *(Yoo-Hoo)*, 11 fl. oz. 40.0
Chocolate flavor drink, canned:
canned, 10 fl. oz.:
    (Sego) 44.0
    all flavors *(Sego* Lite) 21.0
    all flavors *(Sweet Success)* 38.0
    creamy milk *(Nestlé Instant Breakfast)* 37.0
    malt *(Sego)* 44.0
refrigerated *(Sweet Success)*, 12 fl. oz. 45.0
Chocolate flavor drink mix (see also "Cocoa mix"),
    1 pkt., except as noted:
(Nestlé Quik), 2 tbsp. 19.0
(Nestlé Quik No Sugar), 2 tbsp. 7.0
(Pillsbury Instant Breakfast) 28.0
all flavors:
    (Carnation Instant Breakfast) 28.0
    (Carnation Instant Breakfast No Sugar) 12.0
    (Sweet Success) 19.0
shake *(Weight Watchers)* 12.0
Chocolate fruit dip *(Smucker's* Fat Free), 2 tbsp. 31.0
Chocolate milk, 1 cup:
(Crowley's) 29.0
(Nestlé Quik) 31.0
fat free *(Hershey's)* 23.0
low-fat:
    (Hershey's) 30.0
    (Lactaid) 23.0
    (Nestlé Quik) 29.0
    (Nestlé Quik Aseptic) 30.0
    (Parmalat) 28.0
shake, see "Chocolate shake"
Chocolate pastry (see also specific listings), 2 pieces:
dark *(Pepperidge Farm* Clouds) 53.0
milk *(Pepperidge Farm* Clouds) 54.0
Chocolate shake:
(Nestlé Killer), 14 fl. oz. 65.0
(Nestlé Quik), 9 fl. oz. 41.0
Chocolate syrup, 2 tbsp.:
(Fox's No Cal) 0
(Fox's U-Bet) 29.0

Chocolate syrup *(cont.)*
(Hershey's) 24.0
(Smucker's Sundae) 27.0
(Yoo-Hoo) 25.0
dark (Hershey's Special Dark) 27.0
malt (Hershey's) 25.0
Chocolate topping, 2 tbsp.:
(Kraft) 26.0
all varieties (Smucker's Magic Shell) 16.0
caramel (Hershey's) 25.0
cherry Melba (Dickinson's Black Forest) 26.0
dark (Dove) 22.0
double (Hershey's) 26.0
fudge:
    (Smucker's) 28.0
    dark chocolate (Mrs. Richardson's) 20.0
    double (Hershey's) 24.0
    hot (Hershey's) 20.0
    hot (Hershey's Fat Free) 23.0
    hot (Kraft) 24.0
    hot (Mrs. Richardson's) 20.0
    hot (Mrs. Richardson's Fat Free) 25.0
    hot (Smucker's) 24.0
    hot (Smucker's Light) 23.0
    hot (Smucker's Special Recipe) 22.0
milk (Dove) 23.0
mint (Hershey's) 25.0
Chorizo (Goya), 1.6-oz. stick 2.0
Chow mein, see specific entree listings
Chowchow:
(Crosse & Blackwell), 1 tbsp. 1.0
(Stubb's Legendary Original/Spicy), ½ cup 13.0
Chrysanthemum garland:
raw, untrimmed, 1 lb. 19.0
raw, 1″ pieces, ½ cup 5
boiled, drained, 1″ pieces, ½ cup 2.2
Church's Chicken, 1 serving:
chicken, edible portion:
    breast, 2.8 oz. 4.3
    leg, 2 oz. 2.4
    Tender Strip, 1.1 oz. 4.5
    thigh, 2.8 oz. 5.3

wing, 3.1 oz. 7.7
sides:
    biscuit 25.6
    Cajun rice 16.6
    coleslaw. 8.4
    corn on cob 23.5
    fries 28.5
    okra 19.1
    potatoes and gravy 14.0
apple pie 40.5
Churro, cinnamon *(Tio Pepe's),* 1 oz. 14.0
Chutney, 1 tbsp.:
mango *(Patak's* Major Grey's) 12.0
tomato, dried *(Sonoma)* 9.0
tropical fruit and nut *(Patak's)* 12.0
Cilantro, see "Coriander"
Cinnamon, ground:
(McCormick), ¼ tsp. 4
(Tone's), ¼ tsp. 1.1
1 tbsp. 5.4
1 tsp. 2.1
Cisco, without added ingredients 0
Citron, candied:
(S&W), 39 pieces, 1.1 oz. 23.0
diced *(Paradise/White Swan),* 2 tbsp., .9 oz. 19.0
Citrus drink, 8 fl. oz., except as noted:
punch:
    (Goya) 30.0
    (Minute Maid) 31.0
    (Tree Top Juice Rivers Box), 8.45 fl. oz. 33.0
    (Tropicana) 36.0
chilled or frozen* *(Five Alive)* 30.0
chilled or frozen* *(Five Alive* Tropical) 29.0
frozen* *(Minute Maid* Punch) 32.0
frozen* *(Schwan's Vita Sun)* 26.0
Citrus juice blend *(Pet/Season's Best* Medley), 8 fl. oz. . . . 31.0
Citrus salad, in jars, in light syrup *(Sunfresh),* ½ cup 17.0
Clam, meat only:
raw, 4 oz. 2.9
raw, 9 large or 20 small, 6.3 oz. 4.6
boiled, poached, or steamed, 4 oz. 5.8

Clam, canned; ¼ cup or 2 oz.:
baby, whole *(S&W)* 2.0
chopped or minced *(Doxsee)* 2.0
chopped or minced *(S&W)* 1.0
minced *(Progresso)* 2.0
smoked *(S&W)* 2.0
Clam, fried, frozen:
(Gorton's Crunchy), 3 oz. 17.0
(Mrs. Paul's), 28 pieces 28.0
Clam chowder, see "Soup"
Clam dip, 2 tbsp.:
(Breakstone's Chesapeake) 2.0
(Heluva Good New England) 7.0
(Kraft) 3.0
(Kraft Premium) 2.0
(Nalley) 3.0
Clam juice:
(Bookbinder's), 10.5 oz. 1.0
(Doxsee), 1 tbsp. 0
(S&W), 9.6 fl. oz. 0
Clam sauce, canned, ½ cup:
creamy *(Progresso)* 8.0
red *(Progresso)* 8.0
white:
    (Bookbinder's) 4.0
    (Progresso) 1.0
    (Progresso Authentic) 2.0
Clover seeds, sprouted, raw *(Shaw's)*, 2 oz. 0
Clover sprouts *(Jonathan's)*, 1 cup, 3 oz. 3.0
Cloves, ground:
(McCormick), ¼ tsp. 2
1 tbsp. 4.0
1 tsp. 1.3
Cobbler, freeze-dried, apple-blueberry *(AlpineAire)*, ½ cup   46.0
Cobbler, frozen
apple:
    (Marie Callender's), 4¼ oz. 45.0
    (Stilwell), ⅛ pkg. 39.0
    (Stilwell Lite), ⅛ pkg. 22.0
    crumb *(Pet-Ritz)*, ⅙ pkg. 49.0
apple cinnamon *(Pet-Ritz)*, ⅙ pkg. 40.0
apricot *(Stilwell)*, ⅛ pkg. 39.0

berry:
    (Marie Callender's), 4¼ oz. 41.0
    (Stilwell), ⅛ pkg. 42.0
    (Stilwell Lite), ⅛ pkg. 22.0
blackberry:
    (Pet-Ritz), ⅙ pkg. 37.0
    (Stilwell), ⅛ pkg. 39.0
    (Stilwell Lite), ⅛ pkg. 23.0
    crumb *(Pet-Ritz)*, ⅙ pkg. 45.0
blueberry *(Marie Callender's)*, 4 oz. 42.0
cherry:
    (Marie Callender's), 4¼ oz. 50.0
    (Pet-Ritz), ⅙ pkg. 48.0
    (Stilwell), ⅛ pkg. 39.0
    (Stilwell Lite), ⅛ pkg. 23.0
    crumb *(Pet-Ritz)*, ⅙ pkg. 54.0
peach:
    (Marie Callender's), 4¼ oz. 47.0
    (Pet-Ritz), ⅙ pkg. 37.0
    (Stilwell), ⅛ pkg. 38.0
    (Stilwell Lite), ⅛ pkg. 22.0
    crumb *(Pet-Ritz)*, ⅙ pkg. 38.0
strawberry *(Pet-Ritz)*, ⅙ pkg. 40.0
strawberry *(Stilwell)*, ⅛ pkg. 41.0
Cocktail sauce, see "Seafood sauce"
Cocoa, baking, 1 tbsp., except as noted:
unsweetened:
    (Ghirardelli) 5.0
    (Hershey's) 3.0
    (Nestlé Baking) 3.0
sweetened *(Ghirardelli)*, 2½ tbsp. 19.9
Cocoa mix, hot, 1 pkt., except as noted:
(Carnation Fat Free) 4.0
(Carnation No Sugar) 8.0
(Carnation 70) 15.0
(Swiss Miss Diet) 4.0
(Swiss Miss Fat Free) 9.0
(Swiss Miss Lite) 17.5
(Swiss Miss Sugar Free) 10.0
(Weight Watchers) 10.0
almond mocha *(Swiss Miss* Premiere) 28.0

Cocoa mix *(cont.)*
chocolate:
    (Swiss Miss Sensation) 27.0
    all varieties *(Carnation)*, 3 tbsp. 24.0
    all varieties except Irish cream *(Land O Lakes)* 25.0
    almond mocha *(Swiss Miss Premiere)* 28.0
    double *(Ghirardelli)* 21.0
    English toffee *(Swiss Miss Premiere)* 28.5
    hazelnut *(Ghirardelli)* 21.0
    Irish cream *(Land O Lakes)* 28.0
    Irish creme *(Nestlé)*, 3 tbsp. 16.0
    milk *(Swiss Miss)* 22.0
    milk *(Swiss Miss Sugar Free)* 10.0
    milk, with mini marshmallow *(Swiss Miss)* 22.0
    mocha *(Ghirardelli)* 21.0
    raspberry truffle *(Swiss Miss Premiere)* 28.0
    rich *(Swiss Miss)* 23.0
    rich, with or without marshmallow *(Nestlé)* 24.0
    Suisse chocolate truffle *(Swiss Miss Premiere)* 28.0
    Swiss truffle *(Nestlé)*, 3 tbsp. 17.0
    white *(Ghirardelli)*, 2 tbsp. 23.0
    white *(Swiss Miss)* 21.0
and cream *(Swiss Miss)* 25.0
with marshmallows *(Swiss Miss Marshmallow Lovers)* 27.0
with marshmallows *(Swiss Miss Marshmallow Lovers Fat
    Free)* 12.5
with mini marshmallow *(Swiss Miss No Sugar)* 10.0
Coconut:
fresh, in shell, 1 lb. 35.9
fresh, shelled:
    1 piece, 2″ × 2″ × ½″, approx. 1.6 oz. 6.9
    1 oz. 4.3
    shredded or grated, 1 cup not packed 12.2
canned, flaked:
    (Angel Flake), 2 tbsp. 7.0
    (Durkee), 2 tbsp. 6.0
    sweetened, ⅓ cup 10.5
dried, toasted, 1 oz. 12.6
packaged, 2 tbsp., except as noted:
    flaked *(Angel Flake)* 7.0
    flaked *(Mounds)* 8.0
    flaked, and almond bits *(Almond Joy)* 7.0

flaked, sweetened, ⅓ cup 11.8
shredded *(Baker's* Premium) 6.0
Coconut cream, canned, sweetened:
(Coco Casa), 3 tbsp. 35.0
(Coco Goya), 1 tbsp. 22.0
(Coco Lopez), 3 tbsp. 35.0
½ cup 12.4
1 tbsp. 1.6
Coconut milk[1], 1 tbsp. 8
Coconut milk, canned:
(Goya), 1 tbsp. 1.0
(Taste of Thai/Taste of Thai Light), ¼ cup 2.0
Coconut nectar *(R.W. Knudsen),* 8 fl. oz. 26.0
Cod, without added ingredients 0
Cod entree, frozen:
battered *(Schwan's Battercrisp),* 2 oz. 9.0
breaded *(Mrs. Paul's* Premium), 4.25-oz. piece 24.0
breaded *(Van de Kamp's* Light), 3.98-oz. piece 19.0
breaded, nuggets *(Schwan's),* 6 pieces, 3 oz. 18.0
Cod liver oil 0
Codfish fritter, see "Bacalaito"
Coffee:
brewed, 6 fl. oz. 8
instant, regular, 1 rounded tsp. .7
Coffee, flavored, see "Coffee, iced" and "Cappuccino"
Coffee, flavored, mix, 8 fl. oz.*, except as noted:
cafe Amaretto *(General Foods International)* 8.0
cafe Français *(General Foods International)* 7.0
cafe Vienna *(General Foods International)* 11.0
cappuccino:
(Nestlé Instant), 1 pkt. 16.0
(Swiss Miss Sidewalk Cafe), ¼ cup 20.0
cinnamon *(Maxwell House)* 16.0
coffee *(Maxwell House)* 18.0
Italian *(General Foods International)* 10.0
mocha *(Maxwell House)* 17.0
mocha *(Nestlé),* 1 pkt. 21.0
orange *(General Foods International)* 11.0
vanilla *(Maxwell House)* 19.0
chocolate, Viennese *(General Foods International)* 10.0

[1]*Liquid expressed from mixture of grated coconut and water.*

Coffee, flavored *(cont.)*
cinnamon *(Swiss Miss Sidewalk Cafe)*, ¼ cup 20.5
hazelnut, Belgian *(General Foods International)* 12.0
Kahlua cafe *(General Foods International)* 10.0
mocha *(Swiss Miss Sidewalk Cafe)*, ¼ cup 20.0
mocha, cafe *(Carnation Instant Breakfast)* 28.0
mocha, Suisse *(General Foods International)* 8.0
vanilla, French *(General Foods International)* 10.0
vanilla, French *(Swiss Miss Sidewalk Cafe)*, ¼ cup 19.5
Coffee, iced (see also "Cappuccino"):
(Jamaican Gold), 11-oz. can 29.0
(Jamaican Gold Latte), 11-oz. can 27.0
Coffee creamer, see "Creamer, nondairy"
Coffee substitute, cereal grain:
(Natural Touch Kaffree Roma), 1 tsp. 2.0
(Natural Touch Roma Cappuccino), 3 tbsp. 5.0
(Postum Instant), 1 tsp. 3.0
coffee flavor *(Postum* Instant), 1 tsp. 3.0
Cold cuts, see specific listings
Coleslaw, salad mix *(Dole)*, 3 oz. 5.0
Coleslaw dressing, see "Salad dressing"
Collard greens, ½ cup, except as noted:
fresh:
    raw, 1 oz. 2.0
    raw, chopped 1.3
    boiled, drained, chopped 3.9
canned *(Allens/Sunshine)* 5.0
canned *(Stubb's Harvest)* 5.0
frozen, chopped, boiled, drained 6.1
Cookie:
almond:
    (Archway Crescents), 2 pieces, .8 oz. 17.0
    (Frieda's), 2 pieces, 1 oz. 19.0
    (Stella D'Oro Breakfast Treats), .8-oz. piece 16.0
    (Stella D'Oro Chinese Dessert), 1.2-oz. piece 21.0
    (Sunshine Crescents), 4 pieces, 1.1 oz. 22.0
    toast *(Stella D'Oro* Mandel), 2 pieces, 1 oz. 21.0
amaretti di Saronno, chocolate dipped *(Lazzaroni)*, 4 pieces,
    1.1 oz. 22.0
animal:
    (Barnum's Animals), 12 pieces, 1.1 oz. 23.0
    (Sunshine), 14 pieces, 1.1 oz. 24.0

vanilla *(Barbara's)*, 8 pieces, 1 oz. 20.0
anisette:
    (Stella D'Oro Sponge), 2 pieces, 1 oz. 19.0
    (Stella D'Oro Toast), 3 pieces, 1.2 oz. 27.0
    (Stella D'Oro Toast Jumbo), 1 piece, 1.1 oz. 23.0
apple:
    (Newtons Fat Free), 2 pieces, 1 oz. 24.0
    (Sunshine Golden Fruit), .7-oz. piece 15.0
    bar *(Archway* Nonfat), .7-oz. piece 15.0
    bran *(Archway)*, 1.2-oz. piece 27.0
    cinnamon bar *(Tastykake)*, 1.5-oz. bar 29.0
    pastry *(Stella D'Oro* Low Sodium), .7-oz. piece 14.0
    and raisin *(Archway)*, 1.1-oz. piece 20.0
    raisin *(Health Valley* Fat Free Jumbo), 1 piece 19.0
    raisin bar *(Smart Snackers)*, .75 oz. 14.0
    spice *(Health Valley* Fat Free), 3 pieces 24.0
apricot:
    (Health Valley Nonfat), 3 pieces 24.0
    filled *(Archway)*, 1-oz. piece 18.0
    raspberry *(Pepperidge Farm)*, 3 pieces, 1.1 oz. 22.0
(Archway Bells and Stars), 3 pieces, 1 oz. 19.0
(Archway Old Fashion Windmill), .75-oz. piece 15.0
(Archway Party Treats), 3 pieces, 1.1 oz. 20.0
arrowroot *(National)*, .2-oz. piece 3.0
banana bran *(Archway* Low Fat), 1.2-oz. piece 27.0
biscotti:
    all varieties *(Health Valley)*, 2 pieces, 1.1 oz. 23.0
    almond *(Pepperidge Farm Caruso)*, .7-oz. piece 12.0
    anise *(Pepperidge Farm La Scala)*, .7-oz. piece 14.0
    chocolate dipped *(Pepperidge Farm Figaro)*, .8-oz. piece 14.0
    cranberry pistachio *(Pepperidge Farm Tosca)*, .7-oz.
      piece 13.0
biscottini cashews *(Stella D'Oro)*, .7-oz. piece 13.0
blueberry *(Archway)*, 1-oz. piece 19.0
blueberry *(Fruitastic* Bar), 1 bar 13.0
brown edge wafer *(Nabisco)*, 5 pieces, 1 oz. 21.0
butter (see also "shortbread," below):
    (Master Choice Southern Classics), 10 pieces 20.0
    (Peek Freans Petit Beurre), 4 pieces, 1 oz. 22.0
    (Pepperidge Farm Madaillon au Beurre), 4 pieces,
      1.2 oz. 25.0
    (Pepperidge Farm Chessman), 3 pieces, .9 oz. 18.0

Cookie, butter *(cont.)*

   (Sunshine), 5 pieces, 1.1 oz. 21.0

   assorted *(Pepperidge Farm* Toy Chest), 3 pieces, .9 oz.   18.0

   sandwich with fudge *(E.L. Fudge)*, 3 pieces, 1.2 oz. 24.0

butter pecan bites *(Barbara's Small Indulgence)*, 6 pieces . . 16.0

caramel apple *(Barbara's* Fat Free Mini), 6 pieces 22.0

caramel pecan *(Pepperidge Farm)*, .9-oz. piece 16.0

carrot cake *(Archway)*, 1-oz. piece 18.0

cherry cobbler *(Pepperidge Farm)*, .6-oz. piece 11.0

cherry filled *(Archway)*, 1-oz. piece 19.0

cherry nougat *(Archway)*, 3 pieces, 1 oz. 18.0

chocolate:

   (Archway Fat Free), 8-oz. piece 19.0

   (Pepperidge Farm Goldfish), 1.1 oz. 22.0

   (Stella D'Oro Castelets), 2 pieces, 1 oz. 19.0

   (Stella D'Oro Margherite), 2 pieces, 1.1 oz. 18.0

   brownie *(Entenmann's* Fat Free), 2 pieces 20.0

   brownie nut *(Pepperidge Farm)*, 3 pieces, 1.1 oz. 18.0

   caramel center *(Health Valley* Fat Free), 2 pieces 17.0

   covered *(Ritz)*, 3 pieces, 1.1 oz. 17.0

   dark *(Pepperidge Farm* Espirits Noir), .6-oz. piece 10.0

   double *(Barbara's* Fat Free Mini), 6 pieces, 1.1 oz. 20.0

   fudge *(Dare)*, .7-oz. piece 13.0

   fudge, iced *(Tastykake)*, 1.3-oz. piece 25.0

   fudge center *(Health Valley* Fat Free), 2 pieces 17.0

   fudge mint *(Grasshopper)*, 4 pieces, 1.1 oz. 20.0

   laced *(Pepperidge Farm Pirouette)*, 5 pieces, 1.2 oz. . . . 20.0

   milk, peanut butter *(Pepperidge Farm Chocolate Heaven)*,

      2 pieces 15.0

   with nuts *(Pepperidge Farm Geneva)*, 3 pieces, 1.1 oz. . . 19.0

   orange *(Pepperidge Farm* Chocolat a l'Orange), 2 pieces,

      1.1 oz. 23.0

   snaps *(Nabisco)*, 7 pieces, 1.2 oz. 23.0

   wafer *(Nabisco* Famous), 5 pieces, 1.1 oz. 24.0

   wafer, light *(Keebler)*, 8 pieces, 1.1 oz. 25.0

chocolate chip/chunk:

   (Archway), 1-oz. piece 19.0

   (Archway Bag), 3 pieces 17.0

   (Archway Ice Box), 1-oz. piece 19.0

   (Barbara's), 2 pieces, 1.3 oz. 25.0

   (Chip-A-Roos), 3 pieces, 1.3 oz. 23.0

   (Chips Ahoy! Chewy), 3 pieces, 1.3 oz. 23.0

(Chips Ahoy! Chunky), .6-oz. piece 11.0
(Chips Ahoy! Mini), 14 pieces, 1.1 oz. 21.0
(Chips Ahoy! Munch Size), 5 pieces, 1 oz. 18.0
(Chips Ahoy! Real Chocolate), 3 pieces, 1.1 oz. 21.0
(Chips Ahoy! Reduced Fat), 3 pieces, 1.1 oz. 23.0
(Chips Deluxe), .5-oz. piece 9.0
(Chips Deluxe Chocolate Lovers), .6-oz. piece 11.0
(Chips Deluxe Light), .6-oz. piece 11.0
(Chips Deluxe With Peanut Butter Cups), .6-oz. piece . . . 10.0
(Chips Deluxe Rainbow), .6-oz. piece 9.0
(Chips Deluxe Soft 'n Chewy), .6-oz. piece 11.0
(Dare), .5-oz. piece 9.2
(Dare Breaktime), .3-oz. piece 5.0
(Entenmann's), 3 pieces, 1.1 oz. 20.0
(Grandma's Big), 1.4-oz. piece 25.0
(Little Debbie), 2 pieces, 1.3 oz. 24.0
(Pepperidge Farm Old Fashioned), 3 pieces, 1 oz. 18.0
(Pepperidge Farm Chesapeake), .9-oz. piece 15.0
(Pepperidge Farm Goldfish), 1.1 oz. 21.0
(Pepperidge Farm Nantucket), .9-oz. piece 16.0
(Smart Snackers), 2 pieces, 1.06 oz. 22.0
(SnackWell's Reduced Fat), 13 pieces, 1 oz. 22.0
(Tastykake), 1.4-oz. piece 26.0
all varieties *(Health Valley Healthy Chips* Fat Free),
    3 pieces 24.0
bar *(Tastykake)*, 1.5-oz. bar 30.0
chocolate *(Barbara's)*, 2 pieces, 1.3 oz. 23.0
chocolate, walnut, soft *(Pepperidge Farm)*, .9-oz. piece . 16.0
crisps *(Barbara's Small Indulgences)*, 6 pieces, 1 oz. . . . 18.0
drop *(Archway)*, 1-oz. piece 11.0
fudge *(Grandma's* Big), 1.4-oz. piece 27.0
fudge bar *(Grandma's)*, 1.5-oz. bar 29.0
macadamia *(Pepperidge Farm Sausalito)*, .9-oz. piece . . . 16.0
macadamia, soft *(Pepperidge Farm)*, .9-oz. piece 16.0
macadamia, white chunk *(Pepperidge Farm Tahoe)*,
    .9-oz. piece 16.0
mini *(Sunshine)*, 5 pieces, 1.1 oz. 20.0
rainbow *(Chips Deluxe)*, .6-oz. piece 10.0
snaps *(Nabisco)*, 7 pieces, 1.1 oz. 24.0
soft *(Chips Deluxe)*, .5-oz. piece 10.0
soft *(Pepperidge Farm* Chunk), .9-oz. piece 16.0
sprinkled *(Chips Ahoy!)*, 3 pieces, 1.3 oz. 24.0

Cookie, chocolate chip/chunk *(cont.)*

striped *(Chips Ahoy!)*, .6-oz. piece 10.0
and toffee *(Archway)*, 1-oz. piece 19.0
toffee *(Pepperidge Farm Charleston)*, .9-oz. piece 16.0
walnut *(Pepperidge Farm Beacon Hill)*, .9-oz. piece 16.0

chocolate sandwich:

(E.L. Fudge), 2 pieces, .9 oz. 17.0
(Elfin Delights Light), 2 pieces, .9 oz. 19.0
(Hydrox), 3 pieces, 1.1 oz. 21.0
(Hydrox Fat Free), 3 pieces, 1.1 oz. 24.0
(Oreo), 3 pieces, 1.2 oz. 23.0
(Oreo Reduced Fat), 3 pieces, 1.1 oz. 24.0
(Oreo Double Stuf), 2 pieces, 1 oz. 19.0
(Pepperidge Farm Bordeaux), 4 pieces, 1 oz. 20.0
(Pepperidge Farm Brussels), 3 pieces, 1.1 oz. 20.0
(Pepperidge Farm Lido), .6-oz. piece 11.0
(Pepperidge Farm Milano), 3 pieces, 1.2 oz. 21.0
(Smart Snackers), 2 pieces, 1.06 oz. 23.0
(SnackWell's Reduced Fat), 2 pieces, .9 oz. 20.0
(Vienna Fingers Reduced Fat), 2 pieces, 1 oz. 22.0
chocolate fudge *(Keebler Classic Collection)*, .6-oz. piece 12.0
chocolate fudge, double *(Barbara's Cookies & Creme)*,
  2 pieces, .9 oz. 17.0
double *(Pepperidge Farm Milano)*, 2 pieces, 1 oz. 17.0
fudge coated *(Oreo)*, .75-oz piece 14.0
hazelnut *(Pepperidge Farm Milano)*, 2 pieces, .9 oz. 15.0
milk *(Pepperidge Farm Bordeaux)*, 3 pieces, 1.1 oz. 19.0
milk *(Pepperidge Farm Milano)*, 3 pieces, 1.3 oz. 21.0
mint *(Pepperidge Farm Brussels)*, 3 pieces, 1.3 oz. 22.0
mint *(Pepperidge Farm Milano)*, 2 pieces, .9 oz. 16.0
orange *(Pepperidge Farm Milano)*, 2 pieces, .9 oz. 16.0
raspberry *(Barbara's Cookies & Creme)*, 2 pieces, .9 oz. 18.0
vanilla *(Barbara's Cookies & Creme)*, 2 pieces, .9 oz. . . . 18.0
white fudge coated *(Oreo)*, .75-oz. piece 14.0

cinnamon:

apple *(Archway)*, 1-oz. piece 20.0
honey heart *(Archway* Fat Free), 3 pieces, 1.1 oz. 24.0
snaps *(Archway)*, 5 pieces, 1.1 oz. 20.0

cocoa, Dutch *(Archway)*, 1-oz. piece 19.0
cocoa, mocha *(Barbara's* Fat Free Mini), 6 pieces, 1.1 oz. . . 21.0
coconut *(Dare Breaktime)*, .3-oz. piece 5.2
coconut macaroon *(Archway)*, .8-oz. piece 14.0

coffee cake crunch *(Barbara's Small Indulgences)*, 6 pieces,
1 oz. 18.0
cranberry bar:
   (Archway Fat Free), .75-oz. bar 16.0
   (Newtons Fat Free), 2 pieces, 1 oz. 23.0
   (Sunshine Golden Fruit), .7-oz. piece 15.0
Danish *(Nabisco* Import), 5 pieces, 1.2 oz. 22.0
date delight *(Health Valley* Nonfat), 3 pieces 24.0
devil's food cake *(SnackWell's* Fat Free), .6-oz. piece 13.0
egg biscuit (see also "kichel," below):
   (Stella D'Oro Jumbo), 2 pieces, .8 oz. 18.0
   (Stella D'Oro Low Sodium), 3 pieces, 1.1 oz. 20.0
   Roman *(Stella D'Oro)*, 1.2 oz. 21.0
fig:
   (Archway Fat Free), .75-oz. piece 15.0
   (Fig Newtons), 2 pieces, 1.1 oz. 20.0
   (Fig Newtons Fat Free), 2 pieces, 1 oz. 22.0
   (Smart Snackers), .7 oz. 16.0
   (Sunshine Bar), 2 pieces, 1 oz. 20.0
   (Sunshine Golden Fruit Fat Free), .6-oz. piece 13.0
fortune *(Frieda's)*, 4 pieces, 1 oz. 23.0
fortune *(La Choy)*, 4 pieces, 1.1 oz. 26.0
fruit:
   bar *(Archway* Fat Free), ½ piece, 1 oz. 21.0
   cake *(Archway)*, 3 pieces, 1-oz. piece 20.0
   Hawaiian *(Health Valley* Fat Free), 3 pieces 24.0
   honey bar *(Archway)*, 1-oz. piece 18.0
   slices *(Stella D'Oro)*, .6-oz. piece 20.0
   slices *(Stella D'Oro* Fat Free), .6-oz. piece 12.0
fudge:
   (Stella D'Oro Swiss), 2 pieces, .9 oz. 17.0
   bar *(Tastykake)*, 1.5-oz. bar 29.0
   bits *(Grandma's)*, 9 pieces 24.0
   double, cake *(SnackWell's* Fat Free), .6-oz. piece 12.0
   fudge filled *(Keebler* Truffles), 3 pieces, 1.2 oz. 22.0
   mint patties *(Sunshine)*, 2 pieces, .8 oz. 16.0
   nut bar *(Archway)*, 1-oz. piece 17.0
   nutty *(Grandma's* Big), 1.4-oz. piece 25.0
   sandwich *(Grandma's)*, 1 pkg. 41.0
   sandwich *(Grandma's* Value), 3 cookies 31.0
ginger *(Dare Breaktime)*, .3-oz. piece 5.7
ginger *(Pepperidge Farm* Gingerman), 4 pieces, 1 oz. 21.0

Cookie *(cont.)*

ginger snaps:

(Archway), 5 pieces, 1.1 oz. 18.0

(Nabisco), 4 pieces, 1 oz. 22.0

(Sunshine), 7 pieces, 1 oz. 22.0

gingerbread, iced (Archway), 3 pieces, 1.1 oz. 23.0

gingerbread, iced (Sunshine), 5 pieces, 1 oz. 19.0

golden bar (Stella D'Oro), 1-oz. piece 17.0

graham:

(Bugs Bunny), 10 pieces, 1.1 oz. 23.0

(Keebler), 8 pieces, 1 oz. 23.0

(Nabisco), 8 pieces, 1 oz. 22.0

(Pepperidge Farm Goldfish), 1.1 oz. 20.0

amaranth (Health Valley Fat Free), 11 pieces, 1 oz. 23.0

chocolate (Bugs Bunny), 13 pieces, 1.1 oz. 22.0

chocolate (Keebler), 8 pieces, 1.1 oz. 22.0

chocolate (Nabisco Pure), 3 pieces, 1.1 oz. 21.0

chocolate (Teddy Grahams Snacks), 24 pieces, 1.1 oz. . . 22.0

cinnamon (Bugs Bunny), 13 pieces, 1.1 oz. 23.0

cinnamon (Honey Maid), 10 pieces, 1.1 oz. 26.0

cinnamon (Keebler Low Fat), 8 pieces, 1 oz. 24.0

cinnamon (Pepperidge Farm Goldfish), 1.1 oz. 20.0

cinnamon (SnackWell's Fat Free Snacks), 20 pieces,

1.1 oz. 26.0

cinnamon (Sunshine), 2 pieces, 1.1 oz. 22.0

cinnamon (Teddy Grahams Snacks), 24 pieces, 1.1 oz. . . 23.0

French vanilla (Keebler Light), 8 pieces 24.0

fudge coated (Keebler Deluxe), 3 pieces 19.0

fudge coated (Keebler Deluxe Reduced Fat), 3 pieces,

.9 oz. 19.0

fudge coated (Nabisco Family Favorites), 3 pieces, 1 oz. 19.0

fudge coated, marshmallow filled (Keebler S'mores),

3 pieces, 1.1 oz. 21.0

fudge dipped (Sunshine), 4 pieces, 1.2 oz. 21.0

honey (Honey Maid), 8 pieces, 1 oz. 22.0

honey (Keebler Low Fat), 9 pieces, 1.1 oz. 25.0

honey (Sunshine), 2 pieces, 1 oz. 20.0

oat bran (Health Valley Fat Free), 11 pieces, 1 oz. 23.0

granola (Archway Fat Free), 2 pieces, 1 oz. 24.0

granola, soft (Grandma's Bar), 1.5-oz. bar 29.0

hazelnut (Pepperidge Farm), 3 pieces, 1.1 oz. 21.0

hermits (Archway Cookie Jar), 1-oz. piece 19.0

(Heyday Bar), .75-oz. bar 13.0
kichel *(Stella D'Oro* Low Sodium), 21 pieces, 1 oz. 13.0
lemon:
    (Sunshine Coolers), 5 pieces, 1.1 oz. 21.0
    almond *(Barbara's Small Indulgences)*, 6 pieces, 1 oz. . . . 18.0
    creme *(Dare)*, .7-oz. piece 13.0
    drop *(Archway)*, 1-oz. piece 18.0
    frosty *(Archway)*, 1-oz. piece 19.0
    nuggets *(Archway* Fat Free), 5 pieces, 1 oz. 22.0
    nut crunch *(Pepperidge Farm)*, 3 pieces, 1.1 oz. 18.0
    sandwich *(Barbara's Cookies & Creme)*, 2 pieces, .9 oz. 18.0
    snaps *(Archway)*, 5 pieces, 1.1 oz. 20.0
marshmallow:
    chocolate *(Mallomars)*, 2 pieces, .9 oz. 17.0
    chocolate *(Pinwheels)*, 1.1-oz. piece 21.0
    fudge puffs *(Nabisco)*, .75-oz. piece 14.0
    fudge twirls *(Nabisco)*, 1.1-oz. piece 20.0
mint sandwich *(Mystic Mint)*, .6-oz. piece 11.0
molasses:
    (Archway), 1-oz. piece 20.0
    (Archway Low Fat), 1-oz. piece 22.0
    (Archway Old Fashion), 1-oz. piece 20.0
    (Archway Super Pak), 1-oz. piece 20.0
    (Grandma's Old Time Big), 1.4-oz. piece 29.0
    crisps *(Pepperidge Farm)*, 5 pieces, 1.1 oz. 20.0
    dark *(Archway)*, 1-oz. piece 20.0
    drop, soft *(Archway)*, 1-oz. piece 18.0
    iced *(Archway* Iowa), 1-oz. piece 20.0
    iced *(Archway* Ohio), 1-oz. piece 19.0
    iced *(Archway* Super Pak), 1-oz. piece 19.0
mud pie *(Archway)*, 1-oz. piece 18.0
New Orleans cake *(Archway)*, 1-oz. piece 18.0
nut *(Archway* Nutty Nougat), 3 pieces, 1-oz. piece 18.0
nut *(Little Debbie Nutty Bars)*, 2 pieces, 1.2-oz. piece 18.0
oatmeal:
    (Archway), 1-oz. piece 19.0
    (Dare Breaktime), .3-oz. piece 5.0
    (Keebler Classic Collection), 2 pieces, 1 oz. 18.0
    (Nabisco Family Favorites), .6-oz. piece 12.0
    (Ruth's), 1-oz. piece 19.0
    (Ruth's Golden), 1-oz. piece 19.0
    (Sunshine Country), 3 pieces, 1.2 oz. 24.0

Cookie, oatmeal *(cont.)*

apple filled *(Archway)*, 1-oz. piece 18.0
apple spice *(Grandma's* Big), 1.4-oz. piece 26.0
apple spice bar *(Grandma's)*, 1.5-oz. bar 28.0
butterscotch *(Pepperidge Farm)*, 3 pieces, 1.2 oz. 22.0
chewy *(Master Choice)*, .6-oz. piece 9.0
chocolate chip *(Entenmann's* Fat Free), 2 pieces, .8 oz. 19.0
chocolate chip *(Sunshine)*, 3 pieces, 1.3 oz. 23.0
date filled *(Archway)*, 1-oz. piece 18.0
iced *(Archway)*, 1-oz. piece 19.0
iced *(Sunshine)*, 2 pieces, .9 oz. 18.0
Irish *(Pepperidge Farm)*, 3 pieces, 1 oz. 19.0
pecan *(Archway)*, 1-oz. piece 18.0
raspberry *(Archway* Fat Free), 1-oz. piece 24.0
oatmeal raisin:
    (Archway), 1-oz. piece 19.0
    (Archway Bag), 3 pieces, 1 oz. 19.0
    (Archway Fat Free), 1-oz. piece 23.0
    (Barbara's), 2 pieces, 1.3 oz. 24.0
    (Barbara's Fat Free Mini), 6 pieces, 1.1 oz. 22.0
    (Entenmann's Fat Free), 2 pieces, .8 oz. 18.0
    (Health Valley Fat Free), 3 pieces 24.0
    (Little Debbie), 2 pieces, 1.3 oz. 25.0
    (Pepperidge Farm Old Fashioned), 3 pieces, 1.2 oz. . . . 23.0
    (Pepperidge Farm Soft), .9-oz. piece 17.0
    (Pepperidge Farm Santa Fe), .9-oz. piece 18.0
    (Smart Snackers), 2 pieces, 1.06 oz. 22.0
    (SnackWell's Reduced Fat), 2 pieces, 1 oz. 20.0
    (Tastykake Bar), 1.5-oz. bar 28.0
    bran *(Archway)*, 1-oz. piece 19.0
    iced *(Tastykake)*, 1.4-oz. piece 27.0
peach tart *(Pepperidge Farm)*, 2 pieces, 1.1 oz. 23.0
peach-apricot *(Stella D'Oro* Sodium Free), .7-oz. piece 13.0
peanut *(Archway* Jumble), 1-oz. piece 17.0
peanut, crunch *(Archway)*, 6 pieces, 1.1 oz. 18.0
peanut butter:
    (Archway), 1-oz. piece 16.0
    (Archway Ol' Fashion), 1-oz. piece 17.0
    (Grandma's Big), 1.4-oz. piece 22.0
    (Little Debbie Bar), 1.8-oz. bar 30.0
    bits *(Grandma's)*, 9 pieces 21.0
    chip *(Archway)*, 1-oz. piece 16.0

chocolate chip *(Grandma's* Bar), 1.5-oz. bar 24.0
chocolate chip *(Grandma's* Big), 1¼-oz. piece 23.0
chunky *(Tastykake* Bar), 1.5-oz. bar 18.0
fudge *(P.B. Fudgebutters),* 2 pieces, .8 oz. 14.0
graham *(Mr. Peanut P.B. Crisps),* 1 oz. 16.0
graham *(Mr. Peanut P.B. Crisps),* 1.5-oz. pkg. 24.0
nut *(Westbrae* Natural), .9-oz. piece 17.0
patties *(Nutter Butter),* 5 pieces, 1.1 oz. 17.0
sandwich *(Grandma's),* 5 pieces 29.0
sandwich *(Nutter Butter),* 2 pieces, 1 oz. 19.0
sandwich *(Nutter Butter Bites),* 10 pieces, 1.1 oz. 20.0
pecan:
    (Archway Ice Box), 1-oz. piece 17.0
    malted nougat *(Archway),* 3 pieces, 1.1 oz. 17.0
    shortbread, see "shortbread," below
pound cake *(Aunt Bea's),* .9-oz. piece 17.0
prune pastry *(Stella D'Oro* Sodium Free), .7-oz. piece 14.0
raisin *(Dare Sun•Maid),* .5-oz. piece 7.5
raisin *(Health Valley* Fat Free Jumbo), 1 piece 19.0
raisin, oatmeal, see "oatmeal raisin," above
raspberry:
    (Health Valley Fat Free Jumbo), 1 piece 19.0
    (Fruitastic Bar), 1 bar 13.0
    (Newtons Fat Free), 2 pieces, 1 oz. 23.0
    (Sunshine Oh! Berry), 3 pieces, 1 oz. 20.0
    centers *(Health Valley* Fat Free), 1 piece 18.0
    filled *(Archway),* 1-oz. piece 18.0
    filled *(Pepperidge Farm Linzer),* .8-oz. piece 15.0
    filled *(Smart Snackers),* .7 oz. 16.0
    hazelnut *(Pepperidge Farm Chantilly),* .6-oz. piece 12.0
rocky road *(Archway* Iowa), 1-oz. piece 19.0
rocky road *(Archway* Ohio), 1-oz. piece 18.0
sesame *(Stella D'Oro* Regina), 3 pieces, 1-oz. piece 21.0
shortbread:
    (Lorna Doone), 4 pieces, 1 oz. 19.0
    (Pepperidge Farm), 2 pieces, .9 oz. 16.0
    (Simply Sandies), .5-oz. piece 9.0
    butter *(Dare),* .5-oz. piece 7.0
    fudge coated *(Nabisco* Family Favorites), 3 pieces,
        1.1 oz. 22.0
    fudge striped *(Keebler),* 3 pieces, 1.1 oz. 21.0
    fudge striped *(Keebler* Reduced Fat), 3 pieces, 1 oz. 20.0

Cookie, shortbread *(cont.)*

fudge striped *(Sunshine)*, 3 pieces, 1.1 oz. 20.0
pecan *(Pecan Passion)*, .6-oz. piece 9.0
pecan *(Pecan Sandies)*, .6-oz. piece 9.0
pecan *(Pecan Sandies* Reduced Fat), .6-oz. piece 11.0
pecan *(Pepperidge Farm)*, 2 pieces, .9 oz. 14.0
triangles *(Walkers)*, 2 pieces, .7 oz. 12.0
(Social Tea), 6 pieces, 1 oz. 20.0
spice, pfeffernuss *(Archway)*, 2 pieces, 1.3 oz. 32.0
spice, pfeffernuss, drops *(Stella D'Oro)*, 3 pieces, 1 oz. . . . 21.0
sprinkles *(Dare Breaktime)*, .3-oz. piece 5.0
(Stella D'Oro Angel Wings), 2 pieces, .9 oz. 13.0
(Stella D'Oro Angelica Goodies), .8-oz. piece 15.0
(Stella D'Oro Anginetti), 4 pieces, 1.1 oz. 23.0
(Stella D'Oro Como Delights), 1.1 oz. 18.0
(Stella D'Oro Holiday Rings and Stars), 3 pieces, 1.2 oz. . . . 26.0
(Stella D'Oro Holiday Trinkets), 4 pieces, 1.1 oz. 20.0
(Stella D'Oro Hostess with the Mostest), 3 pieces, 1 oz. . . . 19.0
(Stella D'Oro Lady Stella Assortment), 3 pieces, 1 oz. 19.0
(Stella D'Oro Margherite Combination), 2 pieces, 1.1 oz. . . . 22.0
(Stella D'Oro Royal Nuggets), 1.1 oz. 9.0
strawberry:
(Newtons Fat Free), 2 pieces, 1 oz. 23.0
(Pepperidge Farm), 3 pieces, 1.1 oz. 22.0
(Sunshine Oh! Berry Fat Free), 1 oz. 20.0
filled *(Archway)*, .9-oz. piece 16.0
filled *(Archway* Ohio), 1-oz. piece 18.0
sugar:
(Archway), 1-oz. piece 20.0
(Archway Fat Free), .75-oz. piece 17.0
(Dare), .3-oz. piece 6.0
(Keebler Classic Collection), 2 pieces, 1 oz. 18.0
(Pepperidge Farm), 3 pieces, 1.1 oz. 20.0
soft *(Archway)*, 1-oz. piece 18.0
wafer *(Biscos)*, 8 pieces, 1 oz. 21.0
wafer, chocolate *(Sunshine)* 3 pieces, .9 oz. 30.0
wafer, peanut butter *(Sunshine)*, 4 pieces, 1.1 oz. 19.0
wafer, vanilla *(Sunshine)*, 3 pieces, .9 oz. 18.0
waffle *(Biscos)*, 4 pieces, 1.2 oz. 35.0
(Sunshine Jingles), 6 pieces, 1.1 oz. 22.0
vanilla:
(Pepperidge Farm Goldfish), 1.1 oz. 21.0

(Stella D'Oro Margherite), 2 pieces, 1.1 oz. 22.0
bits *(Grandma's)*, 9 pieces 21.0
raspberry tart *(Pepperidge Farm Wholesome Choice)*,
   2 pieces, 1.1 oz. 23.0
wafer *(Archway)*, 5 pieces, 1.1 oz. 22.0
wafer *(Keebler)*, 8 pieces, 1.1 oz. 20.0
wafer *(Keebler* Light), 8 pieces, 1.1 oz. 25.0
wafer *(Nilla)*, 8 pieces, 1.1 oz. 24.0
wafer *(Sunshine)*, 7 pieces, 1.1 oz. 20.0
vanilla sandwich:
   (Cameo), 2 pieces, 1 oz. 21.0
   (Cookie Break), 3 pieces, 1.1 oz. 23.0
   (Grandma's), 1 pkg. 43.0
   (Grandma's Value), 3 pieces 25.0
   (Nabisco Family Favorites), 3 pieces, 1.2 oz. 25.0
   (Smart Snackers), 2 pieces, 1.06 oz. 25.0
   (SnackWell's Reduced Fat), 2 pieces, .9 oz. 21.0
   (Vienna Fingers), 2 pieces, 1 oz. 23.0
   French *(Keebler Classic Collection)*, .6-oz. piece . . . 12.0
   raspberry *(Barbara's Cookies & Creme)*, 2 pieces, .9 oz. 18.0
   vanilla *(Barbara's Cookies & Creme)*, 2 pieces, .9 oz. . . 18.0
wafer:
   fudge *(Grandma's* Value), 4 pieces 25.0
   fudge *(Keebler Fudge Sticks)*, 3 pieces, 1 oz. 20.0
   strawberry or vanilla *(Grandma's* Value), 4 pieces 26.0
walnut, black *(Archway* Ice Box), .8-oz. piece 15.0

Cookie, refrigerated:
bunny, flag, Halloween, holiday, snowman, or valentine
   (Pillsbury), 2 pieces, 1 oz. 16.0
chocolate chip:
   (Nestlé/Nestlé Big Batch), 2 tbsp. or 1 piece* 20.0
   (Nestlé Reduced Fat), 2 tbsp. or 1 piece* 21.0
   (Pillsbury), 1 oz. 17.0
   (Pillsbury Reduced Fat), 1 oz. 18.0
   (Schwan's), 1 piece 17.0
   (SnackWell's), 1 oz. 19.0
   oatmeal *(Pillsbury)*, 1 oz. 17.0
   peanut butter *(Nestlé)*, 2 tbsp. or 1 piece* 19.0
   with walnuts *(Pillsbury)*, 1 oz. 17.0
chocolate chunk *(Pillsbury)*, 1 oz. 18.0
chocolate fudge *(SnackWell's)*, 1 oz. 18.0
Heath (Pillsbury), 1 oz. 17.0

Cookie, refrigerated *(cont.)*
M&M's *(Pillsbury)*, 1 oz. 18.0
oatmeal *(Nestlé Scotchies)*, 2 tbsp. or 1 piece* 20.0
oatmeal raisin *(Schwan's)*, 1 oz. 18.0
peanut butter *(Pillsbury)*, 1 oz. 15.0
Reese's (Pillsbury), 1 oz. 15.0
sugar *(Nestlé)*, ½" slice or 1 piece* 18.0
sugar *(Nestlé)*, 2 pieces 19.0
Cookie crumbs, see "Pie crust"
Cookie mix:
chocolate chip:
    (Arrowhead Mills), 1 piece* 16.0
    (Arrowhead Mills Wheat Free), 1 piece* 14.0
    (Duncan Hines), ½₄ pkg. or 2 pieces* 22.0
    (Robin Hood/Gold Medal Pouch), 2 pieces* 21.0
    oatmeal *(Robin Hood/Gold Medal* Pouch), 2 pieces* ... 20.0
chocolate chunk, double *(Robin Hood/Gold Medal* Pouch),
    2 pieces* 21.0
espresso chip *(Arrowhead Mills)*, 1 piece* 16.0
fudge, candy splash *(Duncan Hines)*, ½₄ pkg. or 2 pieces* 21.0
gingerbread *(Betty Crocker* Fun Kit), 2 pieces* 25.0
oatmeal *(Arrowhead Mills)*, 1 piece* 16.0
peanut butter *(Duncan Hines)*, ½₄ pkg. or 2 pieces* 16.0
peanut butter *(Robin Hood/Gold Medal* Pouch), 2 pieces* .. 19.0
sugar *(Duncan Hines)*, ½₄ pkg. or 2 pieces* 21.0
Cooking sauce, see specific listings
Coquito nut, shelled *(Frieda's)*, 11 pieces, 1.1 oz. 5.0
Coriander, fresh:
untrimmed, 1 lb. 10.0
trimmed, 1 oz. 7
trimmed, ¼ cup 1
Coriander, dried:
(McCormick), ¼ tsp. 1
(Tone's Cilantro), ¼ tsp. 0
ground *(McCormick)*, ¼ tsp. 2
leaf, 1 tbsp. 9
leaf, 1 tsp. 3
seed:
    (McCormick), ¼ tsp. 4
    1 tbsp. 2.8
    1 tsp. 1.0
Corkscrew pasta, see "Pasta"

Corn, fresh:
raw:

(Dole), 1 medium ear, 3.2 oz. 18.0
untrimmed, 1 lb. 31.1
kernels, from 1 ear, approx. 3.2 oz. 17.1
boiled, drained, kernels, ½ cup 20.6
Corn, canned, ½ cup, except as noted:
baby, whole *(Haddon House)* 3.0
baby, whole *(Roland)* 4.0
kernel:

(Del Monte) 18.0
(Del Monte Fiesta) 12.0
(Del Monte Supersweet No Salt/No Sugar) 11.0
(Del Monte Supersweet Vac Pack) 13.0
(Goya) 21.0
(Green Giant) 18.0
(Green Giant Less Salt) 17.0
(Green Giant Niblets), ⅓ cup 15.0
(Green Giant Niblets Extra Sweet), ⅓ cup 10.0
(Green Giant Niblets 50% Less Sodium), ⅓ cup 14.0
(Green Giant Niblets No Salt/Sugar Added), ⅓ cup 13.0
(S&W) 14.0
(S&W Sweet 'n Crisp), ⅓ cup 12.0
(Seneca) 20.0
(Seneca), ⅓ cup 17.0
(Seneca Super Sweet) 21.0
(Seneca Water Pack) 16.0
(Stokely/Stokely No Salt) 14.0
(Stokely Vac Pack), ⅓ cup 14.0
drained 15.2
gold and white *(Del Monte* Supersweet) 18.0
white *(Del Monte)* 17.0
white *(Green Giant),* ⅓ cup 16.0
white *(Stokely/Stokely* No Salt) 14.0
white, sweet *(Green Giant)* 18.0
kernel, with peppers *(Green Giant Mexicorn),* ⅓ cup 14.0
kernel, with peppers *(Stokely),* ⅓ cup 16.0
cream style:

(Del Monte/Del Monte No Salt) 20.0
(Del Monte Supersweet/Supersweet No Salt) 14.0
(Green Giant) 22.0
(S&W) 24.0

Corn, canned, cream style *(cont.)*
   (Seneca) 19.0
   (Stokely) 21.0
   white *(Del Monte)* 21.0
Corn, dried:
(John Cope's), ¼ cup 15.0
freeze-dried *(AlpineAire)*, ½ cup 20.0
freeze-dried *(Mountain House)*, ½ cup 17.0
Corn, freeze-dried, see "Corn, dried"
Corn, frozen, ⅔ cup, except as noted:
on the cob, 1 ear:
   (Green Giant Extra Sweet) 7.0
   (Green Giant Nibblers) 5.0
   (Green Giant Niblets) 11.0
   (John Cope's) 22.0
   (Ore-Ida Mini-Gold) 18.0
   (Schwan's) 36.0
   white *(John Cope's)* 31.0
kernel:
   (Birds Eye Sweet), ⅓ cup 17.0
   (Birds Eye Tendersweet), ⅓ cup 14.0
   (Green Giant Niblets/Green Giant Harvest Fresh Niblets) 17.0
   (Green Giant Niblets Extra Sweet) 13.0
   (Schwan's) 19.0
   white *(Green Giant)*, ¾ cup 20.0
   white *(Green Giant* Extra Sweet) 10.0
   white *(Green Giant Harvest Fresh)*, ½ cup 14.0
   white *(John Cope's)*, ⅓ cup 17.0
cream style *(Green Giant)*, ½ cup 23.0
cream style, white *(John Cope's* Sweet 'N Creamy), ⅓ cup 17.0
in butter sauce *(Green Giant Niblets)* 23.0
in butter sauce, white *(Green Giant)*, ¾ cup 21.0
and broccoli and peppers *(Green Giant American Mixtures)*,
   ¾ cup 13.0
Corn, whole grain:
1 oz. 21.1
1 cup 123.3
Corn bran, crude:
1 oz. 24.3
1 cup 65.1
Corn bread, see "Bread mix"
Corn bread, frozen *(Marie Callender's)*, 1.9-oz. piece 27.0

Corn chips, puffs, and similar snacks (see also "Snack
    chips and crisps"), 1 oz., except as noted:

(Baked Bugles), 1½ cups	23.0
(Baked Bugles Single), 1 bag	30.0
(Barbara's Pinta Chips)	19.0
(Barrel O'Fun Chip), 1.1 oz.	18.0
(Bugles), 1⅓ cups	18.0
(Bugles Original Single), 1½-oz. bag	25.0
(Dipsey Doodles)	16.0
(Fritos Original/Chili Cheese/King Size/Wild N' Mild)	15.0
(Fritos Scoops)	16.0
(Old Dutch Chips), 1.1 oz. or 1¼-oz. bag	16.0
(Old Dutch Puffcorn Curls), 1.1 oz.	14.0
(Planters Chips)	16.0
(Tyson), 12 chips	22.0
all flavors *(Bugles)*, 1⅓ cups	18.0
all flavors *(Sunchips)*	18.0
barbecue:	
(Fritos)	16.0
(Old Dutch), 1.1 oz.	16.0
(Old Dutch), 1¼-oz. bag	19.0
(Smart Snackers Curls)	11.0
blue corn:	
(Barbara's), 1.1 oz.	16.0
(Barbara's Pinta Blues)	17.0
light salt *(Barbara's* Amazing Bakes)	24.0
picante *(Barbara's* Pinta)	17.0
salsa *(Barbara's* Pinta)	19.0
caramel coated *(Old Dutch* Puffcorn)	24.0
cheese:	
(Cheese Doodles)	17.0
(Chee•tos Cheesy Checkers/Puffs)	15.0
(Chee•tos Crunchy)	16.0
cheddar *(Baked Bugles)*, 1½ cups	22.0
fried *(Cheese Doodles)*	16.0
hot *(Chee•tos* Flamin')	16.0
nacho *(Barbara's* Pinta)	18.0
nacho *(Doodle Twisters)*	15.0
nacho *(Tyson)*, 13 chips	19.0
pepperoni *(Combos)*	17.0
pepperoni *(Combos)*, 1.7-oz. bag	30.0

Corn chips, puffs, and similar snacks *(cont.)*
cheese balls:
    (Barrel O'Fun), 1.1 oz. 16.0
    (Planters Cheez) 15.0
    puffed *(Chee•tos)* 13.0
cheese curls:
    (Barrel O'Fun Baked), 1.1 oz. 18.0
    (Barrel O'Fun Crunchy), 1.1 oz. 17.0
    (Chee•tos) 16.0
    (Old Dutch Crunchy) 19.0
    (Planters Cheez) 15.0
    (Planters Cheez), 1¼-oz. pkg. 19.0
    (Smart Snackers), ½ oz. 10.0
cheese puffs:
    (Barbara's Original) 16.0
    (Barbara's Bakes) 13.0
    (Barrel O'Fun Light), 1.1 oz. 24.0
    (Chee•tos) 15.0
    (Jax), 25 pieces, 1.06 oz. 19.0
    cheddar *(No Fries)* 23.0
    cheddar, New York *(Barbara's* Less Fat) 23.0
    jalapeño *(Barbara's)* 18.0
    Monterey Jack and green chili *(Barbara's* Less Fat) 15.0
chili cheese *(Fritos)* 19.0
onion flavor rings *(Borden)*, 1-oz. bag 15.0
pizza *(Smart Snackers* Curls) 11.0
ranch *(Smart Snackers* Curls) 10.0
ranch, puffs *(No Fries)* 23.0
taco *(Taco Bell* Supreme) 18.0
Texas grill *(Fritos* Honey BBQ/Sizzlin' Fajita) 16.0
tortilla:
    (Bachman Original), 12 pieces, 1.06 oz. 20.0
    (Chipitos Black Bean Salsa), 6 pieces, 1.06 oz. 19.0
    (Doritos/Doritos Dunkers) 19.0
    (Mesa) 16.0
    (Nachips) 17.0
    (No Fries Natural) 22.0
    (Old Dutch Restaurant) 18.0
    (Tostitos Baked Original/*Tostitos* Baked Original
      Unsalted) 24.0
    (Tostitos Bite Size/Crispy Round) 17.0
    (Tostitos Restaurant Style/Santa Fe Gold) 19.0

(Tostitos Restaurant Unsalted) 18.0
(Tyson), 12 pieces, 1.2 oz. 22.0
all varieties *(Santitas)* 19.0
crisps *(Mr. Phipps)* 21.0
crisps *(Pepperidge Farm)*, 1.1 oz. 18.0
5 grain *(Kettle* Tias) 18.0
hot *(Doritos* Flamin') 17.0
lime and chili *(Kettle* Tias) 19.0
lime and chili *(Tostitos)* 17.0
pizza *(Doritos* Cravers) 18.0
ranch *(Doritos* Cooler) 18.0
ranch *(Doritos* Cooler Reduced Fat) 19.0
ranch *(No Fries)*, 1.1 oz. 24.0
ranch *(Tostitos* Baked) 21.0
salsa crisps *(Pepperidge Farm)*, 1.1 oz. 18.0
salsa and sour cream *(No Fries)*, 1.1 oz. 25.0
taco *(Doritos* Taco Bell) 18.0
tomato basil *(Kettle* Tias) 18.0
tostados *(Old Dutch)*, 1.1 oz. 19.0
tortilla, blue corn:
    (Barbara's Less Fat) 21.0
    (Kettle Tias) 18.0
    cheddar jalapeño *(No Fries)*, 1.1 oz. 25.0
    hot salsa *(Barbara's* Less Fat) 20.0
tortilla, cheese:
    (Doritos Chester's) 18.0
    cheddar, white *(Barbara's* Less Fat) 20.0
    chili crisps *(Pepperidge Farm)*, 1.1 oz. 18.0
    nacho *(Barrel O'Fun)* 18.0
    nacho *(Borden)* 17.0
    nacho *(Doritos* Cheesier) 18.0
    nacho *(Doritos* Reduced Fat Cheesier) 19.0
    nacho *(Old Dutch)*, 1-oz. bag 17.0
    nacho *(Old Dutch)*, 2¼-oz. bag 39.0
    nacho *(Tyson)*, 13 pieces 19.0
    nacho, crisps *(Mr. Phipps)* 20.0
tortilla, flour:
    cheese and salsa *(Barrel O'Fun)* 19.0
    nacho *(Barrel O'Fun)* 19.0
    white *(Barrel O'Fun)* 20.0
    white, mini rounds *(Barrel O'Fun)* 19.0
    yellow *(Barrel O'Fun* Tostada) 20.0

Corn chips, puffs, and similar snacks, tortilla, flour *(cont.)*
  yellow, mini *(Barrel O'Fun Tostada)* 19.0
tortilla, white corn:
  (Barbara's Less Fat) 21.0
  (Chipitos White Corn Restaurant Style) 18.0
  (Kettle Tias) 18.0
  (Old Dutch), 1.1 oz. 20.0
  (Old El Paso) 16.0
  (Santitas 100%) 19.0
  ranch *(Barbara's Less Fat)* 20.0
Corn dishes, frozen:
scalloped *(Schwan's)*, ½ cup 15.0
soufflé *(Stouffer's)*, 4.8 oz. 21.0
Corn flake crumbs *(Kellogg's)*, 2 tbsp. 9.0
Corn flour:
whole-grain, 1 oz. 21.8
whole-grain, 1 cup 89.9
masa, 1 oz. 21.6
masa, 1 cup 87.0
Corn fritter, frozen *(Mrs. Paul's)*, 1 piece 16.0
Corn grits, dry:
(Albers Quick Hominy), ¼ cup 31.0
(Cee-Leci/Dixie Lily/Jim Dandy), ¼ cup 38.0
(Goya), ¼ cup 39.0
instant, 1-oz. pkt.:
  (Quaker) 22.0
  with bacon bits *(Quaker)* 22.0
  butter flavor *(Quaker)* 21.0
  cheddar flavor *(Quaker)* 21.0
  cheddar, zesty *(Quaker)* 20.0
  with ham bits *(Quaker)* 21.0
  with sausage bits *(Quaker)* 21.0
quick *(Cee-Leci/Dixie Lily/Jim Dandy)*, ¼ cup 35.0
quick, iron fortified *(Jim Dandy)*, ¼ cup 31.0
white, ¼ cup:
  (Arrowhead Mills) 30.0
  (Quaker Hominy) 32.0
  (Quaker Quick Hominy) 29.0
yellow, ¼ cup:
  (Arrowhead Mills) 29.0
  (Dixie Lily/Martha White) 35.0
  (Quaker Quick Hominy) 29.0

Corn pudding mix *(Goya)*, ½ cup* 23.0
Corn relish:
(Green Giant), 1 tbsp. 5.0
(Nance's), 2 tbsp. 6.0
(Pickle Eater's), 1 tbsp. 5.0
Corn syrup, dark or light *(Karo)*, 2 tbsp. 30.0
Cornish hen, without added ingredients 0
Cornmeal (see also "Corn flour" and "Polenta"):
(Frieda's), ¼ cup 23.0
blue *(Arrowhead Mills)*, ¼ cup 25.0
coarse *(Goya)*, 3 tbsp. 25.0
degerminated *(Jim Dandy)*, 3 tbsp. 25.0
fine *(Goya)*, 3 tbsp. 23.0
hi-lysine *(Arrowhead Mills)*, ¼ cup 25.0
masa harina *(Quaker Enriched)*, ¼ cup 25.0
masa harina *(Quaker Preparada Para Tortillas)*, ⅓ cup 27.0
self-rising, 3 tbsp.:
   (Dixie Lily/Martha White/Pekerson's) 23.0
   (Pine Mountain) 22.0
   buttermilk mix *(Dixie Lily/Martha White)* 29.0
   degerminated *(Jim Dandy)* 24.0
   stone ground *(Cabin Home)* 23.0
   white *(Aunt Jemima/Aunt Jemima Degerminated)* 20.0
   white *(Aunt Jemima Mix)* 19.0
   white *(Cee-Leci/Dixie Lily/Hay Market/Mother's
     Best/Omega)* 30.0
   white *(Martha White/Martha White Honey)* 30.0
   white, buttermilk *(Aunt Jemima Mix)* 18.0
   yellow *(Aunt Jemima Mix)* 19.0
   yellow *(Martha White)* 25.0
   yellow, buttermilk *(Martha White Mix)* 31.0
white:
   (Albers), 3 tbsp. 34.0
   (Arrowhead Mills), ¼ cup 23.0
   (Dixie Lily/Hay Market/Martha White/Pekerson's), 3 tbsp. 25.0
   (Goya), 2½ tbsp. 22.0
whole ground *(Cabin Home/Martha White/Pine
   Mountain)*, 3 tbsp. 24.0
yellow:
   (Albers), 3 tbsp. 34.0
   (Arrowhead Mills), ¼ cup 27.0
   (Goya), 2½ tbsp. 25.0

Cornmeal, yellow *(cont.)*
   (Martha White), 3 tbsp. 25.0
Cornstarch *(Argo/Kingsford)*, 1 tbsp. 7.0
Cottonseed kernels, roasted, 1 tbsp. 2.2
Cottonseed meal, partially defatted, 1 oz. 10.9
Country gravy mix:
   (Durkee), 1½ tbsp. 5.0
   (French's), ¼ cup* 5.0
   (Loma Linda Gravy Quik), 1 tbsp. 4.0
Couscous:
dry, ¼ cup, except as noted:
   (Arrowhead Mills) 35.0
   (Fantastic) 43.0
   1 oz. 22.0
   whole wheat *(Fantastic)* 45.0
cooked, ½ cup 20.9
Couscous mix, 1 pkg., except as noted:
almond chicken, vegetarian *(Casbah)* 29.0
asparagus au gratin *(Casbah)* 28.0
cheddar, broccoli, creamy *(Casbah)* 23.0
garlic with red pepper *(Fantastic* Healthy Complements),
   ⅓ cup 41.0
pilaf *(Casbah)*, 1 oz. 20.0
pilaf, savory *(Fantastic)*, ⅓ cup 50.0
royal Thai *(Fantastic* Healthy Complements), ⅓ cup 41.0
tomato Parmesan *(Casbah)* 34.0
Cowpeas, fresh:
(Frieda's Blackeye), ⅓ cup 21.0
raw, in pods, 1 lb. 43.7
raw, trimmed, ½ cup 13.6
boiled, drained, ½ cup 16.7
leafy tips:
   raw, untrimmed, 1 lb. 11.4
   raw, chopped, ½ cup 9
   boiled, drained, 4 oz. 3.2
young pods, with seeds:
   raw, untrimmed, 1 lb. 39.2
   raw, trimmed, ½ cup 4.5
   boiled, drained, ½ cup 3.3
mature, dry, ¼ cup 25.2
mature, boiled, ½ cup 17.9
Cowpeas, canned, see "Black-eyed peas"

Cowpeas, frozen, boiled, drained, ½ cup 20.2
Cowpeas, catjang, see "Catjang"
Crab, meat only, 4 oz.:
Alaska king, raw or cooked, without added ingredients 0
blue, raw 1
blue, boiled, poached, or steamed 0
Dungeness, raw 8
Dungeness, boiled, poached, or steamed 1.1
queen, raw or cooked, without added ingredients 0
Crab, refrigerated or frozen:
chunks, cooked *(Tyson* Delight), 3 oz. 10.0
legs and claws *(Pride of Alaska),* ¾ cup edible 0
Crab, canned, Dungeness *(S&W),* ⅓ cup, 3 oz. 0
"Crab," imitation, frozen or refrigerated:
(Captain Jac Easy Shreds), ½ cup, 3 oz. 11.0
(Peter Pan), 3 oz. 13.0
from surimi, 1 oz. 3.0
flaked, ½ cup, 3 oz.:
   (Captain Jac Crab Tasties) 15.0
   (Pacific Mate Fat Free) 15.0
   (Seafest) 15.0
   or chunk *(Louis Kemp Crab Delights)* 10.0
leg style *(Louis Kemp Crab Delights),* 3 legs, 3 oz. 10.0
leg style, with crab *(Captain Jac Crab Tasties),* 3 legs, 3 oz. 14.0
Crab cake, deviled, frozen:
(Chesapeake Bay), 1.97-oz. piece 7.0
(Mrs. Paul's), 1 piece 17.0
miniature *(Mrs. Paul's),* 6 pieces, 3.5 oz. 25.0
Crabapple, fresh, with peel:
(Frieda's), 1 oz. 5.0
untrimmed, 1 lb. 83.2
trimmed, 1 oz. 5.7
sliced, ½ cup 11.0
Crabapple, canned:
(S&W), 1 piece 8.0
spiced *(Apple Time),* 1 piece, 1.1 oz. 10.0
Cracker:
bacon flavor *(Nabisco),* 15 pieces, 1.1 oz. 19.0
(Barbara's Rite Lite), 5 pieces, .5 oz. 12.0
butter/butter flavor:
   (Hi-Ho), 9 pieces, 1.1 oz. 19.0
   (Keebler Club Partners), 4 pieces, .5 oz. 9.0

Cracker, butter/butter flavor *(cont.)*

   (Ritz/Ritz Low Sodium), 5 pieces, .6 oz. 10.0

   (Ritz Air Crisps Original/Sour Cream & Onion),

      24 pieces, 1.1 oz. 22.0

   (Toasted Complements Buttercrisp), 9 pieces, 1 oz. 19.0

   (Town House), 5 pieces, .6 oz. 9.0

   mini *(Ritz Bits),* 48 pieces, 1.1 oz. 18.0

   thins *(Pepperidge Farm),* 4 pieces, .5 oz. 10.0

   zesty *(SnackWell's),* 32 pieces, 1.1 oz. 23.0

cheese:

   (Appeteasers Original) 18.0

   (Barbara's Bites Original/Hot & Spicy), 26 pieces, 1.1 oz. 24.0

   (Krispy Mild Cheddar), 5 pieces, .5 oz. 10.0

   (Nips), 29 pieces, 1.1 oz. 18.0

   (Nips Air Crisps), 32 pieces 21.0

   (SnackWell's), 38 pieces, 1.1 oz. 23.0

   (Tid-Bit), 32 pieces, 1.1 oz. 17.0

   chili *(Munch 'ems),* 28 pieces, 1.1 oz. 23.0

   garlic herb *(Appeteasers)* 18.0

   Parmesan *(Goldfish),* 60 pieces, 1.1 oz. 19.0

   Swiss *(Nabisco Swiss),* 15 pieces, 1 oz. 18.0

   zesty *(SnackWell's),* 32 pieces, 1.1 oz. 23.0

cheese, cheddar:

   (Better Cheddars/Better Cheddars Low Sodium),

      2 pieces, 1.1 oz. 18.0

   (Better Cheddars Reduced Fat), 24 pieces, 1.1 oz. 19.0

   (Cheez-It/Cheez-It Low Sodium), 27 pieces, 1.1 oz. 16.0

   (Cheez-It Reduced Fat), 30 pieces, 1.1 oz. 19.0

   (Combos) 16.0

   (Combos), 1.7-oz. bag 28.0

   (Goldfish), 55 pieces, 1.1 oz. 19.0

   (Goldfish Reduced Sodium), 60 pieces, 1.1 oz. 18.0

   (Munch 'ems), 30 pieces, 1.1 oz. 21.0

   (Snorkels), 56 pieces, 1.1 oz. 19.0

   double *(Appeteasers),* 1 oz. 17.0

   hot and spicy *(Cheez-It),* 26 pieces, 1.1 oz. 17.0

   white *(Cheez-It),* 26 pieces, 1.1 oz. 17.0

   white *(Wheatables),* 27 pieces, 1.1 oz. 21.0

cheese sandwich:

   (Handi-Snacks Cheez'n Crackers), 1.1-oz. piece 10.0

   (Little Debbie), 1.4 oz. 22.0

   (Ritz), 1.4-oz. pkg. 21.0

(Ritz Bits), 14 pieces, 1.1 oz. 17.0
bacon *(Frito-Lay)*, 1 pkg. 24.0
cheddar *(Frito-Lay)*, 1 pkg. 27.0
cheddar, golden toast *(Frito-Lay)*, 1 pkg. 25.0
cream cheese and chive, golden toast *(Frito-Lay)*, 1 pkg. 25.0
jalapeño cheddar *(Frito-Lay)*, 1 pkg. 24.0
peanut butter, see "peanut butter sandwich," below
wheat *(Frito-Lay)*, 1 pkg. 24.0
(Chicken In A Biskit), 14 pieces, 1.1 oz. 17.0
cracked pepper, see "water or soda," below
croissant *(Carr's)*, 3 pieces, .5 oz. 10.0
flatbread:
  (J.J. Flats Flavorall), .5-oz. piece 11.0
  (Lavosh Hawaii Classic), 8 pieces, 1 oz. 19.0
  (New York), .4-oz. piece 7.0
  (New York Everything), .4-oz. piece 8.0
  all varieties *(New York* Fat Free), .4-oz. piece 8.0
  Cajun *(New York)*, .4-oz. piece 8.0
  caraway rye *(Lavosh Hawaii)*, 8 pieces, 1 oz. 20.0
  garlic *(California Crisps)*, 2 pieces, .5 oz. 8.8
  herb, Italian *(J.J. Flats)*, .5-oz. piece 10.0
  multigrain *(J.J. Flats)*, .5-oz. piece 11.0
  oat bran *(J.J. Flats)*, .5-oz. piece 11.0
  onion *(California Crisps)*, 2 pieces, .5 oz. 10.2
  onion *(J.J. Flats)*, .5-oz. piece 11.0
  onion *(New York)*, .4-oz. piece 7.0
  onion, slightly *(Lavosh Hawaii)*, 8 pieces, 1 oz. 19.0
  peppercorn *(Lavosh Hawaii)*, 8 pieces, 1 oz. 20.0
  poppy *(California Crisps)*, 2 pieces, .5 oz. 10.2
  poppy *(J.J. Flats)*, .5-oz piece 10.0
  poppy *(New York)*, .4-oz. piece 8.0
  pumpernickel onion *(New York)*, .4-oz. piece 7.0
  pumpernickel sesame *(New York)*, .4-oz. piece 8.0
  rosemary garlic *(Lavosh Hawaii)*, 8 pieces, 1 oz. 19.0
  sesame *(J.J. Flats)*, .5-oz. piece 10.0
  sesame *(New York)*, .4-oz. piece 8.0
  10 grain *(California Crisps)*, 2 pieces, .5 oz. 10.2
  10 grain *(Lavosh Hawaii)*, 8 pieces, 1 oz. 19.0
golden *(SnackWell's* Classic), 6 pieces, .5 oz. 11.0
(Goldfish Original), 55 pieces, 1.1 oz. 19.0
(Goya Snack), 11 pieces 21.0
(Goya Tropical), 4 pieces 21.0

Cracker *(cont.)*

graham, see "Cookie"

matzo, 1 oz.:

    (Manischewitz Unsalted) 24.0

    (Manischewitz Everything!) 22.0

    garlic *(Manischewitz* Savory) 23.0

    rye *(Manischewitz)* 23.0

melba rounds/snacks, 5 pieces, .5 oz.:

    plain *(Devonsheer)* 22.0

    bacon *(Old London)* 11.0

    cheese *(Old London)* 10.0

    garlic *(Devonsheer)* 11.0

    garlic *(Old London)* 11.0

    herbs, savory *(Devonsheer)* 11.0

    honey bran *(Devonsheer)* 12.0

    Mexicali corn *(Old London)* 10.0

    onion *(Devonsheer)* 11.0

    onion *(Old London)* 11.0

    rye *(Old London)* 11.0

    sesame *(Devonsheer)* 10.0

    sesame *(Old London)* 9.0

    12 grain *(Devonsheer)* 12.0

    vegetable *(Devonsheer)* 12.0

    white *(Old London)* 11.0

    whole grain *(Old London)* 11.0

melba toast, 3 pieces, .5 oz.:

    plain *(Devonsheer/Devonsheer* No Salt) 11.0

    onion *(Old London)* 11.0

    rye *(Devonsheer)* 11.0

    rye *(Old London)* 11.0

    sesame *(Devonsheer/Devonsheer* No Salt) 10.0

    sesame *(Old London/Old London* No Salt) 10.0

    12 grain *(Devonsheer)* 11.0

    vegetable *(Devonsheer)* 11.0

    wheat *(Devonsheer/Devonsheer* No Salt) 11.0

    wheat *(Old London)* 11.0

    white *(Old London)* 11.0

    whole grain *(Old London/Old London* No Salt) 11.0

milk *(Royal Lunch)*, .4-oz. piece 8.0

multigrain:

    (Hi-Ho), 9 pieces, 1.1 oz. 18.0

    (Wheat Thins), 17 pieces, 1.1 oz. 21.0

5 *(Harvest Crisps)*, 13 pieces, 1.1 oz. 23.0
(Munch 'ems), 30 pieces, 1.1 oz. 20.0
nori maki *(Eden)*, 15 pieces, 1.1 oz. 24.0
oat *(Harvest Crisps)*, 13 pieces, 1.1 oz. 22.0
oat *(Oat Thins)*, 18 pieces, 1.1 oz. 20.0
onion:
   (Toasted Complements), 9 pieces, 1 oz. 19.0
   French *(SnackWell's)*, 32 pieces, 1.1 oz. 23.0
   French *(Wheatables)*, 29 pieces, 1.1 oz. 21.0
peanut butter:
   (Combos), 1 oz. 15.0
   (Handi-Snacks), 1.1-oz. piece 12.0
   grahamstick *(Handi-Snacks)*, 1.1-oz. piece 14.0
peanut butter sandwich:
   (Ritz), 13 pieces, 1.1 oz. 17.0
   cheese *(Frito-Lay)*, 1 pkg. 22.0
   cheese *(Little Debbie)*, 1.4 oz. 22.0
   cheese *(Nabs)*, 6 pieces, 1.4 oz. 24.0
   cheese *(Planters)*, 1.4-oz. pkg. 23.0
   toast *(Frito-Lay)*, 1 pkg. 23.0
   toast *(Little Debbie)*, 1.4 oz. 23.0
   toast *(Nabs)*, 6 pieces, 1.4 oz. 24.0
   toast *(Planters)*, 1.4-oz. pkg. 23.0
   toast *(Sunshine)*, 1.2-oz. pkg. 18.0
pizza:
   (Goldfish), 55 pieces, 1.1 oz. 19.0
   all varieties *(Health Valley)*, 6 pieces 11.0
   bites *(Barbara's)*, 26 pieces, 1.1 oz. 24.0
potato:
   au gratin *(No Fries)*, 1.1 oz. 25.0
   barbecue *(No Fries)*, 1.1 oz. 26.0
   sour cream and chives *(No Fries)*, 1.1 oz. 25.0
(Pretzel Air Crisps), 22 pieces 23.0
ranch *(Munch 'ems)*, 33 pieces, 1.1 oz. 21.0
ranch, Italian *(SnackWell's)*, 32 pieces 23.0
rice, bran *(Health Valley)*, 6 pieces, 1 oz. 19.0
rice, brown *(Eden)*, 5 pieces, 1.1 oz. 22.0
salsa *(Munch 'ems)*, 28 pieces, 1.1 oz. 21.0
saltines, 5 pieces, .5 oz., except as noted:
   (Krispy/Krispy Unsalted Top/Cracked Pepper) 10.0
   (Krispy Fat Free) 12.0
   (Premium/Premium Low Sodium/Unsalted Top) 10.0

Cracker, saltines *(cont.)*

   (Premium Fat Free) 11.0
   (Zesta) 10.0
   mini *(Premium* Bits), 34 pieces, 1.1 oz. 19.0
   multigrain *(Premium)* 10.0
sesame:
   (Breton), 10 pieces, 1.5 oz. 25.0
   (Pepperidge Farm), 3 pieces, .5 oz. 9.0
   (Toasted Complements), 10 pieces, 1 oz. 19.0
sesame cheese *(Twigs)*, 15 pieces, 1.1 oz. 17.0
(Sociables), 7 pieces, .5 oz. 9.0
soup and oyster, .5 oz.:
   (Krispy) 11.0
   (Oysterettes) 10.0
   (Premium) 10.0
sour cream and onion *(Munch 'ems)*, 33 pieces, 1.1 oz. 22.0
(Uneeda), 2 pieces, .5 oz. 11.0
vegetable:
   (Garden Crisps), 15 pieces, 1.1 oz. 22.0
   (Vegetable Thins), 14 pieces, 1.1 oz. 29.0
   (Vivant), 3 pieces, 1/2 oz. 9.0
water or soda:
   (Breton/Breton 50% Less Salt), 10 pieces, 1.5 oz. 26.0
   (Breton Light), 10 pieces, 1.5 oz. 33.0
   (Cabaret), 10 pieces, 1.7 oz. 30.0
   (Carr's Table Water), 5 pieces, .6 oz. 13.0
   (Crown Pilot), .6-oz. piece 13.0
   (Dux), 2 pieces 8.0
   (Hi-Ho), 9 pieces, 1.1 oz. 18.0
   (Pepperidge Farm Original), 5 pieces, .5 oz. 11.0
   (Vivant), 10 pieces, 1.5 oz. 27.0
   cracked pepper *(Carr's Table Water)*, 5 pieces, .6 oz. 13.0
   cracked pepper *(Hi-Ho)*, 9 pieces, 1.1 oz. 18.0
   cracked pepper *(Pepperidge Farm)*, 5 pieces, .5 oz. 12.0
   cracked pepper *(SnackWell's)*, 7 pieces, .5 oz. 13.0
   poppy sesame *(Carr's Table Water)*, 4 pieces, .5 oz. 9.0
   sesame *(Breton)*, 10 pieces, .5 oz. 25.0
   sesame *(Carr's Table Water)*, 5 pieces, .6 oz. 13.0
wheat:
   (SnackWell's Fat Free), 5 pieces, .5 oz. 12.0
   (Stoned Wheat Thins/Stoned Wheat Thins Lower
     Sodium), 2 pieces 10.0

(Toasted Complements), 9 pieces, 1 oz. 19.0
(Triscuit/Triscuit Low Sodium), 7 pieces, 1.1 oz. 21.0
(Triscuit Reduced Fat), 8 pieces, 1.1 oz. 24.0
(Waverly), 5 pieces, .5 oz. 10.0
(Wheat Thins), 16 pieces, 1 oz. 19.0
(Wheat Thins Low Salt), 16 pieces, 1 oz. 20.0
(Wheat Thins Reduced Fat), 18 pieces, 1 oz. 21.0
(Wheat Thins Air Crisps), 24 pieces 21.0
(Wheatables), 26 pieces, 1.1 oz. 18.0
(Wheatsworth), 5 pieces, .6 oz. 10.0
all varieties *(Barbara's* Wheatines), .5-oz. large square . . 11.0
cracked *(Pepperidge Farm),* 2 pieces, .5 oz. 9.0
hearty *(Pepperidge Farm),* 3 pieces, .5 oz. 10.0
herb, garden *(Triscuit),* 6 pieces, 1 oz. 20.0
and rye *(Triscuit* Deli), 7 pieces, 1.1 oz. 22.0
wheat, whole:
   (Carr's), 2 pieces, .6 oz. 11.0
   (Health Valley No Salt), 5 pieces 11.0
   (Hi-Ho), 9 pieces, 1.1 oz. 18.0
   (Krispy), 5 pieces, .5 oz. 10.0
   all varieties *(Health Valley),* 5 pieces 11.0
   and bran *(Triscuit),* 7 pieces, 1.1 oz. 22.0
(Zwieback), .3-oz. piece 5.0
Cracker crumbs and meal:
crumbs *(Ritz),* ⅓ cup 17.0
crumbs, saltine *(Premium* Fat Free), ¼ cup 23.0
matzo meal *(Manischewitz),* ¼ cup 27.0
matzo meal *(Streit's),* ¼ cup 24.0
Cranberry:
fresh, raw:
   whole *(Dole),* ½ cup 6.0
   whole, untrimmed, 1 lb. 54.6
   whole, trimmed, 1 oz. 3.6
   chopped, ½ cup 7.0
dried:
   (Craisins), ⅓ cup 33.0
   (Frieda's), ⅓ cup, 1.4 oz. 28.0
   (Sonoma), ⅓ cup 29.0
Cranberry beans:
dried, ¼ cup 29.5
dried, boiled, ½ cup 21.5
Cranberry beans, canned, with liquid, ½ cup 19.7

Cranberry drink, 8 fl. oz., except as noted:
(Farmer's Market) 31.0
(Tropicana Punch) 34.0
(Tropicana Punch), 11.5 fl. oz. 49.0
(Tropicana Ruby Red) 30.0
juice cocktail *(Seneca)* 35.0
spiced *(J.M.S.* Cooler) 30.0
frozen*, juice cocktail *(Schwan's)* 36.0
frozen, juice cocktail *(Seneca)*, 2 oz. 35.0
Cranberry drink blends, 8 fl. oz.:
hibiscus *(Heinke's)* 30.0
hibiscus *(R.W. Knudsen)* 30.0
lemon *(Santa Cruz)* 29.0
raspberry *(After the Fall)* 23.0
raspberry *(R.W. Knudsen)* 36.0
raspberry-strawberry *(Tropicana Twister)* 31.0
raspberry-strawberry *(Tropicana Twister* Light) 11.0
Cranberry juice, 8 fl. oz., except as noted:
(After the Fall Cape Cod) 24.0
(After the Fall Nantucket) 15.0
(Apple & Eve Naturally Cranberry) 30.0
(Heinke's 100%) 14.0
(R.W. Knudsen Just Cranberry) 14.0
(R.W. Knudsen Yankee) 30.0
(Ocean Spray Cocktail), 6 fl. oz. 25.0
(Season's Best Medley) 29.0
(Snapple), 10 fl. oz. 37.0
concentrate* *(R.W. Knudsen)* 13.0
Cranberry juice blend, 8 fl. oz., except as noted:
apple *(Cranapple)* 40.0
apricot *(Cranicot)* 40.0
blueberry *(Cran•Blueberry)* 41.0
grape *(Apple & Eve)*, 10 fl. oz. 42.0
grape *(Cran•Grape)* 41.0
grapefruit *(After the Fall)* 29.0
kiwi *(After the Fall)* 26.0
mango *(After the Fall)* 26.0
orange *(After the Fall)* 28.0
punch *(Crantastic)* 37.0
raspberry *(After the Fall)* 23.0
strawberry *(After the Fall)* 26.0

strawberry *(Ocean Spray)* 35.0
Cranberry nectar, 8 fl. oz.:
(Heinke's) 30.0
(Santa Cruz) 27.0
guava *(Santa Cruz)* 24.0
bottled or frozen* *(R.W. Knudsen)* 38.0
Cranberry sauce:
(R.W. Knudsen), 1 tbsp. 6.0
whole or jellied:
    (Ocean Spray), 2 oz. 22.0
    (S&W), ¼ cup 26.0
    ½ cup 53.7
Cranberry sauce blends, 2 oz.:
orange *(Cran•Fruit)* 23.0
raspberry *(Cran•Fruit)* 23.0
strawberry *(Cran•Fruit)* 22.0
Cranberry-orange relish, in jars *(New England),* ¼ cup . . . 31.0
Crayfish, without added ingredients 0
Cream, dairy pack:
half-and-half:
    (America's Choice), 2 tbsp. 2.0
    (Crowley's), 1 tbsp. 1.0
    1 cup 10.4
    1 tbsp. 6
light, coffee or table, 1 cup 8.8
light, coffee or table, 1 tbsp. 6
medium (25% fat), 1 cup 8.3
medium (25% fat), 1 tbsp. 5
sour, see "Cream, sour"
whipping[1]:
    light, 1 cup 7.1
    light, 1 tbsp. 4
    heavy *(America's Choice),* 1 tbsp. 1.0
    heavy *(Farmland),* 1 tbsp. 1.0
    heavy, 1 cup 6.6
    heavy, 1 tbsp. 4
whipped topping, see "Cream topping"
Cream, canned, light *(Nestlé Crema),* 1 tbsp. . . . . <1.0
Cream, sour, 2 tbsp., except as noted:
(Breakstone's) 1.0

---

[1]*Unwhipped; volume approximately doubled when whipped.*

Cream, sour *(cont.)*
(Friendship) 2.0
(Heluva Good) 2.0
(Knudsen Hampshire) 1.0
(Land O Lakes) 2.0
(Sealtest) 1.0
1 cup 9.8
1 tbsp. 5
light:
    (Friendship) 2.0
    (Heluva Good) 3.0
    (Knudsen Light) 2.0
    (Land O Lakes Light) 4.0
    (Sealtest Light) 2.0
nondairy, 1 oz. 1.9
nondairy, plain or flavored (Sour Supreme) 1.0
nonfat:
    (Breakstone's/Sealtest Free) 6.0
    (Friendship) 3.0
    (Heluva Good) 3.0
    (Land O Lakes No Fat) 5.0
    (Naturally Yours) 4.0
Cream of tartar *(Tone's)*, 1 tsp. 6
Cream topping, 2 tbsp., except as noted:
(Cool Whip Extra Creamy/Lite/Non-dairy) 2.0
(Kraft Real/Whipped Topping) 1.0
(La Crema Lite) 2.0
(Pet Whip) 2.0
(Rich's) 2.0
pressurized can (Rich's) 2.0
mix*:
    (D-Zerta) 1.0
    (Dream Whip) 2.0
    1 cup 13.0
Creamer, nondairy, 1 tbsp., except as noted:
(Coffee-mate/Coffee-mate Fat Free) 2.0
(Coffee-mate Lite) 1.0
(Rich's Coffee Rich) 3.0
(Rich's Coffee Rich Light) 1.0
(Rich's Farm Rich/Rich's Farm Rich Fat Free/Light) 1.0
powder (Coffee-mate/Coffee-mate Lite), 1 tsp. 1.0
powder (Cremora/Cremora Fat Free/Lite), 1 tsp. 2.0

Creamer, nondairy, flavored:
all flavors:
    liquid *(Coffee-mate),* 1 tbsp. 5.0
    liquid *(International Delight),* 1 tbsp. 7.0
    powdered *(Coffee-mate),* 1⅓ tbsp. 9.0
Crepe, fresh *(Frieda's),* 1 piece 7.0
Cress, garden:
raw, ½ cup 1.4
boiled, drained, ½ cup 2.6
Cress, water, see "Watercress"
Croaker, without added ingredients 0
Croissant, 1 piece, except as noted:
butter:
    (Awrey's), 1.5 oz. 13.0
    (Awrey's), 2 oz. 17.0
    (Awrey's Tip-to-Tip) 26.0
    (Pepperidge Farm Petite) 13.0
dill and onion *(Awrey's)* 24.0
margarine *(Awrey's Tip-to-Tip)* 14.0
margarine, sandwich:
    (Awrey's), 1.8 oz. 17.0
    (Awrey's), 2.5 oz. 23.0
    wheat *(Awrey's)* 22.0
pesto Parmesan *(Awrey's)* 23.0
frozen *(Sara Lee)* 20.0
frozen, petite *(Sara Lee),* 2 pieces 26.0
Crookneck squash:
fresh:
    untrimmed, 1 lb. 18.2
    sliced, raw, ends trimmed, ½ cup 2.6
    sliced, boiled, drained, ½ cup 3.9
canned, cut, drained, no salt, ½ cup 3.2
canned, cut, yellow *(Allens/Sunshine),* ½ cup 5.0
frozen, boiled, sliced, ½ cup 5.3
Croutons (see also "Salad toppers"), ¼ oz. or 2 tbsp.,
    except as noted:
Caesar:
    (Brownberry) 4.0
    (Pepperidge Farm) 4.0
    (Pepperidge Farm Fat Free), 6 pieces, .3 oz. 5.0
cheddar *(Brownberry)* 4.0
cheddar and Romano *(Pepperidge Farm)* 4.0

Croutons *(cont.)*
cheese and garlic:
    (Arnold Crispy) 5.0
    (Brownberry) 5.0
    (Pepperidge Farm) 4.0
cracked pepper and Parmesan *(Pepperidge Farm)* 4.0
garlic *(Old London* Restaurant Style) 4.0
herb, fine *(Arnold* Crispy) 5.0
Italian:
    (Arnold Crispy) 4.0
    (Old London Restaurant Style) 4.0
    spicy *(Pepperidge Farm* Fat Free), 6 pieces, .3 oz. 5.0
    zesty *(Pepperidge Farm)* 4.0
olive oil and garlic *(Pepperidge Farm)* 5.0
onion and garlic:
    (Arnold Crispy) 5.0
    (Brownberry) 4.0
    (Pepperidge Farm) 4.0
ranch:
    (Arnold Crispy) 5.0
    (Brownberry) 4.0
    (Pepperidge Farm) 4.0
seasoned:
    (Arnold Crispy) 5.0
    (Brownberry) 4.0
    (Pepperidge Farm) 4.0
sourdough *(Old London* Restaurant Style) 4.0
sourdough cheese *(Pepperidge Farm)* 4.0
toasted *(Brownberry)* 5.0
Cubanelle chili, see "Pepper, chili"
Cucumber, with peel:
(Dole), ⅓ medium 3.0
untrimmed, 1 lb. 12.8
1 medium, 8¼″ long, 10.9 oz. 8.3
sliced, ½ cup 1.4
hothouse or Japanese *(Frieda's),* ⅔ cup, 3 oz. 2.0
Cucumber, pickled, see "Pickle"
Cucumber dip, creamy *(Kraft* Premium), 2 tbsp. 2.0
Cucumber-garlic dip, see "Tzatziki"
Cucumber salad *(Rosoff/Schorr's),* 1 oz. 3.0
Cucuzza squash *(Frieda's),* ¾ cup, 3 oz. 3.0

Cumin seed, ground:
(McCormick), ¼ tsp. 2
(Tone's), ¼ tsp. 0
1 tbsp. 2.7
1 tsp. 9
Cupcake, see "Cake, snack"
Currant, fresh:
black, European, with stems, 1 lb. 68.4
black, European, ½ cup 8.6
red or white, with stems, 1 lb. 61.3
red or white, ½ cup 7.7
Currant, dried, zante:
(S&W), ¼ cup 31.0
1 oz. 21.0
½ cup 53.3
Curry paste *(Patak's),* 2 tbsp. 4.0
Curry powder:
(Tone's), ¼ tsp. 0
1 tbsp. 3.7
1 tsp. 1.2
Curry sauce, cooking:
(Kylin Thai), ¼ cup 5.0
hot:
   Madras *(Patak's),* ½ cup 17.0
   tikka masala *(Patak's),* ½ cup 14.0
   vindaloo *(Patak's),* ½ cup 16.0
jalfrezzi *(Patak's),* ½ cup 15.0
masala *(Shahi* Cream), ¼ cup 5.0
masala *(Shahi* Curry), ¼ cup 4.0
rogan josh *(Patak's),* ½ cup 12.0
Curry sauce mix *(Knorr),* ⅕ pkg. 4.0
Cusk, without added ingredients 0
Custard, see "Pudding mix"
Custard apple:
untrimmed, 1 lb. 66.3
trimmed, 1 oz. 7.1
Custard marrow, see "Chayote"
Cuttlefish, meat only:
raw, 4 oz. 9
boiled or steamed, 4 oz. 1.0
Cuttlefish, canned, in ink *(Goya),* ¼ cup 2.0

D

FOOD AND MEASURE   CARBOHYDRATE GRAMS

Daikon, see "Radish, Oriental"
Daiquiri mixer:
bottled *(Holland House/Mr & Mrs T)*, 4 fl. oz. 33.0
bottled, strawberry *(Holland House)*, 3.5 fl. oz. 34.0
frozen*:
   banana *(Bacardi)*, 8 fl. oz. 37.0
   peach *(Bacardi)*, 8 fl. oz. 33.0
   strawberry *(Bacardi)*, 8 fl. oz. 33.0
mix *(Bar-Tenders)*, 2 pkts., 1.2 oz. 30.0
Dairy Queen/Brazier, 1 serving:
DQ Homestyle burgers:
   cheeseburger 20.0
   double cheeseburger 35.0
   deluxe double cheeseburger 36.0
   cheeseburger with bacon, double 41.0
   hamburger 29.0
   hamburger, deluxe double 29.0
   Ultimate burger 29.0
sandwiches:
   chicken fillet:
      breaded 37.0
      breaded with cheese 38.0
      grilled 30.0
   fish fillet 39.0
   fish fillet with cheese 40.0
   hot dog:
      plain 19.0
      with cheese 20.0
      with chili 21.0
      with chili and cheese 22.0
chicken strip basket, with BBQ sauce or gravy 88.0
side dishes:
   fries, large 52.0
   fries, regular 40.0
   fries, small 29.0

onion rings, regular 29.0
desserts and shakes:
banana split 96.0
Blizzard:
    Butterfinger, regular 115.0
    Butterfinger, small 80.0
    chocolate chip cookie dough, regular 143.0
    chocolate chip cookie dough, small 99.0
    chocolate sandwich cookie, regular 97.0
    chocolate sandwich cookie, small 79.0
    Heath, regular 119.0
    Heath, small 82.0
    Reese's peanut butter cup, regular 105.0
    Reese's peanut butter cup, small 81.0
    strawberry, regular 95.0
    strawberry, small......................... 66.0
Buster Bar 41.0
cone:
    chocolate, regular 56.0
    chocolate, small 37.0
    chocolate-dipped, regular 63.0
    chocolate-dipped, small 42.0
    vanilla, large............................ 65.0
    vanilla, regular 57.0
    vanilla, small 38.0
DQ cake, undecorated:
    heart, 1/10 cake 41.0
    log, 1/8 cake 43.0
    round 8", 1/8 cake 53.0
    round 10", 1/12 cake 55.0
    sheet, 1/20 cake 54.0
DQ caramel & nut bar 32.0
DQ fudge bar 13.0
DQ sandwich 24.0
DQ Lemon Freez'r, 1/2 cup 20.0
DQ Treatzza Pizza, 1/8 pie:
    Heath 28.0
    M&M's 29.0
    peanut butter fudge 28.0
    strawberry-banana 29.0
DQ vanilla orange bar........................ 17.0

Dairy Queen/Brazier, desserts and shakes *(cont.)*
Dilly bar:
    chocolate 21.0
    chocolate mint 20.0
    toffee with *Heath* pieces 24.0
Fudge Nut Bar 40.0
malt, chocolate, regular .153.0
malt, chocolate, small 111.0
Misty:
    cooler, strawberry 49.0
    slush, regular 74.0
    slush, small 56.0
Peanut Buster parfait 99.0
Queen's Choice Big Scoop, chocolate 28.0
Queen's Choice Big Scoop, vanilla 27.0
shake, chocolate, regular 130.0
shake, chocolate, small 94.0
soft-serve, *DQ,* chocolate or vanilla, ½ cup 22.0
Starkiss 21.0
strawberry shortcake 70.0
sundae, chocolate, regular 73.0
sundae, chocolate, small 51.0
yogurt, *Breeze:*
    Heath, regular 123.0
    Heath, small 85.0
    strawberry, regular 99.0
    strawberry, small 68.0
yogurt, frozen:
    DQ nonfat, ½ cup 21.0
    regular cup 49.0
    cone 59.0
    strawberry sundae 66.0
Dandelion greens:
raw:
  (Frieda's), 2 cups, 3 oz. 3.0
  untrimmed, 1 lb. 41.7
  trimmed, 1 oz. or ½ cup chopped 2.6
boiled, drained, chopped, ½ cup 3.3
Danish, 1 piece:
all varieties *(Awrey's* Petite), 1½ oz. 14.0
apple *(Awrey's),* 2¾ oz. 32.0
apple *(Awrey's* Grande), 4½ oz. 51.0

cake, ring, or twist, see "Cake"
cheese:

    (Awrey's), 2¾ oz. 32.0
    (Awrey's Grande), 4½ oz. 49.0
    (Tastykake Pocket), 3.4 oz. 38.0
    cherry *(Awrey's* Marquise), 3¼ oz. 38.0
    cinnamon *(Awrey's* Marquise), 3¼ oz. 60.0
    lemon *(Awrey's* Marquise), 3¼ oz. 38.0
    raspberry swirl *(Awrey's* Grande), 3¾ oz. 51.0

cherry *(Tastykake* Pocket), 3¼ oz. 45.0
cinnamon swirl *(Awrey's),* 2¾ oz. 32.0
cinnamon swirl *(Awrey's* Grande), 3¾ oz. 57.0
strawberry *(Awrey's),* 2¾ oz. 32.0
strawberry *(Awrey's* Grande), 4½ oz. 53.0

Danish, frozen or refrigerated, 1 piece:
apple *(Pepperidge Farm)* 29.0
cheese *(Pepperidge Farm)* 25.0
raspberry *(Pepperidge Farm)* 29.0

Dasheen, see "Taro"
Date, dehydrated, fine or coarse ground *(Dole),* 1 oz. 27.0
Date, dried, pitted:
(Del Monte), 5–6 pieces., 1.4 oz. 31.0
(Dole), ½ cup 62.0
(Sonoma), 5–6 pieces, 1.4 oz. 30.0
chopped *(Del Monte),* ¼ cup, 1.4 oz. 33.0
chopped *(Dole),* ½ cup 56.0
Date nut pastry *(Awrey's),* 1 piece 20.0
De Arbol chili, see "Pepper, chili"
Delicata squash *(Frieda's),* ¾ cup, 3 oz. 7.0
Demi-glacé sauce mix *(Knorr),* 1 tbsp. 4.0
Denny's, 1 serving:
breakfast, without bread:
    All American Slam 24.0
    Belgian waffle, plain 23.0
    Belgian waffle supreme, without bacon or sausage 50.0
    chicken fried steak and eggs 31.0
    French Slam 58.0
    French toast, plain, 2 pieces 51.0
    ham 'n' cheddar omelette 24.0
    Moons Over My Hammy, without potato 46.0
    Original *Grand Slam,* without syrup or margarine 65.0
    pancakes, plain, 3 pieces 95.0

Denny's, breakfast *(cont.)*

pork chop and eggs	21.0
porterhouse steak and eggs	21.0
Scram Slam	30.0
Senior Belgian Waffle Slam, without syrup or margarine	12.0
Senior Omelette	27.0
Senior Starter, without bacon or sausage	36.0
Senior Triple Play, without bacon or sausage	64.0
sirloin steak and eggs	21.0
Slim Slam, with syrup, without topping	98.0
Southern Slam	47.0
Super/Play It Again Slam	98.0
T-bone steak and eggs	21.0
Ultimate Omelette	29.0
veggie-cheese omelette	29.0

breakfast, junior:

basic breakfast	38.0
Belgian waffle	20.0
Junior French Slam, without syrup or margarine	18.0
Junior Grand Slam, without syrup or margarine	33.0

breakfast items:

apple juice, 10 oz.	33.0
applesauce	15.0
bacon, 4 slices	1.0
bagel, dry, whole	46.0
banana	29.0
banana/strawberry medley	27.0
biscuit, plain	40.0
biscuit and sausage gravy	45.0
cantaloupe, 3 oz.	8.0
cereal, dry, average, 1 oz.	23.0
cream cheese, 1 oz.	1.0
egg, 1	1.0
egg substitute, *Sunny Fresh*	1.0
fresh fruit mix	9.0
grapefruit, half	16.0
grapefruit juice, 10 oz.	29.0
grapes, 3 oz.	15.0
grits, 4 oz.	18.0
ham, 3 oz.	2.0
hashed browns	20.0
hashed browns, covered	21.0

hashed browns, covered and smothered 26.0
honeydew. 8.0
margarine, whipped, .5 oz. 0
muffin, blueberry 42.0
muffin, English, plain, dry 24.0
oatmeal, 4 oz. 18.0
orange juice, 10 oz. 31.0
sausage, 4 links 0
strawberries, frozen, with sugar, 3 oz. 26.0
syrup, 1.5 oz. 36.0
syrup, reduced calorie, 1.5 oz. 6.0
toast, dry, 1 slice 17.0
tomato juice, 10 oz. 11.0
topping, blueberry, 3 oz. 26.0
topping, strawberry, 3 oz. 26.0
salad, without dressing, except as noted:
   fried chicken 30.0
   garden chicken delite 14.0
   grilled chicken Caesar, with dressing 23.0
   Oriental chicken, with dressing 49.0
   side Caesar, with dressing 20.0
   side garden 16.0
dressings, 1 oz.:
   blue cheese 4.0
   Caesar 1.0
   French 3.0
   French, reduced calorie 8.0
   honey mustard, fat free 9.0
   Italian, creamy 4.0
   Italian, reduced calorie 3.0
   Oriental 6.0
   ranch 1.0
   Thousand Island 2.0
condiments, 1.5 oz.:
   BBQ sauce 11.0
   horseradish sauce 3.0
   sour cream 2.0
soup, 8 oz.:
   cheese 13.0
   chicken noodle 8.0
   clam chowder 22.0
   cream of broccoli 15.0

Denny's, soup *(cont.)*

    cream of potato............................. 23.0
    split pea................................. 18.0
    vegetable beef............................ 11.0

sandwiches, without fries or substitutes:

    bacon, lettuce, and tomato 37.0
    bacon Swiss burger....................... 27.0
    Charleston Chicken 53.0
    chicken melt............................. 43.0
    club 62.0
    Delidinger.............................. 62.0
    deluxe grilled cheese 44.0
    Denny Burger 26.0
    French dip, without horseradish sauce 53.0
    fried fish 74.0
    grilled chicken........................... 60.0
    Humdinger Hamburger 30.0
    patty melt 36.0
    Super Bird 48.0

sandwiches, lunch combinations:

    ham and Swiss on rye, without soup or salad 40.0
    turkey breast on multigrain, without soup or salad 39.0

sandwiches, senior, sandwich only:

    half grilled cheese 21.0
    ham and Swiss, without fries or substitutes 34.0
    turkey, without fries or substitutes 39.0

appetizers, without condiments, except as noted:

    Buffalo chicken strips 43.0
    Buffalo wings, 12 pieces 1.0
    chicken quesadilla 43.0
    chicken strips, 5 pieces 56.0
    mozzarella sticks, 8 pieces, with sauce 56.0
    onion rings, 7 pieces 44.0
    Sampler...............................104.0

entrees[1]:

    battered cod, with tartar sauce 48.0
    Charleston Chicken 16.0
    chicken fried steak........................ 14.0
    chicken strip, with honey-mustard dressing 55.0

---

[1] *Add bread; choice of salad, soup, or fruit; choice of potato or rice pilaf; and choice of vegetable.*

Denny Cut Prime Rib, 8 oz., with au jus and horseradish . 8.0
grilled Alaskan salmon 1.0
grilled breast of chicken 0
liver with bacon and onions 13.0
pork chop dinner 0
porterhouse steak 0
roast turkey and stuffing 63.0
shrimp 49.0
steak and shrimp 31.0
T-bone steak dinner 0
junior meals, without fries or substitutes:
  burger 16.0
  fried fish 25.0
  grilled cheese 35.0
  shrimp basket 27.0
senior meals[1]:
  battered cod, without potato or pilaf 25.0
  chicken fried steak 29.0
  grilled chicken breast 16.0
  liver with bacon and onions 20.0
  pork chop 0
  pot roast 6.0
  turkey and stuffing 61.0
sides:
  broccoli in butter sauce, 4 oz. 7.0
  carrots in honey glaze, 4 oz. 12.0
  corn in butter sauce, 4 oz. 19.0
  corn bread stuffing, 2 oz. 20.0
  french fries, unsalted, 4 oz. 44.0
  fries, seasoned, 4 oz. 35.0
  gravy, brown, chicken, or country, 1 oz. 2.0
  green beans with bacon, 4 oz. 6.0
  green peas in butter sauce, 4 oz. 14.0
  potato, baked, plain, 6 oz. 43.0
  potato, mashed, plain, 6 oz. 21.0
  rice pilaf, 3 oz. 21.0
  sliced tomatoes, 3 slices 3.0
pies, "Mother Butler," 1/6 pie:
  apple 59.0
  apple, with *Equal* 43.0

[1] *Add bread; choice of soup, salad, or fruit; and choice of vegetable.*

Denny's, pies *(cont.)*
   cheesecake pie 48.0
     blueberry topping, 3 oz. 26.0
     cherry topping, 3 oz. 26.0
   cherry 83.0
   chocolate pecan 107.0
   coconut cream 58.0
   Dutch apple 65.0
   French silk 60.0
   German chocolate 66.0
   key lime 79.0
   lemon meringue 71.0
   pecan 81.0
other desserts:
   banana split sundae, 19 oz. 121.0
   chocolate cake, 4 oz. 53.0
   hot fudge cake sundae, 8 oz. 83.0
   sundae, double scoop, without topping, 6 oz. . . . 29.0
   sundae, single scoop, 3 oz., without topping 14.0
   tapioca, 4 oz. 21.0
   toppings, 2 oz.:
     blueberry 17.0
     chocolate 27.0
     fudge 30.0
     strawberry 17.0
coffee, flavored, 8 oz.:
   French vanilla 16.0
   hazelnut 14.0
   Irish cream 16.0
raspberry iced tea, 16 oz. 21.0
Dessert, see specific listings
Dessert bar mix, see "Cake, snack, mix"
Dessert filling, see "Pastry filling" and "Pie filling"
Dessert mix, chilled, no-bake:
banana cream *(Betty Crocker)*, 1/9 pkg. 31.0
banana cream *(Betty Crocker)*, 1/9 dessert* 35.0
chocolate French silk *(Betty Crocker)*, 1/8 pkg. 35.0
chocolate French silk *(Betty Crocker)*, 1/8 dessert* 39.0
coconut cream *(Betty Crocker)*, 1/9 pkg. 34.0
coconut cream *(Betty Crocker)*, 1/9 dessert* 38.0
cookies 'n creme *(Betty Crocker)*, 1/6 pkg. 49.0
cookies 'n creme *(Betty Crocker)*, 1/6 dessert* 52.0

Sunkist lemon supreme *(Betty Crocker)*, 1/9 pkg. 51.0
Sunkist lemon supreme *(Betty Crocker)*, 1/9 dessert* 52.0
Diable sauce *(Escoffier)*, 1 tbsp. 4.0
Dill dip, 2 tbsp.:
(Bernstein's Zesty) 2.0
(Heluva Good) 2.0
(Marie's) 3.0
Dill seed:
(McCormick), 1/4 tsp. 4
1 tbsp. 3.6
1 tsp. 1.2
Dill weed:
fresh, 5 sprigs 1
fresh, 1/2 cup loosely packed 3
dried:
   (McCormick), 1/4 tsp. 1
   (Tone's), 1/4 tsp. 0
   1 tbsp. 1.7
   1 tsp. 6
Dock, boiled, drained, 4 oz. 3.3
Dolphinfish, without added ingredients 0
Domino's Pizza:
cheese pizza, 12" medium pie:
   deep dish, 2 of 8 slices 51.8
   hand-tossed, 2 of 8 slices 48.9
   thin crust, 1/4 pie 30.1
   "Add a Topping":
      anchovies 0
      bacon 1
      beef, pre-cooked 0
      cheddar cheese 2
      extra cheese 3
      ham 3
      mushrooms, fresh 7
      mushrooms, canned 9
      olives, green 1
      olives, ripe 6
      onion 5
      pepperoni 2
      peppers, banana or green 6
      pineapple tidbits 2.5
      sausage, Italian 1.6

Domino's Pizza (cont.)

cheese pizza, 14″ large pie:

    deep dish, 2 of 12 slices 54.8

    hand-tossed, 2 of 12 slices 44.2

    thin crust, 1/6 pie 54.8

    "Add a Topping":

        anchovies 0

        bacon 1

        beef, pre-cooked 0

        cheddar cheese 2

        extra cheese 3

        ham 3

        mushrooms, fresh 5

        mushrooms, canned 6

        olives, green 1

        olives, ripe 5

        onion 7

        pepperoni 2

        peppers, banana or green 5

        pineapple tidbits 2.0

        sausage, Italian 1.3

cheese pizza, 6″ deep dish, 1 pie:

    plain 65.5

    "Add a Topping":

        anchovies 0

        bacon 1

        beef, pre-cooked 0

        cheddar cheese 3

        extra cheese 4

        ham 3

        mushrooms, fresh or canned 4

        olives, green 1

        olives, ripe 5

        onion 6

        pepperoni 2

        peppers, banana or green 5

        pineapple tidbits 1.2

        sausage, Italian 1.3

Buffalo wings:

    barbecue, 1 piece 1.6

    hot, 1 piece 5

breadstick, 1 piece 10.7

cheesy bread, 1 piece	10.8
salad, small	4.0
salad, large	7.6
Marzetti salad dressings, 1.5 oz.:	
blue cheese	2.0
Caesar, creamy	2.0
French, honey	14.0
Italian, house	1.0
Italian, light	2.0
ranch	1.0
ranch, fat free	10.0
Thousand Island	5.0

Donut, 1 piece, except as noted:

plain:

(Awrey's), 1.5 oz.	19.0
(Awrey's), 2 oz.	21.0
(Hostess)	15.0
(Tastykake Assorted)	19.0
blueberry *(Hostess)*	21.0
cinnamon *(Tastykake* Assorted)	24.0
cinnamon sugar *(Entenmann's* Variety Pack)	32.0
coconut top *(Awrey's)*	25.0

crumb:

(Entenmann's)	34.0
(Entenmann's Variety Pack)	52.0
(Hostess Donettes), 6 pieces, 3 oz.	53.0
crunch *(Awrey's)*	35.0
crunch top *(Awrey's)*	19.0
devil's food crumb *(Entenmann's)*	33.0

frosted/iced, chocolate:

(Awrey's), 1.75 oz.	23.0
(Awrey's), 2.5 oz.	31.0
(Hostess)	19.0
(Hostess Donettes), 6 pieces, 3 oz.	42.0
chocolate *(Awrey's)*, 1.75 oz.	25.0
chocolate *(Awrey's)*, 2.5 oz.	34.0
custard Bismark *(Awrey's)*	36.0
mini *(Entenmann's)*, 2 pieces	23.0
rich *(Entenmann's)*	27.0
rich *(Entenmann's* Variety Pack)	37.0
rich *(Tastykake)*	30.0
rich, mini *(Entenmann's Popettes)*, 3 pieces	29.0

Donut, frosted/iced, chocolate *(cont.)*
    rich, mini *(Tastykake)*, 4 pieces 29.0
    rich, with raspberry *(Entenmann's)* 31.0
    ring *(Awrey's)* 33.0
    sour creme *(Awrey's)* 52.0
glazed:
    (Entenmann's Popems), 6 pieces 33.0
    (Hostess) 35.0
    buttermilk *(Entenmann's)* 36.0
    chocolate *(Entenmann's Popems)*, 4 pieces 29.0
    honey, devil's food *(Awrey's)* 43.0
    honey, ring *(Awrey's)* 30.0
    orange *(Tastykake)* 33.0
    sour creme *(Awrey's)* 42.0
honey wheat *(Tastykake)* 33.0
honey wheat, mini *(Tastykake)*, 6 pieces 39.0
powdered sugar:
    (Awrey's), 1.5 oz. 19.0
    (Awrey's), 2.25 oz. 44.0
    (Entenmann's Softee) 27.0
    (Hostess Donettes), 6 pieces, 3 oz. 47.0
    (Tastykake Assorted) 24.0
    cinnamon *(Hostess)* 19.0
    jelly Bismark *(Awrey's)* 35.0
    mini *(Tastykake)*, 6 pieces 40.0
raspberry filled *(Hostess O's)* 34.0
sour creme, plain *(Awrey's)* 41.0
sprinkle topped *(Awrey's)* 19.0
stick, see "Cake, snack"
vanilla iced *(Awrey's Long John)* 44.0
vanilla iced, jelly Bismark *(Awrey's)* 35.0
white, iced *(Awrey's)* 24.0
Donut, frozen, glazed *(Rich's)*, 1 piece 16.0
Dressing, see "Salad dressing" and specific listings
Drum, freshwater, without added ingredients 0
Duck, domesticated or wild, without added ingredients 0
Duck sauce, see "Sweet and sour sauce"
Dumpling entree, Oriental, frozen *(Lean Cuisine)*, 9 oz. . . . 52.0

E

FOOD AND MEASURE   **CARBOHYDRATE GRAMS**

Eclair, chocolate, frozen, 1 piece:
(Rich's) 24.0
(Weight Watchers) 25.0
triple (Weight Watchers) 25.0
Eel, without added ingredients 0
Egg, chicken:
raw, 1 large:
   whole 6
   white only 3
   yolk only[1] 3
cooked, hard-boiled, chopped, 1 cup 1.5
cooked, poached, 1 large 6
dried, 1 oz.:
   whole 1.4
   whole, stabilized 7
   white, stabilized, flakes 1.2
   yolk 1
Egg, substitute or imitation, 1/4 cup:
(Egg Beaters) 1.0
(Egg Watchers) 1.0
(Morningstar Farms Better 'n Eggs) 0
(Morningstar Farms Scramblers) 2.0
(Second Nature) 3.0
Egg, duck, 1 egg 1.0
Egg, goose, 1 egg 1.9
Egg, quail, 1 egg . . . . <.1
Egg, turkey, 1 egg 9
Egg breakfast, freeze-dried, 1/2 cup:
with bacon (Mountain House) 5.0
omelet, cheese (Mountain House) 7.0
Egg breakfast, frozen (see also specific listings), 1 pkg.:
omelet, ham and cheese (Weight Watchers) 30.0

[1]Includes a small portion of white.

Egg breakfast, frozen *(cont.)*
patty:
 with Canadian bacon *(Swanson Great Starts* Low Fat/
  Low Cholesterol) 33.0
 and pancake *(Swanson Great Starts* Low Fat/Low
  Cholesterol) 30.0
 and sausage, home fries *(Swanson Great Starts* Low Fat/
  Low Cholesterol) 18.0
scrambled:
 and bacon *(Swanson Great Starts)* 17.0
 with home fries *(Swanson Great Starts)* 15.0
 and sausage *(Swanson Great Starts)* 21.0
Egg breakfast sandwich, frozen, 1 pkg.:
biscuit, see "Sausage biscuit"
with cheese *(Swanson Great Starts)* 30.0
muffin:
 (Weight Watchers) 28.0
 with bacon and cheese *(Swanson Great Starts)* 25.0
 with Canadian bacon, cheese *(Hormel Quick Meal)* 29.0
 with ham *(Schwan's)* 24.0
 with sausage, cheese *(Hormel Quick Meal)* 28.0
omelet *(Weight Watchers* Classic) 26.0
vegetarian *(Morningstar Farms)*:
 bagel, with scrambler, patty, and cheese 40.0
 muffin, with scrambler and patty 32.0
 muffin, with scrambler, patty, and cheese 35.0
Egg roll, frozen:
(Empire Kosher), 3-oz. roll 28.0
(Empire Kosher Mini), 6 rolls 43.0
chicken:
 (Chun King/La Choy), 3-oz. roll 25.0
 (Schwan's), 2 rolls, 4 oz. 28.0
 mini *(Chun King)*, 12 rolls 58.0
 mini *(La Choy)*, 14 rolls 67.0
 sweet and sour *(La Choy)*, 3-oz. roll 29.0
pork:
 (Chun King/La Choy), 3-oz. roll 23.0
 (Schwan's), 2 rolls, 4 oz. 14.0
 moo shu *(La Choy)*, 3-oz. roll 25.0
pork and shrimp:
 bite size *(La Choy)*, 15 rolls 31.0
 mini *(Chun King)*, 12 rolls 56.0

mini *(La Choy)*, 14 rolls 65.0
shrimp:
    (Chun King/La Choy), 3-oz. roll 24.0
    mini *(Chun King)*, 12 rolls 57.0
    mini *(La Choy)*, 14 rolls 68.0
vegetable with lobster, mini *(La Choy)*, 14 rolls 65.0
" 'Egg' roll, vegetarian, frozen *(Worthington)*, 1 roll 20.0
Egg roll entree, frozen, vegetable *(Lean Cuisine)*, 9 oz. . . . 59.0
Egg roll wrapper:
(Frieda's), 2 pieces, 1.7 oz. 28.0
(Nasoya), 1.5 oz. 23.7
Eggnog, dairy, ½ cup:
(Borden) 17.0
(Borden Light) 23.0
(Crowley) 23.0
(Crowley Light) 22.0
(Crowley Nonfat) 25.0
Eggplant, fresh, with peel:
raw:
    untrimmed, 1 lb. 23.0
    trimmed, 1" pieces, ½ cup 2.5
    Japanese *(Frieda's)*, ⅔ cup, 3 oz. 5.0
boiled, drained, 1" cubes, ½ cup 3.2
Eggplant appetizer, 2 tbsp., except as noted:
(Progresso Caponata) 2.0
roasted *(Peloponnese)* 11.0
stuffed, baby *(Krinos)*, 1.1 oz., about 2 pieces 0
stuffed, rolettes *(Paesana)*, 3¾ oz. 9.0
Eggplant dip *(Victoria)*, 2 tbsp. 2.0
Eggplant entree, frozen:
cutlets *(Celentano)*, 5 oz. 23.0
parmigiana:
    (Celentano), 10-oz. pkg. 30.0
    (Celentano 14 oz.), ½ pkg. 22.0
    (Celentano Value Pack), 1 cup, 8 oz. 19.0
    (Mrs. Paul's), ½ cup 19.0
rollettes *(Celentano)*, 10 oz. 27.0
rollettes *(Celentano* Great Choice), 10 oz. 39.0
Eggplant pickle relish *(Patak's* Brinjal), 1 tbsp. 10.0
Elderberry, fresh:
4 oz. 20.8
½ cup 13.3

Empanadilla, frozen:

plain *(Goya),* 2 pieces 58.0

plain, cocktail size *(Goya),* 7 pieces 56.0

pizza flavor *(Goya),* 2 pieces 56.0

Enchilada, canned *(Gebhardt),* 2 pieces 20.0

Enchilada dinner, frozen:

(Amy's), 10 oz. 41.0

(Chi-Chi's Baja), 15.4 oz. 82.0

beef:

    (Patio), 12 oz. 52.0

    (Swanson), 1 pkg. 60.0

    with chili sauce *(Banquet* Family), 1 piece, 4.7 oz. 19.0

cheese *(Patio),* 12 oz. 52.0

chicken:

    (Chi-Chi's Suprema), 14.9 oz. 71.0

    (Healthy Choice Suprema), 11.3 oz. 45.0

    (Patio), 12 oz. 48.0

Enchilada entree, frozen:

beef:

    (Banquet), 11 oz. 54.0

    (Patio Chili 'n Beans Large), 2 pieces, 7¾ oz. 35.0

    (Patio Family), 2 pieces, 5.7 oz. 31.0

    and tamale, chili gravy with *(Morton),* 10 oz. 40.0

beef and cheese *(Patio* Chili 'n Beans Large), 2 pieces,

    7¾ oz. 35.0

black bean *(Amy's* Family), 4.38 oz. 18.0

black bean and vegetable *(Amy's),* 4.75 oz. 20.0

cheese:

    (Amy's), 4.75 oz. 16.0

    (Amy's Family), 4.38 oz. 15.0

    (Banquet), 11 oz. 56.0

    (Patio Family), 2 pieces, 5.7 oz. 26.0

    and rice *(Stouffer's),* 9¾ oz. 48.0

chicken:

    (Banquet), 11 oz. 54.0

    (Stouffer's 57 oz.), 4.75 oz. 25.0

    and rice *(Stouffer's),* 10 oz. 45.0

chicken Suiza:

    (Healthy Choice), 10 oz. 43.0

    (Weight Watchers), 9 oz. 33.0

    with rice *(Lean Cuisine),* 9 oz. 47.0

Enchilada sauce, ¼ cup:
(Chi-Chi's) 3.0
(Gebhardt) 3.5
(La Victoria) 3.0
(Las Palmas Original) 2.0
(Old El Paso Mild/Medium/Hot) 4.0
(Rosarita Mild) 3.0
green chili *(Las Palmas)* 3.0
green chili *(Old El Paso)* 3.0
hot *(Las Palmas)* 3.0
Enchilada seasoning mix:
(Durkee), 1½ tsp. 2.0
(Lawry's), 2 tsp. 4.0
(Old El Paso), 2 tsp. 0
Endive:
untrimmed, 1 lb. 13.1
chopped, ½ cup 8
Endive, Belgian, see "Chicory, witloof"
Entree mix, frozen:
Alfredo, creamy *(Green Giant Create A Meal!),* 2 cups[1] 31.0
Alfredo, creamy *(Green Giant Create A Meal!),* 1¼ cups[2] . . . 33.0
beef, Oriental, with vegetables and rice *(Schwan's Meal Kit),*
   1½ cups[1] or 1 cup[2] 29.0
broccoli stir-fry *(Green Giant Create A Meal!),* 2⅓ cups[1]
   or 1⅓ cups[2] 16.0
cacciatore *(Birds Eye Easy Recipe Meal Starter),* 2 cups[1] . . 22.0
cheddar, creamy *(Green Giant Create A Meal!),* 1¾ cups[1] . . 26.0
cheddar, creamy *(Green Giant Create A Meal!),* 1½ cups[2] . . 29.0
cheese and herb primavera *(Green Giant Create A Meal!),*
   1¾ cups[1] or 1¼ cups[2] 27.0
chicken:
   with fried rice and vegetables *(Schwan's Meal Kit),*
      1½ cups[1] or 1 cup[2] 40.0
   noodle, creamy *(Green Giant Create A Meal!),* 1½ cups[1] 31.0
   noodle, creamy *(Green Giant Create A Meal!),* 1¼ cups[2] 34.0
   stir-fry, with rice and vegetables *(Schwan's*
      Meal Kit),* 1½ cups[1] or 1 cup[2] 35.0
garlic herb *(Green Giant Create A Meal!),* 2⅓ cups[1] 29.0
garlic herb *(Green Giant Create A Meal!),* 1¼ cups[2] 30.0

[1]*Entree mix as packaged.*
[2]*Prepared according to package directions, with meat and oil.*

Entree mix, frozen *(cont.)*
lemon herb *(Green Giant Create A Meal!)*, 1½ cups[1]
    or 1½ cups[2] 37.0
lo mein *(Green Giant Create A Meal!)*, 2⅓ cups[1] or
    1¼ cups[2] 35.0
mushroom and wine *(Green Giant Create A Meal!)*,
    1¾ cups[1] or 1¼ cups[2] 31.0
primavera *(Birds Eye Easy Recipe Meal Starter)*, 1¾ cups[1]   17.0
stir-fry, Asian *(Birds Eye Easy Recipe Meal Starter)*,
    2¼ cups[1] 45.0
stir-fry, Oriental *(Birds Eye Easy Recipe Meal Starter)*,
    2¼ cups[1] 23.0
sweet and sour *(Green Giant Create A Meal!)*, 1¾ cups[1]
    or 1¼ cups[2] 29.0
Szechuan *(Green Giant Create A Meal!)*, 1¾ cups[1] or
    1¼ cups[2] 22.0
teriyaki *(Green Giant Create A Meal!)*, 1¾ cups[1] or
    1¼ cups[2] 18.0
vegetable almond stir-fry *(Green Giant Create A Meal!)*,
    1¾ cups[1] or 1⅓ cups[2] 22.0
vegetable stew, hearty *(Green Giant Create A Meal!)*,
    1¼ cups[1] or 1¼ cups[2] 25.0
Entree sauce, see specific listings
Eppaw:
1 oz. 9.0
½ cup 15.8
Escarole, see "Endive"
Etouffee dinner mix *(Luzianne)*, ¼ pkg. 42.0

---

[1]*Entree mix as packaged.*
[2]*Prepared according to package directions, with meat and oil.*

F

FOOD AND MEASURE   **CARBOHYDRATE GRAMS**

Fajita, canned, beef or chicken *(Nalley* Superba), 1 cup . . . 30.0
Fajita entree, chicken, frozen:
(Healthy Choice Fiesta), 7 oz. 36.0
(Schwan's), 4-oz. piece 16.0
Fajita mix *(Old El Paso),* 2 pieces* 47.0
Fajita sauce:
(S&W Southwestern), 1 tbsp. 2.0
and marinade *(World Harbors* Guadalupe), 2 tbsp. 10.0
skillet *(Lawry's),* 2 tbsp. 2.0
Fajita seasoning mix:
(Lawry's), 2 tsp. 3.0
(Old El Paso), 1 tbsp. 0
beef *(Durkee* Easy), ⅙ pkg. 4.0
Falafel mix:
(Casbah), ⅛ pkg. 20.0
(Fantastic Falafil), ½ cup 42.0
Farina, whole-grain (see also "Cereal"):
dry, 1 oz. 22.1
cooked, 1 cup 24.6
Fat, see specific listings
Fava beans, see "Broad beans"
Feijoa, raw:
(Frieda's), 5 oz. 15.0
with skin, 1 medium, 2.3 oz. 5.3
pureed, ½ cup 12.0
Fennel, bulb, raw, trimmed:
(Frieda's), ¾ cup, 3 oz. 6.0
1 bulb, 8.3 oz. 17.1
trimmed, 1 oz. 2.1
sliced, ½ cup 6.3
Fennel seed:
1 tbsp. 3.0
1 tsp. 1.1
Fenugreek seed:
1 tbsp. 6.5

Fenugreek seed *(cont.)*
1 tsp.............................. 2.2
Fettuccine, plain, dry, see "Pasta"
Fettuccine, refrigerated:
(Contadina), 1¼ cups 45.0
(Di Giorno), 2.5 oz. 39.0
artichoke *(Tutta Pasta),* 2 oz............... 38.0
black squid *(Tutta Pasta),* 2 oz............. 37.0
spinach *(Contadina),* 1¼ cups 45.0
spinach *(Di Giorno),* 2.5 oz................. 38.0
Fettuccine entree, frozen:
Alfredo:
    (Banquet), 10.5 oz. 39.0
    (Healthy Choice), 8 oz. 39.0
    (Lean Cuisine), 9 oz. 45.0
    (Marie Callender's), 1 cup 29.0
    (Stouffer's), 10 oz...................... 50.0
    with broccoli *(Weight Watchers),* 8.5 oz. 34.0
    with four cheeses *(The Budget Gourmet* Special
        Selections), 11.5 oz..................... 47.0
    with broccoli and chicken *(Marie Callender's),* 1 cup ... 30.0
    chicken, see "Chicken entree"
    and meatballs, in wine sauce *(The Budget Gourmet*
        Italian Originals), 10¼ oz. 40.0
primavera:
    (Lean Cuisine), 9 oz. 36.0
    (Marie Callender's), 1 cup 25.0
    (Stouffer's), 10 oz...................... 49.0
    in herb sauce, with chicken *(The Budget Gourmet* Italian
        Originals), 10 oz. 35.0
Fettuccine entree mix, approx. 1 cup*, except as noted:
with Alfredo sauce *(Pasta Roni)* 48.0
broccoli, au gratin *(Pasta Roni)* 39.0
cheddar, mild *(Pasta Roni)* 39.0
chicken sauce *(Pasta Roni)* 41.0
with creamy basil sauce *(Knorr* Cup), 1 pkg........... 41.0
Romanoff *(Pasta Roni)* 46.0
Stroganoff *(Pasta Roni)*......................... 48.0
Fig:
fresh:
    untrimmed, 1 lb. 86.1
    1 large, 2.3 oz. 12.3

1 medium, 1.8 oz. 9.6
California, 4 figs, 2 oz. 38.8
Calimyrna *(Frieda's)*, 1 oz. 5.8
canned:
   in heavy syrup, ½ cup 29.7
   in heavy syrup, Kadota *(Oregon)*, ½ cup 30.0
   in heavy syrup, Kadota *(S&W)*, 5 figs 32.0
dried:
   10 figs, 6.6 oz. 122.2
   Calamata string *(Agora)*, ½ cup 58.0
   California, 4 figs, 2 oz. 38.8
   Calimyrna or mission *(Blue Ribbon/SunMaid)*, 4 figs,
     1½ oz. 28.0
   white/mission *(Sonoma)*, 3–4 figs, 1.4 oz. 26.0
Filbert, shelled:
dried:
   1 oz. 4.4
   chopped, 1 cup 17.6
   blanched, 1 oz. 4.5
dry-roasted, salted or unsalted, 1 oz. 5.1
oil-roasted, salted or unsalted, 1 oz. 5.4
Fillo pastry, frozen *(Apollo)*, ⅛ pkg. 35.0
Finnan haddie, without added ingredients 0
Finocchio, see "Fennel"
Fish, see specific listings
"Fish," vegetarian:
frozen *(Worthington)*, 2 fillets 8.0
mix *(Loma Linda* Ocean Platter), ⅓ cup 8.0
Fish batter mix, see "Fish seasoning and coating mix"
Fish dinner, frozen (see also specific fish listings):
baked, herb *(Healthy Choice)*, 10.9 oz. 54.0
battered portions, with chips *(Swanson)*, 1 pkg. 55.0
breaded sticks *(Swanson* Budget), 1 pkg. 51.0
lemon pepper *(Healthy Choice)*, 10.7 oz. 47.0
Fish entree, frozen (see also specific fish listings):
(Van de Kamp's Fish 'n Fries), 6.5 oz. 41.0
baked, with shells *(Lean Cuisine)*, 9 oz. 28.0
cakes *(Mrs. Paul's)*, 2 pieces 23.0
and chips *(Swanson)*, 1 pkg. 38.0
fillets, baked:
   breaded *(Mrs. Paul's* Crisp & Healthy), 2 pieces 20.0
   breaded *(Van de Kamp's* Crisp & Healthy), 2 pieces . . . 20.0

Fish entree, fillets, baked *(cont.)*

garlic and pepper *(Mrs. Paul's/Van de Kamp's)*, 1 piece   17.0
lemon pepper *(Mrs. Paul's/Van de Kamp's)*, 1 piece ...   17.0

fillets, battered:

(Gorton's), 2 pieces 16.0
(Mrs. Paul's), 1 piece 13.0
(Van de Kamp's), 1 piece 12.0
lemon pepper *(Gorton's)*, 2 pieces 18.0

fillets, breaded:

(Gorton's Crunchy), 2 pieces 17.0
(Mrs. Paul's), 2 pieces 20.0
(Van de Kamp's), 2 pieces 17.0
cornmeal *(Mrs. Paul's/Van de Kamp's)*, 1 piece 15.0
garlic and herb *(Gorton's Crunchy)*, 2 pieces 20.0
hot and spicy *(Gorton's Crunchy)*, 2 pieces 19.0
potato *(Gorton's)*, 2 pieces 17.0
Southern fried *(Gorton's Crunchy)*, 2 pieces 20.0

fillets, grilled, 1 piece:

all varieties *(Mrs. Paul's/Van de Kamp's)* 0
Italian herb *(Gorton's)* 2.0
lemon pepper *(Gorton's)*........................ 1.0

fillets, in butter-flavored sauce *(Mrs. Paul's)*, 1 piece 4.0
grilled, with vegetables *(Lean Cuisine Cafe Classics)*, 8⅞ oz.   14.0
with macaroni and cheese *(Stouffer's Homestyle)*, 9 oz. ... 37.0
with macaroni and cheese *(Swanson)*, 1 pkg. 38.0
nuggets *(Van de Kamp's)*, 8 pieces 20.0
portions, battered *(Gorton's)*, 1 piece 12.0
portions, battered *(Van de Kamp's)*, 2 pieces 26.0
portions, breaded *(Mrs. Paul's)*, 2 pieces 16.0
portions, breaded *(Van de Kamp's)*, 3 pieces 23.0
sticks *(Kid Cuisine Funtastic)*, 8¼-oz. pkg. 55.0
sticks *(Swanson Fun Feast Frenzied)*, 1 pkg. 47.0

sticks, battered:

(Gorton's), 5 pieces 16.0
(Mrs. Paul's), 6 pieces 19.0
(Van de Kamp's), 6 pieces 18.0

sticks, breaded:

(Gorton's Crunchy), 6 pieces 16.9
(Gorton's Value Pack), 6 pieces 18.0
(Mrs. Paul's), 6 pieces 20.0
(Mrs. Paul's Crisp & Healthy), 6 pieces 26.0
(Mrs. Paul's Value Pack), 6 pieces 19.0

  (Van de Kamp's), 6 pieces 23.0
  (Van de Kamp's Crisp & Healthy), 6 pieces 26.0
  (Van de Kamp's Snack/Value Pack), 6 pieces 21.0
  mini *(Van de Kamp's),* 13 pieces 19.0
  potato *(Gorton's),* 6 pieces 22.0
Fish roe, see "Caviar" and "Roe"
Fish sandwich, fillet, frozen, 1 piece:
(Hormel Quick Meal) 48.0
with cheese *(Mrs. Paul's)* 38.0
Fish sauce mix, lemon butter *(Weight Watchers),* ¼ cup* . 1.0
Fish seasoning:
batter seasoning, Cajun *(Tone's),* 1 tsp. 2.6
seafood *(Old Bay),* ½ tsp. 0
seafood *(Tone's),* 1 tsp. 9
Fish seasoning and coating mix:
(Shake'n Bake), ¼ pkt. 14.0
lemon butter *(Durkee/French's* Roasting Bag), ¼ pkg. 6.0
lemon pepper dill *(Durkee Easy),* ⅙ pkg. 4.0
tomato basil *(Durkee Easy),* ⅐ pkg. 4.0
Flatbread, see "Cracker"
Flatfish, without added ingredients 0
Flavor enhancer *(Ac'cent),* ½ tsp. 0
Flax seeds *(Arrowhead Mills),* 3 tbsp. 11.0
Flounder:
fresh, without added ingredients 0
frozen *(Van de Kamp's),* 4 oz. 0
Flounder entree, fillets, frozen:
breaded *(Mrs. Paul's* Premium), 3-oz. piece 16.0
breaded *(Van de Kamp's* Light), 4-oz. piece 19.0
Flour, see "Wheat flour" and specific listings
Flying fish, without added ingredients 0
Fra diavolo sauce, see "Pasta sauce"
Frankfurter, 1 link, except as noted:
(Boar's Head) 0
(Hormel 10), 1.6 oz. 2.0
(Hormel 8), 2 oz. 2.0
(Hormel Big 8), 2 oz. 1.0
(Hormel Light & Lean 97), 1.6 oz. 4.0
(Hormel Light & Lean 97 Jumbo), 2 oz. 5.0
(John Morrell Fat Free), 1.4 oz. 6.0
(John Morrell Lite) 5.0
(Louis Rich Wieners) 3.0

Frankfurter *(cont.)*

(Oscar Mayer Wieners)	1.0
(Oscar Mayer Wieners Light)	2.0
(Oscar Mayer Wieners, Little), 6 links, 2 oz.	2.0
(Oscar Mayer Wieners, Little Hot & Spicy), 6 links, 2 oz.	1.0
(Oscar Mayer Big & Juicy Wieners)	1.0
(Oscar Mayer Bun-Length Wieners)	2.0
(Oscar Mayer Fat Free)	2.0
(Schwan's Old Fashioned Wieners)	2.0
(Schwan's Skinless)	2.0

beef:

(Boar's Head Giant)	1.0
(Boar's Head Lite)	0
(Boar's Head Skinless)	0
(Hebrew National/Hebrew National Reduced Fat), 1.7 oz.	1.0
(Hebrew National 8 oz./Quarter Pound/Jumbo)	1.0
(Hebrew National Bulk), 2.7 oz.	1.0
(Hebrew National Family Pack), 2 oz.	0
(Hebrew National Picnic Pack), 1.6 oz.	1.0
(Hebrew National Reduced Fat 3 lb.), 2.7 oz.	0
(Hormel 8)	1.0
(Hormel Light & Lean 97)	4.0
(Louis Rich)	3.0
(Oscar Mayer)	1.0
(Oscar Mayer Light)	2.0
(Oscar Mayer Big & Juicy), 2.7 oz.	1.0
(Oscar Mayer Big & Juicy Deli), 2.7 oz.	1.0
(Oscar Mayer Big & Juicy Quarter Pound), 4 oz.	2.0
(Oscar Mayer Bun-Length)	2.0
(Oscar Mayer Fat Free)	2.0
(Wranglers)	1.0

cocktail:

(Hormel), 5 links	1.0
beef *(Boar's Head)*, 5 links	0
beef *(Hebrew National)*, 4 links	0
beef *(Hebrew National* 32 oz.), 6 links	0
smoked *(Hormel Smokies)*, 5 links	1.0

cheese *(Oscar Mayer)*	1.0
cheese *(Wranglers)*	1.0
hot and spicy *(Oscar Mayer Big & Juicy)*	1.0
smoked *(Oscar Mayer Big & Juicy* Smokie)	1.0
smoked *(Wranglers)*	1.0

turkey, see "Turkey frankfurter"
"Frankfurter," vegetarian, 1 link:
(NewMenu VegiDog) 1.0
canned:
   (Loma Linda Big) 2.0
   (Loma Linda Linketts) 1.0
   (Worthington Veja-Links) 1.0
   (Worthington Veja-Links* Low Fat) 1.0
   (Worthington Super-Links) 2.0
frozen:
   (Morningstar Farms Deli Franks) 3.0
   (Natural Touch Vege) 2.0
   (Worthington Leanies) 2.0
   corn battered *(Loma Linda* Corn Dog) 18.0
refrigerated, chili *(Yves Veggie Cuisine* Dogs) 5.0
refrigerated, tofu *(Yves Veggie Cuisine* Weiners) 4.0
Frankfurter sandwich, frozen, 1 piece, except as noted:
(Hormel Quick Meal Jumbo Dog) 28.0
bagel wrapped *(Hebrew National* Bagel Dog) 47.0
bagel wrapped, with cheese *(Schwan's),* 4.5-oz. piece 34.0
on bun *(Swanson Fun Feast),* 1 pkg. 47.0
with cheese *(Hormel Quick Meal* Cheesey Dog) 29.0
chili with cheese *(Hormel Quick Meal)* 30.0
corn dog:
   (Hormel/Hormel Quick Meal) 25.0
   (Schwan's), 2.3-oz. piece 16.0
   mini *(Hormel Quick Meal),* 5 pieces 23.0
Franks and beans, see "Beans and franks"
French toast, frozen, 2 pieces, except as noted:
(Aunt Jemima Original) 38.0
(Downyflake) 43.0
apple cinnamon stick *(Schwan's),* 5 pieces 58.0
cinnamon *(Aunt Jemima)* 37.0
cinnamon swirl *(Downyflake)* 45.0
French toast breakfast, frozen, 1 pkg.:
cinnamon swirl *(Swanson Great Starts)* 34.0
with sausage *(Swanson Great Starts)* 33.0
sticks, with syrup *(Swanson Kids Breakfast Blast)* 50.0
Frosting, ready-to-spread, 2 tbsp., except as noted:
banana creme *(Pillsbury Creamy Supreme)* 23.0
butter cream *(Betty Crocker Creamy Deluxe)* 25.0
butter pecan *(Betty Crocker Creamy Deluxe)* 25.0

Frosting *(cont.)*
buttercream *(Duncan Hines)* 22.0
butterscotch *(Duncan Hines)* 22.0
caramel *(Duncan Hines)* 22.0
caramel chocolate chip *(Betty Crocker Creamy Deluxe)* 21.0
caramel pecan *(Pillsbury Creamy Supreme)* 19.0
cherry *(Betty Crocker Creamy Deluxe)* 24.0
chocolate:
   (Betty Crocker Creamy Deluxe) 24.0
   (Betty Crocker Creamy Deluxe Low Fat) 27.0
   (Betty Crocker Sweet Rewards), 1 tbsp. 26.0
   (Betty Crocker Whipped Deluxe) 14.0
   (Duncan Hines) 20.0
   (Pillsbury Creamy Supreme) 21.0
   (Pillsbury Creamy Supreme Funfetti) 22.0
   buttercream *(Duncan Hines)* 20.0
   chip *(Betty Crocker Creamy Deluxe)* 25.0
   chip cookie dough *(Betty Crocker Creamy Deluxe)* 25.0
   chocolate chip *(Betty Crocker Creamy Deluxe)* 23.0
   dark *(Betty Crocker Creamy Deluxe)* 22.0
   dark *(Duncan Hines)* 20.0
   dark *(Pillsbury Creamy Supreme)* 20.0
   with dinosaurs *(Betty Crocker Creamy Deluxe Party)* . . . 24.0
   fudge *(Pillsbury Creamy Supreme)* 21.0
   fudge *(SnackWell's)* 22.0
   fudge, hot *(Pillsbury Creamy Supreme)* 21.0
   milk *(Betty Crocker Creamy Deluxe)* 24.0
   milk *(Betty Crocker Creamy Deluxe Low Fat)* 27.0
   milk *(Betty Crocker Sweet Rewards),* 1 tbsp. 26.0
   milk *(Betty Crocker Whipped Deluxe)* 27.0
   milk *(Duncan Hines)* 20.0
   milk *(Pillsbury Creamy Supreme)* 21.0
   milk *(SnackWell's)* 22.0
   milk, swirl with fudge glaze *(Pillsbury Creamy Supreme)* 22.0
   mocha *(Duncan Hines)* 20.0
   mocha *(Pillsbury Creamy Supreme)* 22.0
   sour cream *(Betty Crocker Creamy Deluxe)* 23.0
   Swiss almond *(Betty Crocker Creamy Deluxe)* 25.0
coconut pecan *(Betty Crocker Creamy Deluxe)* 18.0
coconut pecan *(Pillsbury Creamy Supreme)* 17.0
cookie *(Pillsbury Creamy Supreme Oreo)* 23.0

cream cheese:
    (Betty Crocker Creamy Deluxe) 24.0
    (Betty Crocker Whipped Deluxe) 16.0
    (Duncan Hines) 22.0
    (Pillsbury Creamy Supreme) 24.0
lemon:
    (Betty Crocker Creamy Deluxe) 24.0
    (Betty Crocker Whipped Deluxe) 16.0
    cream *(Duncan Hines)* 22.0
    creme *(Pillsbury Creamy Supreme)* 24.0
rainbow, chip *(Betty Crocker Creamy Deluxe)* 25.0
raspberries n' cream *(Duncan Hines)* 22.0
strawberry:
    (Betty Crocker Whipped Deluxe) 16.0
    'n cream *(Duncan Hines)* 22.0
    cream cheese *(Betty Crocker Creamy Deluxe)* 26.0
    creme *(Pillsbury Creamy Supreme)* 24.0
vanilla:
    (Betty Crocker Creamy Deluxe Low Fat) 28.0
    (Betty Crocker Sweet Rewards), 1 tbsp. 26.0
    (Betty Crocker Whipped Deluxe) 16.0
    (Duncan Hines) 22.0
    (Pillsbury Creamy Supreme) 23.0
    (Pillsbury Creamy Supreme Funfetti) 25.0
    (SnackWell's) 25.0
    all varieties *(Betty Crocker Creamy Deluxe)* 24.0
    with bears *(Betty Crocker Creamy Deluxe Party)* 24.0
    French *(Pillsbury Creamy Supreme)* 25.0
    pink *(Pillsbury Creamy Supreme Funfetti)* 24.0
    swirl, with fudge glaze *(Pillsbury Creamy Supreme)* 25.0
    wild cherry *(Duncan Hines)* 22.0
white:
    (Betty Crocker Whipped Deluxe) 16.0
    chocolate *(Betty Crocker Creamy Deluxe)* 24.0
    sour cream *(Betty Crocker Creamy Deluxe)* 25.0
Frosting mix:
chocolate *(Robin Hood)*, 2 tbsp. dry or 2 tbsp.* 24.0
chocolate fudge *(Betty Crocker)*, 3 tbsp. dry or 2 tbsp.* . . . 24.0
coconut pecan *(Betty Crocker)*, 3 tbsp. dry or 2 tbsp.* 21.0
vanilla *(Betty Crocker)*, 3 tbsp. dry or 2 tbsp.* 24.0
white *(Betty Crocker)*, 3 tbsp. dry 24.0
Fructose *(Estee)*, 1 tsp. 4.0

Fruit, see specific listings
Fruit, candied, see specific listings
Fruit, mixed, candied:
(S&W Glace), 2 tbsp. 25.0
(White Swan), 1 tbsp., .8 oz. 18.0
(White Swan Deluxe), 2 tbsp., 1.2 oz. 25.0
fruit and peel mix *(Paradise* Old English), 1 tbsp., .8 oz. . . . 18.0
cake mix *(Queen Anne/Paradise* Extra Fancy), 2 tbsp.,
   1.2 oz. 25.0
Fruit, mixed, canned or in jars (see also "Fruit cocktail"),
   ½ cup, except as noted:
in juice:
   (Del Monte Naturals Snack Cup), 4-oz. cup 13.0
   chunky *(Del Monte* Naturals) 15.0
   chunky *(Libby's* Lite) 14.0
   chunky *(S&W* Natural) 19.0
in extra light syrup, chunky *(Del Monte* Lite) 15.0
in light syrup *(Del Monte* Lite Snack Cup), 4-oz. cup 13.0
in heavy syrup:
   (Del Monte Snack Cup), 4-oz. cup 20.0
   chunky *(Del Monte)* 24.0
salad, in light syrup *(Sunfresh)* 22.0
salad, in light syrup *(Sunfresh* Ambrosia) 16.0
salad, tropical, in light syrup:
   (Del Monte) 21.0
   (Dole) 20.0
   (Sunfresh) 20.0
Fruit, mixed, dried:
(Del Monte), ⅓ cup, 1.4 oz. 30.0
(Dole Sun Giant), 1.5 oz. 24.0
(Sonoma), 1.4 oz. 30.0
diced *(Sonoma),* ⅓ cup 31.0
and nuts, see "Trail mix"
Fruit, mixed, frozen:
(Big Valley), ⅔ cup 14.0
(Schwan's), 1¼ cups 17.0
(Stilwell), 1 cup 20.0
Fruit bar, frozen (see also "Ice bar" and "Yogurt bar"),
   1 bar:
all flavors:
   (Dole Fruit Juice) 11.0
   (Dole Fruit Juice No Sugar) 6.0

(Minute Maid Fruit Juice), 2.25 oz. 15.0
(Minute Maid Juice), 1.75 oz. 12.0
(Popsicle All Natural) 12.0
(Popsicle Junior) 26.0
(Popsicle Rainbow Jets) 12.0
(Popsicle Fantastic Fruity) 14.0
(Starburst 12-Pack) 12.0
(Starburst Singles) 20.0
(Starburst No Sugar Added) 6.0
banana cream *(Frozfruit)* 20.0
cantaloupe *(Frozfruit)* 15.0
cherry *(Frozfruit)* 18.0
coconut:
    (Dole Fruit 'n Juice), 4 oz. 33.0
    (Edy's/Dreyer's) 27.0
    cream *(Frozfruit)* 17.0
cranberry-apple *(Frozfruit)* 20.0
guava pineapple *(Frozfruit)* 20.0
kiwi-strawberry *(Frozfruit)* 23.0
lemon *(Frozfruit)* 22.0
lemon iced tea *(Frozfruit)* 19.0
lemonade *(Dole* Fruit 'n Juice), 4 oz. 24.0
lime:
    (Dole Fruit 'n Juice), 4 oz. 24.0
    (Edy's/Dreyer's) 23.0
    (Frozfruit) 21.0
orange *(Frozfruit)* 21.0
orange *(Minute Maid),* 3.75 oz. 24.0
peach *(Dole* Fruit 'n Juice), 2.5 oz. 17.0
peach *(Edy's/Dreyer's)* 35.0
piña colada, cream *(Frozfruit)* 23.0
pine-coconut *(Dole* Fruit 'n Juice), 4 oz. 27.0
pine-orange-banana *(Dole* Fruit 'n Juice), 2.5 oz. 16.0
pine-orange-banana *(Dole* Fruit 'n Juice), 4 oz. 26.0
pineapple *(Frozfruit)* 19.0
raspberry *(Dole* Fruit 'n Juice), 2.5 oz. 16.0
raspberry *(Frozfruit)* 20.0
raspberry-kiwi *(Edy's/Dreyer's)* 23.0
strawberry:
    (Dole Fruit 'n Juice), 2.5 oz. 17.0
    (Dole Fruit 'n Juice), 4 oz. 26.0
    (Edy's/Dreyer's) 23.0

Fruit bar, frozen, strawberry *(cont.)*
    (Frozfruit) 20.0
    (Minute Maid), 3.75 oz. 31.0
    (Schwan's) 12.0
    banana cream *(Frozfruit)* 21.0
    cream *(Frozfruit)* 21.0
tropical *(Frozfruit)* 23.0
watermelon *(Frozfruit)* 13.0
Fruit cocktail, canned, ½ cup:
(Del Monte Very Cherry) 22.0
(Hunt's) 23.0
in water 10.4
in juice:
    (Del Monte Naturals) 15.0
    (Libby's Lite) 15.0
    (S&W Natural) 20.0
in extra light syrup *(Del Monte* Lite) 15.0
in light syrup 18.0
in heavy syrup *(Del Monte)* 24.0
in heavy syrup *(S&W)* 23.0
honey flavor *(Del Monte* Natural) 20.0
Fruit dip, see "Caramel dip" and "Chocolate fruit dip"
Fruit drink blends (see also "Soft drinks" and specific
    listings):
(Capri Sun Mountain Cooler), 6.75 fl. oz. 26.0
(Capri Sun Pacific Cooler), 6.75 fl. oz. 29.0
(Capri Sun Surfer Cooler), 6.75 fl. oz. 27.0
(Dole Fruit Fiesta), 16 fl. oz. 68.0
(Dole Lanai), 16 fl. oz. 59.0
(Dole Tropical Breeze), 16 fl. oz. 59.0
(Hi-C Ecto Cooler), 8 fl. oz. 32.0
(Hi-C Ecto Cooler Box), 8.45 fl. oz. 34.0
(Lincoln Party), 8 fl. oz. 34.0
(Snapple Bali Blast), 8 fl. oz. 30.0
(Snapple Samoan Splash), 8 fl. oz. 29.0
(Tropicana), 8 fl. oz. 32.0
(Veryfine Avalanche), 8 fl. oz. 26.0
(Veryfine Tropical Breeze), 8 fl. oz. 30.0
nectar *(Kern's* Tropical), 11.5 fl. oz. 48.0
punch:
    (Capri Sun), 6.75 fl. oz. 26.0
    (Capri Sun Maui), 6.75 fl. oz. 28.0

(Capri Sun Safari), 6.75 fl. oz.	25.0
(Dole Paradise), 10 fl. oz.	38.0
(Dole Tropical), 10 fl. oz.	33.0
(Farmer's Market Tropical), 8 fl. oz.	29.0
(Heinke's California), 8 fl. oz.	28.0
(Heinke's Macchu Pichu), 8 fl. oz.	30.0
(Heinke's Paradise), 8 fl. oz.	28.0
(Hi-C), 8 fl. oz.	29.0
(Hi-C 16 oz.), 8 fl. oz.	32.0
(Hi-C Box), 8.45 fl. oz.	34.0
(Hi-C Tropical Box), 8 fl. oz.	32.0
(Hi-C Blue Cooler), 8 fl. oz.	31.0
(Hi-C Blue Cooler Box), 8.45 fl. oz.	33.0
(R.W. Knudsen Rain Forest), 8 fl. oz.	29.0
(R.W. Knudsen Tropical/Tropical Aseptic), 8 fl. oz.	29.0
(Minute Maid), 8 fl. oz.	31.0
(Minute Maid Box), 8 fl. oz.	33.0
(Snapple), 8 fl. oz.	28.0
(Tree Top), 8 fl. oz.	32.0
(Tree Top Juice Rivers Box), 8.45 fl. oz.	33.0
tropical *(Minute Maid* Premium), 8 fl. oz.	30.0
tropical *(Minute Maid* Premium Box), 8 fl. oz.	31.0

frozen*, 8 fl. oz.:

(Dole Fruit Fiesta)	34.0
(Dole Lanai)	30.0
(Dole Tropical Breeze)	30.0
punch *(R.W. Knudsen* Tropical)	29.0
punch *(Minute Maid* Premium)	31.0
punch *(Schwan's Vita-Sun)*	24.0
punch, tropical *(Minute Maid* Premium)	29.0

Fruit glacé, see "Fruit, mixed, candied" and specific listings

Fruit glaze, see "Glaze"

Fruit juice, see specific fruit listings

Fruit juice blends (see also specific listings), 8 fl. oz., except as noted:

(Ceres Medley)	31.0
(R.W. Knudsen Morning Blend/Vita)	31.0
(R.W. Knudsen Natural Breakfast)	29.0
(Season's Best Medley)	32.0
(Snapple Vitamin Supreme), 10 fl. oz.	38.0

punch:

(After the Fall Maui)	23.0

Fruit juice blends, punch *(cont.)*
   (After the Fall Sangria de la Noche) 30.0
   (Apple & Eve Nothin' But Juice) 29.0
   (Juicy Juice) 32.0
   (Tree Top), 10 fl. oz. 37.0
   (Tree Top), 11.5 fl. oz. 43.0
   (Tree Top Box), 8.45 fl. oz. 32.0
   (Veryfine Juice-Ups) 36.0
   citrus *(R.W. Knudsen* Aseptic) 29.0
tropical fruit:
   (Dole), 10 fl. oz. 44.0
   (Juicy Juice) 29.0
   chilled or frozen* *(Dole)* 34.0
frozen* *(R.W. Knudsen* Natural Breakfast) 27.0
Fruit and nut mix, see "Trail mix"
Fruit pectin:
(Sure•Jell), ¼ tsp. 1.0
unsweetened, 1¾-oz. pkg. 45.2
Fruit protector *(Ever-Fresh),* ¼ tsp. 1.0
Fruit snack, all varieties, 1 oz., except as noted:
all varieties:
   (Betty Crocker Tazmanian Devil), 1 pouch 21.0
   (Fruit By the Foot), 1 roll 17.0
   (Fruit Roll Ups), 2 rolls 24.0
   (Fruit Roll Ups Pouch), 1 roll 12.0
   (Gushers), 1 pouch 20.0
   (Smart Snackers), .5 oz. 13.0
apple *(Stretch Island)* 25.0
apple, organic *(Stretch Island)* 24.0
apricot *(Stretch Island)* 23.0
blackberry *(Stretch Island)* 24.0
cherry *(Stretch Island)* 24.0
grape, regular or organic *(Stretch Island)* 24.0
raspberry, organic *(Stretch Island)* 25.0
tropical *(Stretch Island)* 22.0
Fruit spreads (see also "Jam and preserves"), 1 tbsp.:
all varieties:
   (R.W. Knudsen) 13.0
   (Kraft Reduced Calorie) 5.0
   (Polaner) 10.0
   (Simply Fruit) 13.0
   (Slenderella Reduced Calorie) 5.0

(Smucker's Homestyle) 11.0
and peanuts *(Smucker's* Super Spreaders) 10.0
Fruit syrup (see also specific listings), ¼ cup:
(Smucker's) 52.0
light *(Smucker's)* 33.0
and maple *(R.W. Knudsen)* 38.0
Fruit-nut mix, see "Trail mix"
Fudge, see "Candy"
Fudge topping, see "Chocolate topping"
Fusilli, plain, dry, see "Pasta"
Fusilli, refrigerated *(Tutta Pasta),* 1 cup 58.0
Fusilli pasta mix, with creamy pesto *(Knorr),* ⅔ cup 47.0

G

Gai choy, see "Cabbage, mustard"
Gai lan, see "Kale, Chinese"
Garbanzo beans, see "Chickpeas"
Garbanzo flour *(Arrowhead Mills),* ¼ cup 15.0
Garden salad, ½ cup:
dill *(S&W)* 14.0
marinated *(S&W)* 13.0
Garlic:
trimmed, 1 oz. 9.4
1 clove, approx. .1 oz. 1.0
crushed *(Christopher Ranch),* 1 tsp. 1.0
crushed *(Frieda's),* 1 oz. 8.7
granulated, 1 tsp. 2.9
granulated *(Tone's),* ¼ tsp. 1.0
Garlic, elephant *(Frieda's),* 1 tbsp. 1.0
Garlic, pickled *(Christopher Ranch),* 3 pieces, ¼ oz. 0
Garlic dip, 2 tbsp.:
(Nalley) 2.0
Italian *(Marie's)* 3.0
roasted, and onion *(Marie's* Fat Free) 7.0
Garlic dressing *(Christopher Ranch),* 1 tbsp. 1.0
Garlic pepper:
(Tone's), ¼ tsp. 0
(Lawry's), ¼ tsp. 0
1 tsp. 1.8
Garlic pickle relish *(Patak's),* 1 tbsp. 4.0
Garlic powder:
(McCormick), ¼ tsp. 5
(Tone's), ¼ tsp. 1.0
1 tbsp. 6.1
1 tsp. 2.3
Garlic salt:
(Durkee California), ½ tsp. 0
(Lawry's), ¼ tsp. 0
(Morton), ½ tsp. . . . . <1.0

(Tone's), ¼ tsp. 0
1 tsp. 5
Garlic spread:
(Lawry's Concentrate), 2 tsp. 1.0
(Lawry's Ready-to-Spread), 1 tbsp. 2.0
Garlic sprouts *(Jonathan's),* 1 cup, 4 oz. 14.0
Garlic-basil, chopped *(Paesana),* 1 tsp. 0
Gefilte fish, drained:
(Manischewitz Gold/Jelled Broth), 1 ball with jell 10.0
(Manischewitz Gold Vegetable Medley), 1 ball and ⅙ carrot . 5.0
(Manischewitz Gold with Olives/Carrots), 1 ball and ¼ carrot . 3.0
zesty *(Manischewitz* Gold/Brine), 1 ball 4.0
Gelatin, unflavored *(Knox),* 1 pkt. 0
Gelatin dessert, all flavors, 1 cont.:
(Hunt's Snack Pack) 25.0
(Jell-O Snacks) 18.0
(Jell-O Sugar Free Snacks) 0
(Kraft Handi-Snacks) 20.0
(Swiss Miss Gels) 18.0
Gelatin dessert mix*, ½ cup, except as noted:
all flavors *(Jell-O Sugar Free)* 0
all flavors, except black raspberry *(Jell-O)* 19.0
black raspberry *(Jell-O)* 20.0
strawberry *(D-Zerta)* 0
strawberry *(Jell-O 1-2-3),* ⅔ cup 26.0
Gelatin drink mix, orange *(Knox),* 1 pkt. 4.0
Ghee, see "Butter"
Gardiniera, see "Vegetables, mixed, pickled"
Gil choy, see "Chives, Chinese"
Ginger, root:
(Frieda's), 1 tbsp. 1.0
untrimmed, 1 lb. 63.6
trimmed, 1 oz. 4.3
chopped *(Christopher Ranch),* 1 tsp. 3.0
5 slices, ⅛″ × 1″ diam. 1.7
sliced, ¼ cup 3.6
Ginger, candied or crystallized:
(Frieda's), 9 pieces, 1.1 oz. 26.0
(Paradise/White Swan), 3 pieces, 1 oz. 26.0
Ginger, ground:
(McCormick), ¼ tsp. 4
1 tbsp. 3.8

Ginger, ground *(cont.)*
1 tsp. 1.3
Ginger, pickled:
(Eden), 1 tbsp. 3.0
Japanese, 1 oz. 2.1
Ginger drink *(Santa Cruz Hawaiian),* 8 fl. oz. 27.0
Gingerbread, see "Bread mix, sweet"
Ginkgo nut:
in shell:
   raw, 1 lb. 129.6
   raw, 4 oz. 32.4
   dried, 4 oz. 62.5
shelled, raw, 1 oz. 10.7
shelled, dried, 1 oz. 20.6
canned, 1 oz., approx. 22 small, 11 medium, or 9 large 6.3
canned, 1 cup 34.3
Glacé, cake, see "Fruit, mixed, candied"
Glaze, fruit, 2 tbsp.:
for banana, creamy *(Marie's)* 8.0
for blueberries, peaches, or strawberries *(Marie's)* 10.0
pie, strawberry *(Smucker's)* 21.0
Glaze, ham, see "Ham glaze"
Glaze mix, see "Seasoning and coating mix"
Gluten, see "Wheat flour"
Goa beans, see "Winged beans"
Goat, without added ingredients 0
Goatfish, without added ingredients 0
Gobo root, see "Burdock root"
Godfather's Pizza, 1 slice:
cheese, original crust:
   mini, ¼ pie 19.0
   medium, ⅛ pie 34.0
   large, ¹⁄₁₀ pie 36.0
   jumbo, ¹⁄₁₀ pie 53.0
cheese, golden crust:
   medium, ⅛ pie 26.0
   large, ¹⁄₁₀ pie 28.0
combo, original crust:
   mini, ¼ pie 21.0
   medium, ⅛ pie 36.0
   large, ¹⁄₁₀ pie 38.0
   jumbo, ¹⁄₁₀ pie 56.0

combo, golden crust:
    medium, ⅛ pie 28.0
    large, ⅒ pie 31.0
Golden nugget squash *(Frieda's)*, ¾ cup, 3 oz. 7.0
Goose, without added ingredients 0
Goose fat 0
Goose liver, see "Liver" and "Pâté"
Gooseberry:
fresh:
    untrimmed, 1 lb. 46.2
    trimmed, 1 oz. 7.6
    green *(Frieda's)*, 1 oz. 2.7
canned, in light syrup *(Comstock)*, ½ cup 20.0
canned, in light syrup, ½ cup 23.6
Gorgonzola sauce, refrigerated *(Monterey Pasta Company)*,
    4 oz. 3.0
Goulash seasoning mix *(Knorr* Recipe), 1⅓ tbsp. 6.0
Gourd:
dishcloth:
    raw, untrimmed, 1 lb. 14.4
    raw, 1 medium, approx. 8.5 oz. 7.8
    boiled, drained, 1″ slices, ½ cup 12.8
white-flower:
    raw, untrimmed, 1 lb. 10.8
    raw, 1 medium, approx. 2.5 lb. 26.1
    boiled, drained, 1″ cubes, ½ cup 2.7
Gourd strips, see "Kanpyo"
Grains, see specific listings
Granadilla, see "Passion fruit"
Granola, see "Cereal"
Granola and cereal bar (see also "Snack bar"), 1 bar,
    except as noted:
(Rice Krispies Treats) 18.0
all varieties:
    (Health Valley Fat Free Granola) 35.0
    (Health Valley Healthy Breakfast Bakes Fat Free) 26.0
    (Health Valley Healthy Cereal Bars No Fat) 26.0
    (Health Valley Healthy Energy Bars) 40.0
    (Kellogg's Low Fat) 16.0
    (Nature's Choice Fat Free Granola) 23.0
    (Nature's Choice Real Fruit), 2 bars 26.0
    (Nutri-Grain) 27.0

Granola and cereal bar, all varieties *(cont.)*
    (Quaker Chewy Lowfat) 22.0
    except oatmeal raisin and orchard blend *(Nature Valley*
       Low Fat) 21.0
    scones *(Health Valley)* 43.0
with almonds, chewy *(Little Debbie)* 25.0
apple filled *(Nature's Choice* Fat Free Cereal) 27.0
blueberry filled *(Nature's Choice* Fat Free Cereal) 27.0
carob chip *(Nature's Choice* Granola) 16.0
chocolate chip:
    (Carnation Chewy) 22.0
    (Kudos Enrobed) 19.0
    (Little Debbie) 33.0
    (Nature's Choice Grrr-Nola Treats) 15.0
    (Quaker Chewy) 21.0
    (Rice Krispies) 20.0
    chunk *(Carnation* Granola) 22.0
cinnamon *(Nature Valley)*, 2 bars 35.0
cinnamon and oats *(Barbara's* Granola) 31.0
cinnamon raisin *(Nature's Choice* Granola) 16.0
coconut almond *(Barbara's* Granola) 23.0
cranberry filled *(Nature's Choice* Fat Free Cereal) 27.0
fudge:
    (Kudos) 19.0
    dipped, macaroon *(Little Debbie)* 34.0
    dipped, with peanuts *(Little Debbie)* 33.0
(Kudos M&M's) 17.0
(Kudos Snickers) 16.0
oatmeal raisin:
    (Little Debbie) 33.0
    (Nature Valley Low Fat) 22.0
    (Sweet Success) 23.0
oats and honey:
    (Carnation Granola) 23.0
    (Little Debbie) 32.0
    (Nature's Choice Granola) 15.0
oats 'n honey *(Nature Valley)*, 2 bars 35.0
orchard blend *(Nature Valley* Low Fat) 22.0
peach filled *(Nature's Choice* Fat Free Cereal) 27.0
peanut butter:
    (Barbara's Granola) 28.0
    (Kudos) 18.0

(Nature Valley), 2 bars 33.0
(Nature's Choice Granola) 14.0
chocolate chip (Carnation Chewy) 21.0
chocolate chip (Quaker Chewy) 19.0
and jelly (Nature's Choice Grrr-Nola) 14.0
raspberry filled (Nature's Choice Fat Free Cereal) 27.0
strawberry filled (Nature's Choice Fat Free Cereal) 27.0
Grape, fresh:
(Dole), 1½ cups 24.0
(Frieda's), 4.9 oz. 25.0
American type (slipskin):
   untrimmed, 1 lb. 45.1
   10 medium 4.1
   peeled and seeded, ½ cup 7.9
European type (adherent skin):
   untrimmed, 1 lb. 72.0
   seedless, 10 medium 8.9
   seedless or seeded, ½ cup 14.2
Grape, canned, seedless, ½ cup:
in water 12.6
in heavy syrup:
   (Comstock) 23.0
   (S&W) 23.0
   (S&W Fancy Jubilee) 33.0
   ½ cup 25.2
Grape drink, 8 fl. oz., except as noted:
(Capri Sun), 6.75 fl. oz. 28.0
(Dole), 10 fl. oz. 38.0
(Hi-C) 32.0
(Hi-C Box), 8.45 fl. oz. 34.0
(Lincoln) 32.0
(Veryfine Glacial) 28.0
grapeade (Snapple) 28.0
punch (Tree Top Juice Rivers Box), 8.45 fl. oz. 36.0
punch, chilled or frozen* (Minute Maid) 32.0
frozen*:
   (Bright & Early) 34.0
   (Minute Maid) 33.0
   (Schwan's Vita-Sun) 26.0
   juice cocktail (Schwan's) 26.0
   white cocktail (Seneca) 32.0

Grape drink mix, 8 fl. oz.*:
(Kool-Aid) 25.0
(Kool-Aid with Sugar) 16.0
Grape juice, 8 fl. oz., except as noted:
(After the Fall Concord) 31.0
(Goya) 36.0
(Juicy Juice) 32.0
(R.W. Knudsen Aseptic) 35.0
(R.W. Knudsen Concord) 40.0
(Lucky Leaf) 34.0
(Minute Maid Box), 8.45 fl. oz. 32.0
(Season's Best) 39.0
(Veryfine) 37.0
(Veryfine Juice-Ups) 32.0
purple *(Seneca)* 40.0
white *(Seneca)* 41.0
bottled or frozen* *(R.W. Knudsen)* 37.0
frozen *(Seneca)*, 2 oz. 40.0
Grape leaves, in jars *(Krinos)*, 1 leaf 0
Grape leaves, stuffed:
(Cedar's), 6 pieces, 5 oz. 22.0
in jars *(Perfecta* Dolmadakia), 4.4 oz. 19.9
Grapefruit, fresh:
(Dole), ½ medium 18.0
pink or red:
   California or Arizona, ½ medium, 3¾″ diam. 11.9
   California or Arizona, sections with juice, ½ cup 11.1
   Florida, ½ medium, 3¾″ diam. 9.2
   Florida, sections with juice, ½ cup 8.6
white:
   California, ½ medium, 3¾″ diam. 10.7
   California, sections with juice, ½ cup 10.5
   Florida, ½ medium, 3¾″ diam. 9.7
   Florida, sections with juice, ½ cup 9.4
Grapefruit, canned or chilled:
(S&W Natural Style), ⅔ cup 14.0
in water, ½ cup 11.2
in juice, ½ cup 11.4
in juice, pink or white *(Sunfresh)*, ½ cup 9.0
Grapefruit drink, 8 fl. oz., except as noted:
pink:
   (Ocean Spray) 28.0

(Tree Top Desert Ice) 29.0
(Tropicana Twister) 29.0
(Tropicana Twister), 11.5 fl. oz. 40.0
(Tropicana Twister Light). 10.0
frozen* *(Schwan's)* 27.0
ruby red *(Ocean Spray)* 33.0
ruby red and tangerine *(Ocean Spray)* 32.0
Grapefruit juice, 8 fl. oz., except as noted:
fresh 22.4
fresh, juice from 3¾″ fruit 18.0
(Dole), 10 fl. oz. 29.0
(Goya) 36.0
(Ocean Spray) 24.0
(S&W), 6 fl. oz. 18.0
(S&W) 25.0
(Tree Top) 25.0
(Tree Top), 10 fl. oz. 30.0
(Tree Top), 11.5 fl. oz. 35.0
(Veryfine) 20.0
blend *(Dole* Sunripe) 31.0
blend, cranberry *(Apple & Eve* Ruby Red) 30.0
golden *(Tropicana)* 23.0
pink *(R.W. Knudsen)* 23.0
red *(R.W. Knudsen* Rio) 35.0
red, ruby *(Tropicana* Carton/Plastic) 25.0
white *(R.W. Knudsen)* 23.0
frozen* *(Minute Maid)* 24.0
Gravy, see specific listings
Great northern beans:
dried, ¼ cup 29.3
dried, boiled, ½ cup 18.6
canned, ½ cup:
    (Allens) 19.0
    (Eden Organic Jars) 23.0
    (Goya) 18.0
    (Green Giant/Joan of Arc) 18.0
    (Seneca) 26.0
    (Stokely) 19.0
    (Sun-Vista) 17.0
    with liquid 27.6
    with sausage *(Trappey's)* 18.0

Green beans, fresh:

raw:

    (Dole), ¾ cup, 3 oz. 5.0

    untrimmed, 1 lb. 28.5

    trimmed, ½ cup 3.9

boiled, drained, ½ cup 4.9

Green beans, canned, ½ cup, except as noted:

(Allens Shells Out) 6.0

(Goya) 4.0

(Green Giant Kitchen Sliced) 4.0

(Green Giant Kitchen Sliced Less Sodium) 3.0

(Seneca) 5.0

(Stokely/Stokely No Salt) 4.0

all varieties, except Italian cut *(Del Monte/Del Monte* No

    Salt) 4.0

whole *(Green Giant)* 5.0

whole, cut, or French *(S&W)* 4.0

cut:

    (Allens/Sunshine/Alma/Crest Top) 6.0

    (Allens No Salt) 3.0

    (Green Giant/Green Giant Less Sodium) 4.0

    with wax beans *(S&W)* 4.0

French style *(Allens)* 3.0

French style *(Green Giant)* 4.0

Italian cut *(Allens/Sunshine)* 7.0

Italian cut *(Del Monte)* 6.0

dilled *(S&W)*, 1 oz. 5.0

with potatoes *(Allens/Sunshine)* 7.0

Green beans, freeze-dried *(Mountain House)*, ⅔ cup 5.0

Green beans, frozen:

(Seabrook), 1 cup 4.0

whole *(Birds Eye)*, 3 oz. 5.0

cut:

    (Green Giant), ¾ cup 5.0

    (Green Giant Harvest Fresh), ⅔ cup 5.0

    (Schwan's), ⅔ cup 6.0

    or French cut *(Birds Eye)*, ½ cup 6.0

Italian *(Birds Eye)*, ½ cup 8.0

sliced *(Stilwell)*, ⅔ cup 4.0

with blue cheese *(Birds Eye)*, ½ cup 6.0

with toasted almonds *(Birds Eye)*, ¾ cup 7.0

Green bean combinations, frozen:
and almonds *(Green Giant Harvest Fresh),* ⅔ cup 5.0
mushroom casserole *(Stouffer's),* 3.8 oz. 13.0
potatoes, onions, and peppers *(Green Giant American
   Mixtures)* ¾ cup 8.0
Green peas, see "Peas, green"
Green pepper, see "Pepper, sweet"
Greens (see also specific listings), mixed, canned *(Allens/
   Sunshine),* ½ cup 8.0
Grenadine syrup, 2 tbsp.:
(Mr & Mrs T) 18.0
(Rose's) 22.0
Grilling sauce (see also specific listings), 2 tbsp., except as
   noted:
Chardonnay *(Knorr)* 2.0
herb, Tuscan *(Knorr)* 2.0
mandarin ginger *(Knorr* Microwave) 3.0
Parmesano *(Knorr* Microwave), 3 tbsp. 3.0
plum, spicy *(Knorr)* 9.0
tequila lime *(Knorr)* 5.0
Grits, see "Corn grits"
Ground cherry:
in husk, 1 lb. 47.8
trimmed, ½ cup 7.8
Grouper, without added ingredients 0
Guacamole dip (see also "Avocado dip"), *(Nalley),* 2 tbsp. . 2.0
Guacamole seasoning *(Lawry's),* ½ tsp. 1.0
Guanabana, frozen, chunks *(Goya),* ⅓ pkg. 13.0
Guanabana nectar, canned *(Goya),* 12 fl. oz. 57.0
Guava:
common:
   untrimmed, 1 lb. 43.1
   1 medium, 4 oz. 10.7
   ½ cup 9.8
strawberry, untrimmed, 1 lb. 66.0
strawberry, ½ cup 21.2
Guava drink, 8 fl. oz.:
(Mauna La'l) 32.0
(Snapple Guava Mania) 29.0
Guava juice *(After the Fall* Maya), 8 fl. oz. 28.0
Guava nectar:
(Goya), 12 fl. oz. 59.0

Guava nectar *(cont.)*

(Kern's), 8 fl. oz. 38.0

(Libby's/Kern's), 11.5 fl. oz. 54.0

Guava paste *(Goya)*, ¾″ slice 24.0

Guava sauce, cooked, ½ cup 11.3

Guavadilla, see "Passion fruit"

Guinea hen, without added ingredients 0

Gumbo dinner mix *(Luzianne)*, ⅕ pkg. 33.0

Gyro mix *(Casbah)*, ¹⁄₁₀ pkg. 12.0

H

FOOD AND MEASURE   **CARBOHYDRATE GRAMS**

Häagen-Dazs Ice Cream Shop:
ice cream, ½ cup:
- butter pecan 20.0
- *Brownies a la Mode (Exträas)* 26.0
- *Cappuccino Commotion (Exträas)* 25.0
- *Caramel Cone Explosion (Exträas)*............. 27.0
- chocolate 22.0
- chocolate chip............................. 24.0
- chocolate chocolate, Belgian 29.0
- chocolate chocolate chip 26.0
- chocolate chocolate mint................... 25.0
- chocolate peanut butter, deep 27.0
- coffee 21.0
- coffee chip 25.0
- *Cookie Dough Dynamo (Exträas)* 29.0
- cookies & cream 23.0
- macadamia brittle 25.0
- macadamia nut 20.0
- *Midnight Cookies and Cream* 29.0
- pralines & cream 27.0
- rum raisin 22.0
- strawberry 23.0
- *Strawberry Cheesecake Craze (Exträas)* 27.0
- Swiss chocolate almond 23.0
- vanilla 21.0
- vanilla fudge 26.0
- vanilla Swiss almond 23.0
ice cream bar, 1 bar:
- chocolate, uncoated 16.0
- coffee 15.0
- vanilla, uncoated 15.0
sorbet, ½ cup:
- banana strawberry 34.0
- chocolate 30.0
- mango 30.0

Häagen-Dazs, sorbet *(cont.)*
    orchard peach 35.0
    raspberry 30.0
    strawberry 33.0
    Zesty Lemon 31.0
sorbet, soft-serve, mango or raspberry, ¹/₂ cup 25.0
yogurt, soft-serve, ¹/₂ cup:
    chocolate, nonfat 23.0
    chocolate mousse, nonfat 24.0
    coffee 20.0
    vanilla, nonfat 22.0
    vanilla mousse, nonfat 23.0
Habaneros chili, see "Pepper, chili"
Haddock, without added ingredients 0
Haddock, frozen, raw, fillet *(Schwan's),* 4 oz. 0
Haddock entree, frozen:
battered *(Van de Kamp's),* 2 pieces 18.0
breaded:
    (Mrs. Paul's Premium), 1 piece 17.0
    (Van de Kamp's), 2 pieces 19.0
    (Van de Kamp's Light), 1 piece 19.0
    squares *(Schwan's),* 1 piece, 4 oz. 17.0
    sticks *(Schwan's),* 3 pieces, 3 oz. 13.0
Hake, see "Blue hake" and "Whiting"
Halibut, Atlantic or Pacific, without added ingredients 0
Halibut, frozen *(Peter Pan),* 4 oz. 0
Halibut entree, frozen, battered *(Van de Kamp's),* 3 pieces 22.0
Halvah, chocolate *(Joyva),* 1.75 oz. 16.0
Ham, fresh, without added ingredients 0
Ham, cured:
whole leg, unheated, 4 oz. 1
whole leg, roasted, 4 oz. or 1 cup chopped or diced 0
boneless:
    (11% fat), unheated, 4 oz. 3.5
    (11% fat), roasted, 4 oz. or 1 cup chopped or diced 0
    extra lean (5% fat), unheated, 4 oz. 1.1
    extra lean (5% fat), roasted, 4 oz. 1.7
    extra lean (5% fat), roasted, chopped or diced, 1 cup . . . 2.1
Ham, canned or refrigerated, 3 oz., except as noted:
(Black Label Refrigerated/Shelf) 0
(Curemaster Half) 0
(Hormel Light & Lean) 2.0

(John Morrell Boneless) 2.0
(Jones Dairy Farm Country Carved Family) 0
(Oscar Mayer Slice/Steak) 0
(Schwan's Haugin's Farm), 2 oz. 1.0
(Swift Premium) 1.0
all varieties *(Jones Dairy Farm)* 0
baked *(Louis Rich Dinner),* 3.3-oz. slice 1.0
Black Forest *(Boar's Head Baby)* 3.0
chunk *(Hormel),* 2 oz. 0
honey *(Patrick Cudahy ReaLean)* 5.0
maple *(Boar's Head Baby Honey Coat)* 4.0
maple *(Jones Dairy Farm Country Carved Family)* 1.0
maple glaze *(Boar's Head Sweet Slice)* ....<1.0
minced, 1 oz. 5
smoke flavor *(Patrick Cudahy ReaLean)* 4.0
smoked *(Boar's Head Sweet Slice)* ....<1.0
smoked, semi-boneless *(Boar's Head)* 1.0
spiral sliced *(Spiral Cure 81 Half)* 1.0
steak:
   (Jones Dairy Farm Lean Choice/Rock River) 0
   honey *(Patrick Cudahy)* 4.0
   smoke flavor *(Patrick Cudahy)* 1.0
Virginia *(Boar's Head Ready-to-Eat)* 3.0
Virginia, smoked *(Boar's Head Baby Gourmet)* ... 1.0
"Ham," vegetarian, frozen, sliced *(Worthington Wham),*
  2 slices 1.0
Ham bologna *(Boar's Head),* 2 oz. 2.0
Ham glaze:
(Crosse & Blackwell), 1 tbsp. 8.0
(Marzetti), 2 tbsp. 9.0
Ham lunch meat (see also "Prosciutto"), 2 oz., except as
  noted:
(Boar's Head Deluxe) 2.0
(Boar's Head Lower Sodium Extra Lean) ....<1.0
(Healthy Deli Cinnamon Apple Grove) 4.0
(Healthy Deli Deluxe/Less Sodium/Old Tyme Taverne) 1.0
(Hormel Light & Lean 97), 1-oz. slice 0
(Hormel Light & Lean 97 Deli) 0
(Jones Dairy Farm Lean Choice), 2 slices 0
(Menumaster), 1 oz. 1.0
(Old Tyme), 1 oz. 0
(Oscar Mayer Lower Sodium), 3 slices 2.0

Ham lunch meat *(cont.)*
baked:
    (Louis Rich Carving Board), 2 slices 1.0
    (Oscar Mayer), 3 slices, 2.2 oz. 2.0
    (Oscar Mayer Fat Free), 3 slices, 1.7 oz. 1.0
baked, Virginia *(Healthy Deli/Healthy Deli Less Sodium)* 3.0
Black Forest *(Boar's Head)* 2.0
Black Forest *(Healthy Deli)* 1.0
boiled:
    (Oscar Mayer), 3 slices, 2.2 oz. 0
    (Oscar Mayer Deli-Thin), 4 slices 1.0
    (Patrick Cudahy), 1-oz. slice . . . . <1.0
cappacola *(Boar's Head Cappy)* 3.0
cappacola *(Healthy Deli Cappi)* 2.0
chopped *(Black Label)* 3.0
chopped *(Oscar Mayer)*, 1-oz. slice 1.0
cooked:
    (Alpine Lace) 1.0
    (Hormel Deli) 2.0
    (Hormel Low Salt) 1.0
    (Patrick Cudahy Less Sodium), 1-oz. slice 0
honey:
    (Healthy Deli Honey Valley Farms) 2.0
    (Louis Rich Fat Free), 2 slices 2.0
    (Louis Rich Carving Board Thin), 6 slices 2.0
    (Louis Rich Carving Board Traditional) 1.0
    (Oscar Mayer), 3 slices, 2.2 oz. 2.0
    (Oscar Mayer Deli-Thin), 4 slices 2.0
    (Oscar Mayer Fat Free), 3 slices, 1.7 oz. 2.0
    (Patrick Cudahy), 1-oz. slice 1.0
hot *(Healthy Deli Rodeo)* 1.0
jalapeño *(Healthy Deli)* 3.0
maple:
    (Boar's Head Honey Coat) 3.0
    (Healthy Deli Vermont) 3.0
    (Patrick Cudahy), 1-oz. slice 2.0
pepper *(Boar's Head)* 3.0
pepper *(Healthy Deli)* 2.0
smoked:
    (Boar's Head Gourmet) 2.0
    (Hormel Light & Lean 97 Deli) 2.0
    (Louis Rich Fat Free), 2 slices 1.0

    (Louis Rich Carving Board), 2 slices 0
    (Oscar Mayer), 3 slices, 2.2 oz. 0
    (Oscar Mayer Deli-Thin), 4 slices 0
    double *(Healthy Deli)* 1.0
spiced *(Boar's Head)* 1.0
Virginia *(Boar's Head)* 3.0
Virginia *(Healthy Deli)* 2.0
Ham patty *(Hormel)*, 2-oz. patty 1.0
Ham salad spread *(Libby's Spreadables)*, ⅓ cup 8.0
Ham spread:
deviled:
    (Cure 81), 2 oz. 1.0
    (Underwood), ¼ cup 0
    with crackers *(Red Devil Snackers)*, 1 pkg. 18.0
honey *(Underwood)*, ¼ cup 3.0
honey, with crackers *(Red Devil Snackers)*, 1 pkg. 20.0
Ham and asparagus entree, bake, frozen *(Stouffer's)*,
    9½ oz. 32.0
Ham and cheese loaf *(Oscar Mayer)*, 1 oz. 1.0
Ham and cheese patty *(Hormel)*, 2-oz. patty 0
Ham and cheese sandwich, frozen, 1 piece:
(Croissant Pockets), 4.5-oz. piece 39.0
(Deli Stuffs), 4.5-oz. piece 42.0
(Hormel Quick Meal) 46.0
(Hot Pockets), 4.5-oz. piece 37.0
(Schwan's), 4.4-oz. piece 33.0
(Totino's Big & Hearty), 4.8-oz. piece 32.0
bologna and salami *(Schwan's Ranchero)*, 5.5-oz. piece . . . 42.0
and Swiss *(Sara Lee)* 27.0
and turkey *(Schwan's Croissant)*, 4-oz. piece 23.0
Hamburger, see "Beef, frozen," "Beef sandwich," and
    specific restaurant listings
"Hamburger," vegetarian:
(NewMenu VegiBurger), 3 oz. 12.0
canned:
    (LaLoma Redi-Burger), ⅝" slice 5.0
    (Loma Linda Vege-Burger), ¼ cup 2.0
    (Worthington), ¼ cup 2.0
frozen, 1 patty:
    (Amy's California) 17.0
    (Amy's Chicago) 20.0
    (Green Giant Harvest Burgers Original) 8.0

"Hamburger," vegetarian, frozen *(cont.)*

   (Ken & Robert's Veggie Burger) 19.0
   (Morningstar Farms Prime Patties) 5.0
   (Morningstar Farms Better'n Burger) 6.0
   (Morningstar Farms Grillers) 5.0
   (Natural Touch Vegan Burger) 6.0
   (Natural Touch Vege Burger) 4.0
   black bean, Southwestern *(Fantastic Nature's Burger),*
     2.5 oz. 20.0
   black bean, spicy *(Morningstar Farms)* 16.0
   black bean, spicy *(Natural Touch)* 15.0
   garden grain *(Morningstar Farms)* 18.0
   garden vegetable *(Morningstar Farms)* 9.0
   garden vegetable *(Natural Touch)* 8.0
   grilled *(Fantastic Nature's Burger),* 2.5 oz. 23.0
   Italian *(Green Giant Harvest Burgers)* 8.0
   red pepper and garlic *(Fantastic Nature's Burger),* 2.5 oz. 20.0
   Southwestern *(Green Giant Harvest Burgers)* 9.0
   tofu *(Natural Touch* Okara) 4.0
frozen, ground:
   (Green Giant Harvest Burger For Recipes), ²/₃ cup 8.0
   (Morningstar Farms Burger Style Recipe Crumbles),
     ²/₃ cup 4.0
   (Natural Touch Crumbles), ½ cup 4.0
   (Worthington), ½ cup 3.0
refrigerated *(Hempeh Burger),* 1 patty 12.0
refrigerated *(Yves Veggie Cuisine),* 1 patty 9.0
mix, dry, ¼ pkg., except as noted:
   (Morningstar Farms Garden Grille Veggie Burger Kit) 6.0
   (Morningstar Farms Southwestern Veggie Burger Kit) ... 9.0
   (Natural Touch Original Veggie Kit) 6.0
   (Natural Touch Southwestern Veggie Kit) 9.0
   (Worthington Granburger), 3 tbsp. 3.0
   chunks *(Loma Linda Vita-Burger)* 6.0
   granules *(LaLoma Vita-Burger),* 3 tbsp. 6.0
mix *(Fantastic Nature's Burger* BBQ), 1 patty* 34.0
mix *(Fantastic Nature's Burger* Original), 1 patty* 30.0
Hamburger entree mix, dry, except as noted:
beef pasta *(Hamburger Helper),* ²/₃ cup mix or 1 cup* 23.0
beef Romanoff *(Hamburger Helper),* ²/₃ mix dry or 1 cup* .. 28.0
beef stew *(Hamburger Helper Homestyle),* ½ cup mix
   or 1 cup* 26.0

beef taco *(Hamburger Helper)*, ½ cup mix or 1 cup* 30.0
beef teriyaki *(Hamburger Helper)*, ¼ cup mix or 1 cup* . . . 34.0
cheddar and bacon *(Hamburger Helper)*, ⅔ cup 25.0
cheddar and bacon *(Hamburger Helper)*, 1 cup* 28.0
cheddar melt *(Hamburger Helper)*, ¾ cup 29.0
cheddar melt *(Hamburger Helper)*, 1 cup* 31.0
cheese, three *(Hamburger Helper)*, ½ cup 28.0
cheese, three *(Hamburger Helper)*, 1 cup* 31.0
with cheese *(Hamburger Mate)*, ⅕ pkg. 30.0
cheeseburger macaroni *(Hamburger Helper)*, ⅓ cup 28.0
cheeseburger macaroni *(Hamburger Helper)*, 1 cup* 31.0
chili *(Hamburger Mate)*, ⅕ pkg. 31.0
chili macaroni *(Hamburger Helper)*, ⅓ cup mix or 1 cup* . . 30.0
fettuccine Alfredo *(Hamburger Helper)*, ½ cup 24.0
fettuccine Alfredo *(Hamburger Helper)*, 1 cup* 26.0
Italian, cheesy *(Hamburger Helper)*, ½ cup 26.0
Italian, cheesy *(Hamburger Helper)*, 1 cup* 29.0
Italian, zesty *(Hamburger Helper)*, ⅓ cup mix or 1 cup* . . . 34.0
Italian rigatoni *(Hamburger Helper Homestyle)*, ⅓ cup mix
   or 1 cup* 29.0
lasagna *(Hamburger Helper)*, ⅔ cup mix or 1 cup* 30.0
meat loaf *(Hamburger Helper)*, 1½ tbsp. 10.0
meat loaf *(Hamburger Helper)*, ⅙ loaf* 11.0
Mexican, zesty *(Hamburger Helper)*, ⅔ cup 31.0
Mexican, zesty *(Hamburger Helper)*, 1 cup* 32.0
mushroom and wild rice *(Hamburger Helper)*, ¼ cup 28.0
mushroom and wild rice *(Hamburger Helper)*, 1 cup* 30.0
nacho cheese *(Hamburger Helper)*, ½ cup 28.0
nacho cheese *(Hamburger Helper)*, 1 cup* 30.0
with noodles *(Hamburger Mate)*, ⅕ pkg. 27.0
with pasta and tomato sauce *(Hamburger Mate)*, ⅕ pkg. . . . 32.0
pizza *(Hamburger Helper Pizzabake)*, ⅓ cup mix or ⅙ pan* 28.0
pizza pasta *(Hamburger Helper)*, ½ cup 30.0
pizza pasta *(Hamburger Helper)*, 1 cup* 31.0
potato au gratin *(Hamburger Helper)*, ⅔ cup 23.0
potato au gratin *(Hamburger Helper)*, 1 cup* 24.0
potato Stroganoff *(Hamburger Helper)*, ⅔ cup 24.0
potato Stroganoff *(Hamburger Helper)*, 1 cup* 25.0
rice Oriental *(Hamburger Helper)*, ¼ cup mix or 1 cup* . . . 35.0
Salisbury *(Hamburger Helper Homestyle)*, ¾ cup mix
   or 1 cup* 26.0
shells, cheesy *(Hamburger Helper)*, ½ cup 27.0

Hamburger entree mix *(cont.)*

shells, cheesy *(Hamburger Helper)*, 1 cup* 29.0
spaghetti *(Hamburger Helper)*, ½ cup mix or 1 cup* 29.0
stew *(Hamburger Helper)*, ⅔ cup mix or 1 cup* 22.0
Stroganoff *(Hamburger Helper)*, ⅔ cup 30.0
Stroganoff *(Hamburger Helper)*, 1 cup* 33.0
Swedish meatball *(Hamburger Helper Homestyle)*, ⅔ cup
  mix or 1 cup* 24.0

Hardee's, 1 serving:

breakfast items:

  Big Country Breakfast, bacon 62.0
  Big Country Breakfast, sausage 62.0
  biscuit:

    Apple Cinnamon 'N' Raisin 30.0
    bacon and egg 45.0
    bacon, egg, and cheese 45.0
    country ham 45.0
    ham 47.0
    ham, egg, and cheese 48.0
    jelly 57.0
    Rise 'N' Shine 44.0
    sausage 44.0
    sausage and egg 45.0
    Ultimate Omelet 45.0
  Biscuit 'N' Gravy 55.0
  Frisco Breakfast Sandwich, ham 46.0
  Hash Rounds, regular 24.0
  pancakes, 3 cakes 56.0

burgers and sandwiches:

  Big Roast Beef sandwich 35.0
  The Boss 42.0
  Cravin' Bacon cheeseburger 38.0
  cheeseburger 30.0
  cheeseburger, mesquite bacon 32.0
  cheeseburger, quarter pound double 31.0
  chicken fillet sandwich 54.0
  Fisherman's Fillet 54.0
  Frisco burger 43.0
  grilled chicken sandwich 38.0
  hamburger 29.0
  hamburger, the works 41.0
  Hot Ham 'N' Cheese 34.0

Mushroom 'N' Swiss burger 39.0
roast beef sandwich, regular 26.0
fried chicken:
    breast 29.0
    leg 15.0
    thigh 30.0
    wing 23.0
sides:
    baked beans, 5 oz. 32.0
    coleslaw, 4 oz. 13.0
    fries, small 33.0
    fries, medium 49.0
    fries, large 59.0
    gravy, 1.5 oz. 3.0
    mashed potato, 4 oz. 14.0
salads:
    garden 11.0
    grilled chicken 11.0
    side salad 4.0
dressings:
    French, fat free 17.0
    ranch 6.0
    Thousand Island 9.0
desserts and shakes:
    Big Cookie 41.0
    cone, *Cool Twist,* vanilla/chocolate 34.0
    cone, chocolate 34.0
    cone, vanilla 34.0
    peach cobbler, 6 oz. 60.0
    shake, chocolate 67.0
    shake, peach 77.0
    shake, strawberry 83.0
    shake, vanilla 65.0
    sundae, hot fudge 51.0
    sundae, strawberry 43.0
Hash (see also specific hash listings), canned
    (Mary Kitchen Fiesta), 1 cup 29.0
Hazelnut, see "Filbert"
Hazelnut butter *(Roaster Fresh),* 1 oz. 5.0
Head cheese *(Oscar Mayer),* 1-oz. slice 0
Heart, braised or simmered, 4 oz.:
beef 5

Heart *(cont.)*
chicken, broiler-fryer 1
lamb 2.2
pork 5
turkey 2.3
veal 1
Hearts of palm, see "Palm"
Herbs, see specific listings
Herbs, mixed *(Lawry's* Pinch of Herbs), ¼ tsp. 0
Herring, fresh, kippered, or smoked, without added
   ingredients 0
Herring, canned, see "Sardine"
Herring, in jars, drained, 2 oz., except as noted:
(Vita Homestyle) 5.0
(Vita Party Snacks) 10.0
lunch, sliced *(Vita)* 5.0
in sour cream *(Vita),* ¼ cup, 2¼ oz. 8.0
roll mops *(Vita),* 2½ oz., about 1 piece 9.0
Herring, pickled, 4 oz. 10.9
Herring salad *(Vita),* ¼ cup 15.0
Hickory nut, dried, shelled, 1 oz. 5.2
Hoisin sauce:
(House of Tsang), 1 tsp. 3.0
(Ka•Me), 2 tbsp. 10.0
(Lee Kum Kee), 2 tbsp. 25.0
Hollandaise grilling sauce *(Knorr* Microwave), 2 tbsp. 1.0
Hollandaise sauce mix:
(Durkee), ¹/₁₀ pkg. 2.0
(French's), 2 tbsp. 2.0
(Knorr), ¹/₁₀ pkg. 2.0
Homestyle gravy mix, ¼ cup*:
(Durkee) 3.0
(French's) 3.0
(Pillsbury) 3.0
Hominy, canned, ½ cup:
golden:
   (Allens/Uncle William) 27.0
   (Goya) 27.0
   (Sun-Vista) 19.0
   (Van Camp's) 17.0
Mexican *(Allens/Uncle William)* 25.0

white:
  (Allens/Uncle William) 22.0
  (Goya) 22.0
  (Sun-Vista) 18.0
  (Van Camp's) 16.0
Hominy grits, dry, see "Corn grits"
Honey *(Aunt Sue's/Grandma's/Sue Bee),* 1 tbsp. 17.0
Honey bun, see "Bun, sweet"
Honey butter *(Downey's),* .5 oz. 8.0
Honey Dijon marinade *(World Harbors),* 2 tbsp. 7.0
Honey hickory sauce *(World Harbors* Ember Wisp), 2 tbsp. 10.0
Honey loaf *(Oscar Mayer),* 1-oz. slice 1.0
Honey mustard sauce, California style *(Rice Road),* 1 tbsp. . 4.0
Honey roll sausage, beef, 1 oz. 6
Honeycomb, strained *(Frieda's),* 1 oz. 23.3
Honeydew melon:
untrimmed, 1 lb. 19.2
1/10 melon, 7" × 2" slice, approx. 8 oz. 11.8
trimmed *(Dole),* 1/10 melon, 4.8 oz. 14.0
pulp, cubed, 1/2 cup 7.8
Horned melon *(Frieda's),* 1 melon, 3.5 oz. 0
Hors d'oeuvre kit, frozen, 1 filled sheet, except as noted:
(Pepperidge Farm), 7 sheets 41.0
beef Stroganoff *(Pepperidge Farm)* 27.0
chicken à la king *(Pepperidge Farm)* 28.0
shrimp Newburg *(Pepperidge Farm)* 31.0
Horseradish, fresh, 1/2 cup, except as noted:
(Frieda's), 1 tbsp. 1.0
leafy tips:
  raw, untrimmed, 1 lb. 23.3
  raw, chopped 8
  boiled, drained, chopped 2.3
pods:
  raw, untrimmed, 1 lb. 20.1
  raw, sliced 4.3
  boiled, drained, sliced 4.8
Horseradish, prepared, 1 tsp., except as noted:
(Boar's Head) 0
(Heluva Good) 0
(Kraft Original/Cream Style) 0
red (with beets):
  (Gold's) 0

Horseradish, prepared, red (with beets) *(cont.)*
   (Hebrew National), ½ cup 4.0
   (Rosoff), 1 tbsp. 2.0
white *(Rosoff),* 1 tbsp. 1.0
Horseradish sauce:
(Heinz), 1 tsp. 1.0
(Heluva Good), 1 tsp. 0
(Reese), 2 tbsp. 4.0
(Sauceworks), 2 tbsp. . . . . <1.0
Hot dog, see "Frankfurter"
Hot dog sauce, see "Chili sauce"
Hot fudge sauce, see "Chocolate topping"
Hot sauce, see "Pepper sauce" and specific listings
Hubbard squash:
(Frieda's), ¾ cup, 3 oz. 7.0
raw, untrimmed, 1 lb. 25.3
raw, cubed, ½ cup 5.1
baked, cubed, ½ cup 11.0
boiled, drained, mashed, ½ cup 7.6
Hummus:
(Casbah), 1 oz. 7.5
all varieties *(Cedar's* Hommus), 2 tbsp. 5.0
dip *(Cedar's* Sports), 2 tbsp. 4.0
Hummus mix:
(Casbah), 1 oz. 14.0
dip *(Fantastic),* 2 tbsp. 9.0
Hungarian chili, see "Pepper, chili"
Hush puppies, frozen:
(Schwan's), 3 pieces, 2.25 oz. 29.0
(Stilwell), 3 pieces 19.0
Hush puppy mix *(Martha White),* ¼ cup 25.0
Hyacinth beans, fresh:
raw, untrimmed, 1 lb. 38.8
raw, trimmed, ½ cup 3.7
boiled, drained, ½ cup 4.1
Hyacinth beans, mature:
dried, ¼ cup 31.9
dried, boiled, ½ cup 20.1

FOOD AND MEASURE   **CARBOHYDRATE GRAMS**

Ice, Italian:
cherry *(Luigi's)*, 6 fl. oz. 28.0
cherry *(Marino's)*, 4.7 oz. 26.0
chocolate fudge *(Luigi's)*, 6 fl. oz. 38.0
cocoa, Dutch *(Marino's)*, 4.7 oz. 29.0
grape *(Luigi's)*, 6 fl. oz. 26.0
lemon *(Luigi's)*, 6 fl. oz. 25.0
lemon *(Marino's)*, 4.7 oz. 26.0
strawberry *(Luigi's)*, 6 fl. oz. 26.0
Ice bar, see also "Fruit bar, frozen," 1 bar:
all flavors:
    (Popsicle) 11.0
    (Popsicle Sugar Free/Tropical Sugar Free) 3.0
    (Popsicle Super Twin) 16.0
bubble gum swirl *(Popsicle)* 13.0
cappuccino *(Frozfruit)* 18.0
cherry:
    (Good Humor Bubble Play) 25.0
    (Good Humor Torpedo) 8.0
    (Popsicle Bubble Play) 19.0
    (Super Mario Bros.) 28.0
cherry, lemon, and raspberry:
    (Good Humor Hyper Stripe) 21.0
    (Popsicle Firecracker) 10.0
    (Supersicle Firecracker) 20.0
cherry and pineapple *(Popsicle Big Stick)* 12.0
(Cool Creations Ice Pop) 13.0
(Cool Creations Surprise Pop) 14.0
cotton candy swirl *(Popsicle)* 13.0
(Ghoulie) 25.0
(Good Humor Jumbo Jet Star) 20.0
lemon *(Great White)* 18.0
lemon and cherry *(Mighty Morphin Power Rangers Zeo)* . . . 25.0
orange, pineapple, and lemon *(Good Humor Shoot Hoops!)*   23.0
(Popsicle Lick-A-Color), 2 oz. 13.0

Ice bar *(cont.)*
(Popsicle Lick-A-Color), 3.5 oz. 22.0
(Popsicle Rainbow), 1.75 oz. 11.0
(Popsicle Rainbow), 3.5 oz. 22.0
(Popsicle Squeeze Ups) 22.0
(Popsicle Tingle Twister) 11.0
raspberry *(Spider-Man)* 26.0
(Schwan's Pop) 3.0
(Schwan's Twin Pop) 16.0
strawberry *(Street Sharks)* 26.0
(Supersicle Candy Stripe/Sour Tower) 20.0
watermelon *(Good Humor)*. 20.0
Ice cone, 1 cone:
(Good Humor Snow Cone) 14.0
cherry *(Screwball)* 22.0
Ice cream, ½ cup:
almond:
    butter *(Breyers* All Natural) 15.0
    praline *(Edy's/Dreyer's* Grand) 21.0
    Swiss, fudge twirl *(Breyers* Light/Lowfat) 23.0
    toasted *(Dreyer's* Grand) 15.0
amaretto *(Häagen-Dazs DiSaronno)* 26.0
apple pie *(Edy's* Limited Edition) 19.0
banana cream pie *(Edy's* Homemade) 19.0
banana split *(Edy's* Grand) 19.0
bananas Foster *(Healthy Choice)* 21.0
(Ben & Jerry's Chubby Hubby) 32.0
(Ben & Jerry's Chunky Monkey) 30.0
(Ben & Jerry's Cool Britannia) 29.0
(Ben & Jerry's Holy Cannoli) 27.0
(Ben & Jerry's Phish Food) 41.0
(Ben & Jerry's Rainforest Crunch) 24.0
(Ben & Jerry's Wavy Gravy) 29.0
Black Forest *(Healthy Choice)* 23.0
brownie, blond, sundae *(Ben & Jerry's* Low Fat) 38.0
brownie, fudge:
    (Breyers Blends Sara Lee) 23.0
    (Healthy Choice) 22.0
    à la mode *(Healthy Choice)* 22.0
    chocolate *(Ben & Jerry's)* 33.0
    double *(Edy's* Grand) 19.0
    double chocolate *(Schwan's)* 22.0

marble *(Breyers* Light/Lowfat) 24.0
butter crunch *(Schwan's)* 17.0
butter crunch *(Schwan's* Lowfat) 19.0
butter pecan:
    (Ben & Jerry's) 20.0
    (Breyers All Natural) 15.0
    (Breyers Light/Lowfat) 19.0
    (Edy's Homemade) 17.0
    (Edy's/Dreyer's No Sugar) 12.0
    (Edy's/Dreyer's Grand) 15.0
    (Edy's/Dreyer's Grand Light) 16.0
    (Häagen-Dazs) 20.0
    (Schwan's) 15.0
    (Sealtest) 16.0
    crunch *(Healthy Choice)* 22.0
butterscotch ripple *(Schwan's)* 18.0
cappuccino:
    (Breyers Blends Maxwell House) 19.0
    chocolate chunk *(Healthy Choice)* 22.0
    mocha fudge *(Healthy Choice)* 23.0
caramel cream, dreamy *(Edy's* Grand Light) 17.0
caramel praline:
    almond *(Breyers* All Natural) 21.0
    crunch *(Breyers* Fat Free) 27.0
    crunch *(Edy's/Dreyer's* Fat Free) 26.0
cherry:
    blackjack *(Schwan's)* 19.0
    chocolate chip *(Ben & Jerry's* Cherry Garcia) 25.0
    chocolate chip *(Edy's* Grand) 18.0
    chocolate chunk *(Edy's/Dreyer's* Grand) 17.0
    chocolate chunk *(Healthy Choice)* 19.0
    dark sweet *(Schwan's)* 17.0
    nut *(Schwan's)* 16.0
cherry vanilla:
    (Breyers All Natural) 17.0
    (Schwan's) 17.0
    black, swirl *(Edy's/Dreyer's* No Sugar) 12.0
    black, vanilla swirl *(Edy's* Fat Free) 23.0
Chiquita 'n chocolate *(Edy's/Dreyer's* Grand Light) 13.0
chocolate:
    (Breyers All Natural) 19.0
    (Breyers Fat Free) 20.0

Ice cream, chocolate *(cont.)*

   (Edy's/Dreyer's Grand) 25.0
   (Häagen-Dazs) 22.0
   (Häagen-Dazs Fat Free) 29.0
   (Schwan's) 17.0
   (Sealtest) 19.0
   chunk, triple *(Healthy Choice)* 21.0
   chunky *(Schwan's)* 18.0
   triple *(Edy's/Dreyer's* No Sugar) 13.0

chocolate almond:

   (Breyers Blends Hershey's Almond) 23.0
   (Schwan's) 17.0
   fudge *(Edy's/Dreyer's Grand* Light) 15.0

chocolate brownie chunk *(Edy's/Dreyer's* Fat Free) 28.0

chocolate chip:

   (Breyers All Natural) 18.0
   (Edy's Homemade) 20.0
   (Edy's/Dreyer's Grand Chips!) 18.0
   (Schwan's) 17.0
   (Sealtest) 18.0
   chocolate *(Häagen-Dazs)* 26.0

chocolate chip, mint:

   (Breyers All Natural) 18.0
   (Breyers Light/Lowfat) 21.0
   (Breyers No Sugar Added) 13.0
   (Edy's/Dreyer's Grand Chips!) 18.0
   (Healthy Choice) 21.0
   (Schwan's Chip and Mint) 17.0
   (Sealtest) 17.0

chocolate chip cookie dough:

   (Ben & Jerry's) 30.0
   (Breyers All Natural) 20.0
   (Breyers Light/Lowfat) 22.0
   (Schwan's) 19.0
   (Sealtest) 20.0

chocolate chunk, double *(Edy's* Homemade) 23.0
chocolate cookie, mint *(Ben & Jerry's)* 27.0

chocolate fudge:

   (Edy's/Dreyer's Fat Free) 26.0
   (Edy's/Dreyer's Fat Free/No Sugar) 21.0
   mousse *(Edy's Grand)* 19.0
   mousse *(Edy's/Dreyer's Grand* Light) 17.0

mousse *(Healthy Choice)* 21.0
ripple *(Schwan's)*. 18.0
sundae *(Edy's Grand)* 19.0
chocolate marshmallow ripple *(Schwan's)*. 21.0
chocolate mumbo jumbo *(Edy's/Dreyer's Grand)* 18.0
chocolate peanut butter crunch *(Edy's/Dreyer's Fat Free)* . . . 27.0
coffee (see also "cappuccino" and "espresso"):
   (Ben & Jerry's Coffee Coffee Buzz Buzz Buzz). 27.0
   (Breyers All Natural). 15.0
   (Edy's/Dreyer's Grand) 16.0
   (Häagen-Dazs) 21.0
   (Starbuck's Biscotti Bliss) 30.0
   caffe almond fudge *(Starbuck's)* 30.0
   Italian roast *(Starbuck's)*. 27.0
   java chip *(Starbuck's)*. 30.0
   latte *(Starbuck's Low Fat)* 31.0
   mocha *(Starbuck's Low Fat)* 32.0
   vanilla mocha swirl *(Starbuck's)*. 31.0
   and biscotti *(Ben & Jerry's Low Fat)* 33.0
coffee fudge:
   (Edy's/Dreyer's Fat Free) 25.0
   (Edy's/Dreyer's Fat Free/No Sugar) 21.0
   (Häagen-Dazs Fat Free). 32.0
coffee toffee crunch *(Ben & Jerry's Heath)* 28.0
cookie chunk *(Edy's/Dreyer's Fat Free)* 26.0
cookie creme de mint *(Healthy Choice)* 24.0
cookie dough *(Edy's/Dreyer's Grand)* 20.0
cookie dough *(Edy's/Dreyer's Grand Light)* 18.0
cookie jar *(Edy's Toll House Limited Edition)* 19.0
cookies 'n cream:
   (Breyers All Natural) 19.0
   (Edy's/Dreyer's Grand) 18.0
   (Edy's/Dreyer's Grand Light) 16.0
   (Häagen-Dazs) 23.0
   (Healthy Choice) 21.0
   (Schwan's). 18.0
   mint *(Breyers Fat Free)* 22.0
   mint *(Dreyer's Grand Light)*. 16.0
cream, sweet, and cookies *(Ben & Jerry's Low Fat)* 31.0
(Edy's Butterfinger Blast Limited Edition) 19.0
(Edy's Championship Sundae Limited Edition) 19.0
(Edy's Slammin' Sundae Light Limited Edition) 18.0

Ice cream *(cont.)*

egg nog *(Edy's Toll House* Limited Edition) 18.0
espresso:
   chip *(Edy's Grand)* 17.0
   fudge chip *(Dreyer's Grand* Light) 17.0
   swirl, dark roast *(Starbuck's)* 29.0
French silk *(Edy's/Dreyer's Grand* Light) 18.0
fudge:
   chunk *(Ben & Jerry's* New York) 28.0
   marble *(Edy's/Dreyer's* Fat Free) 25.0
   marble *(Edy's/Dreyer's* No Sugar) 13.0
   mint *(Dreyer's* Fat Free) 25.0
   royal *(Sealtest)* 19.0
fudge brownie, double *(Edy's/Dreyer's* No Sugar) 13.0
fudge toffee parfait *(Breyers* Light/Lowfat) 24.0
heavenly hash *(Sealtest)* 20.0
ice cream sandwich *(Edy's Grand)* 14.0
Irish cream *(Häagen-Dazs Baileys)* 23.0
macadamia brittle *(Häagen-Dazs)* 25.0
maple nut *(Schwan's)* 15.0
(Milky Way) 22.0
mocha, see "coffee," above
mocha fudge:
   (Edy's/Dreyer's No Sugar) 13.0
   almond *(Dreyer's Grand)* 18.0
   almond *(Dreyer's Grand* Light) 16.0
   almond *(Schwan's)* 19.0
mud pie *(Dreyer's Grand)* 19.0
Neapolitan *(Dreyer's Grand)* 16.0
Neapolitan *(Schwan's)* 17.0
orange cream bar *(Edy's* Limited Edition) 19.0
peach *(Breyers* All Natural) 18.0
peach *(Schwan's)* 17.0
peanut butter:
   (Breyers Blends Reese's Pieces) 24.0
   caramel *(Breyers Blends NutRageous)* 22.0
   cup *(Ben & Jerry's)* 30.0
   cup *(Breyers Blends Reese's)* 24.0
   cup *(Edy's Grand* Light Cups!) 17.0
   fudge ripple *(Schwan's)* 18.0
pecan praline sundae *(Schwan's)* 19.0
peppermint *(Edy's* Limited Edition) 17.0

praline:
   almond crunch *(Breyers Light/Lowfat)* 21.0
   almondine sundae *(Schwan's Lowfat)* 21.0
   caramel or caramel cluster *(Healthy Choice)* 25.0
   pecan *(Breyers No Sugar)* 18.0
pumpkin *(Edy's Limited Edition)* 17.0
raspberry ripple *(Schwan's)* 18.0
raspberry rumble *(Schwan's)* 21.0
raspberry vanilla swirl *(Edy's/Dreyer's Fat Free/No Sugar)* . . 19.0
rocky road:
   (Breyers Light/Lowfat) 23.0
   (Edy's/Dreyer's Grand) 17.0
   (Edy's/Dreyer's Grand Light) 16.0
   (Healthy Choice) 28.0
   (Schwan's) 21.0
   deluxe *(Breyers All Natural)* 24.0
root beer float *(Edy's Limited Edition)* 19.0
rum raisin *(Häagen-Dazs)* 22.0
(Schwan's Summer's Dream) 19.0
(Snickers) 26.0
strawberries and cream *(Edy's Homemade)* 18.0
strawberry:
   (Breyers All Natural) 15.0
   (Breyers Fat Free) 19.0
   (Edy's/Dreyer's Grand Real) 17.0
   (Edy's/Dreyer's No Sugar) 11.0
   (Häagen-Dazs) 23.0
   (Häagen-Dazs Fat Free) 29.0
   (Schwan's) 16.0
   (Schwan's Fat Free/No Sugar Added) 23.0
   (Sealtest) 19.0
strawberry shortcake *(Healthy Choice)* 23.0
tin roof sundae *(Schwan's)* 19.0
toffee bar crunch *(Breyers All Natural)* 18.0
turtle fudge cake *(Healthy Choice)* 25.0
vanilla:
   (Ben & Jerry's) 21.0
   (Breyers All Natural) 15.0
   (Breyers Fat Free) 21.0
   (Breyers Light/Lowfat) 18.0
   (Breyers No Sugar) 11.0
   (Edy's Homemade) 17.0

Ice cream, vanilla *(cont.)*

 (Edy's/Dreyer's Fat Free) 23.0
 (Edy's/Dreyer's Fat Free/No Sugar) 19.0
 (Edy's/Dreyer's No Sugar) 11.0
 (Edy's/Dreyer's Grand) 14.0
 (Edy's/Dreyer's Grand Avalanche) 17.0
 (Edy's/Dreyer's Grand Light) 15.0
 (Häagen-Dazs) 21.0
 (Häagen-Dazs Fat Free) 29.0
 (Healthy Choice) 18.0
 (Schwan's) 16.0
 (Schwan's Fat Free/No Sugar Added) 22.0
 (Schwan's Lowfat) 17.0
 (Sealtest) 16.0
 bean *(Edy's/Dreyer's Grand)* 15.0
 French *(Breyers* All Natural) 15.0
 French *(Breyers* Light/Lowfat) 17.0
 French *(Edy's/Dreyer's Grand)* 16.0
 French *(Schwan's)* 20.0
 French *(Sealtest)* 16.0
vanilla and black cherry *(Breyers Take Two* All Natural) 16.0
vanilla caramel:
 (Edy's/Dreyer's Fat Free/No Sugar) 21.0
 (Edy's/Dreyer's No Sugar) 17.0
 fudge swirl *(Ben & Jerry's)* 33.0
vanilla and chocolate *(Breyers Take Two* All Natural) 17.0
vanilla and chocolate *(Edy's/Dreyer's Grand)* 16.0
vanilla and chocolate mint patty *(Ben & Jerry's* Low Fat) . . 33.0
vanilla chocolate swirl *(Edy's/Dreyer's* Fat Free/No Sugar) . . 19.0
vanilla-chocolate-strawberry combination:
 (Breyers All Natural) 16.0
 (Breyers Fat Free) 19.0
 (Breyers No Sugar Added) 11.0
 (Edy's Grand) 16.0
 (Sealtest) 18.0
vanilla fudge *(Häagen-Dazs)* 25.0
vanilla fudge twirl:
 (Breyers All Natural) 19.0
 (Breyers Fat Free) 24.0
 (Breyers No Sugar Added) 14.0
vanilla and orange sherbet *(Breyers Take Two* All Natural) . . 21.0
vanilla and strawberry *(Breyers Take Two* Fat Free) 21.0

vanilla Swiss almond *(Häagen-Dazs)* 23.0
vanilla with toffee crunch *(Ben & Jerry's Heath)* 28.0
"Ice cream," nondairy, ½ cup, except as noted:
all flavors *(Tofutti Soft Serve/Soft Serve Lite)* 20.0
all fruit flavors *(Tofutti Fruitti)* 20.0
bar, 1 piece:
    chocolate *(Rice Dream)* 32.0
    nutty chocolate *(Rice Dream)* 23.0
    nutty vanilla *(Rice Dream)* 23.0
    strawberry *(Rice Dream)* 31.0
    vanilla *(Rice Dream)* 33.0
better pecan *(Tofutti)* 22.0
cappuccino *(Rice Dream)* 23.0
carob *(Rice Dream)* 24.0
carob almond *(Rice Dream)* 24.0
cherry almond *(Rice Dream)* 24.0
chocolate:
    (Rice Dream) 24.0
    (Tofutti) 18.0
    cake *(Tofutti)* 26.0
    fudge *(Tofutti Low Fat)* 25.0
chocolate chip *(Rice Dream)* 26.0
cocoa marble fudge *(Rice Dream)* 25.0
coffee marshmallow *(Tofutti Low Fat)* 24.0
cookies n' dream *(Rice Dream)* 26.0
mint carob chip *(Rice Dream)* 26.0
mint chocolate chip *(Rice Dream)* 26.0
Neapolitan *(Rice Dream)* 24.0
orange vanilla swirl *(Rice Dream)* 23.0
passion island fruit *(Tofutti Low Fat)* 21.0
peach mango *(Tofutti Low Fat)* 23.0
pie, 1 piece:
    cookie, chocolate *(Rice Dream)* 39.0
    cookie, mint *(Rice Dream)* 39.0
    cookie, mocha *(Rice Dream)* 40.0
    cookie, vanilla *(Rice Dream)* 40.0
    vanilla, chocolate covered *(Tofutti Cutie)* 18.0
sandwich, 1 piece:
    chocolate *(Tofutti Cutie)* 16.0
    vanilla *(Tofutti Cutie)* 17.0
    wildberry *(Tofutti Cutie)* 17.0

"Ice cream," nondairy *(cont.)*

stick, 1 piece:

    chocolate *(Tofutti Fruitti)* 15.0

    fudge *(Tofutti* Teddy) 19.0

    fudge *(Tofutti* Treats) 6.0

strawberry *(Rice Dream)* 24.0

strawberry banana *(Tofutti* Low Fat) 23.0

vanilla:

    (Rice Dream) 23.0

    (Tofutti) 20.0

    (Tofutti Cutie Slice), 1 slice 15.0

    almond bark *(Tofutti)* 21.0

    fudge *(Tofutti)* 25.0

    fudge *(Tofutti* Low Fat) 24.0

    Swiss almond *(Rice Dream)* 25.0

wildberry:

    (Tofutti) 24.0

    (Tofutti Slice), 1 slice 18.0

    chocolate covered *(Tofutti* Slice), 1 slice 18.0

Ice cream bar, 1 bar, except as noted:

all flavors *(Fudgsicle* Pop Variety Pack), 1.75 oz. 12.0

almond:

    (Breyers), 4 oz. 28.0

    (DoveBar), 2.8 oz. 23.0

    (DoveBar Singles), 3.5 oz. 29.0

    (Good Humor), 3 oz. 25.0

    (Good Humor), 3.75 oz. 31.0

    (Klondike) 26.0

(Ben & Jerry's Chunky Monkey) 32.0

(Butterfinger) 16.0

caramel creme swirl with toffee chips *(DoveBar)* 31.0

caramel crunch *(Klondike)* 31.0

cherry royale *(Dove Bite Size)*, 5 bars 35.0

chocolate:

    (Fudgsicle Bar), 2.5 oz. or 2.7 oz. 17.0

    (Fudgsicle Bar Fat Free), 1.75 oz. 13.0

    (Fudgsicle Bar Sugar Free), 1.75 oz. 8.0

    (Klondike) 22.0

    (Nestlé Crunch) 17.0

    (3 Musketeers), 1.6 oz. 17.0

    (3 Musketeers Singles), 2.2 oz. 22.0

    (Weight Watchers Chocolate Treat) 20.0

chocolate dipped *(Good Humor* Choco Taco) 38.0
dark chocolate coated *(DoveBar)*, 2.8 oz. 27.0
dark chocolate coated *(DoveBar)*, 3.5 oz. 34.0
dark chocolate coated *(Häagen-Dazs)*, 3.2 oz. 27.0
dark chocolate coated *(Häagen-Dazs* Single), 4 oz. 33.0
dip *(Weight Watchers)* 11.0
double *(Dove Bite Size)*, 5 bars 34.0
milk chocolate coated *(Milky Way)* 24.0
milk chocolate coated *(Milky Way* Reduced Fat) 19.0
chocolate candy center *(Good Humor* Crunch) 21.0
chocolate cookie dough *(Ben & Jerry's)* 44.0
chocolate eclair:
   (Col. Crunch) 21.0
   (Good Humor Eclair), 3 oz. 21.0
   (Good Humor), 3.75 oz. 28.0
chocolate malt *(Schwan's Push-Ems)* 15.0
chocolate mousse *(Weight Watchers)* 9.0
chocolate pudding *(Schwan's)* 18.0
chocolate sundae crunch *(Schwan's)* 22.0
coffee *(Klondike)* 25.0
coffee and almond crunch *(Häagen-Dazs)*, 3 oz. 22.0
coffee and almond crunch *(Häagen-Dazs* Single), 3.7 oz. . . . 27.0
cookies 'n cream *(Edy's/Dreyer's)* 22.0
(Cool Creations Mickey Mouse), 2.5 oz. 10.0
(Cool Creations Mickey Mouse), 4 oz. 17.0
fudge double *(Supersicle)* 29.0
fudge stick *(Schwan's)* 22.0
fudge stick *(Schwan's Trim Creations)* 13.0
(Good Humor WWF) 25.0
Irish creme cordial with dark chocolate *(Dove Bite Size)*,
   5 bars 33.0
(Klondike Krispy) 28.0
(Klondike Krunch), 3 oz. 19.0
(Klondike Krunch), 3.75 oz. 24.0
mint, green, and chocolate fudge truffle swirl *(DoveBar)* . . . 31.0
mocha cashew crunch *(DoveBar)* 25.0
(Nestlé Crunch Crunch King) 21.0
(Nestlé Crunch Reduced Fat) 14.0
peanut butter *(Reese's NutRageous)* 22.0
peanut butter *(Schwan's P-Nut Butter Creme)* 14.0
peanut stick *(Schwan's)* 16.0

Ice cream bar *(cont.)*

peppermint with dark chocolate *(Dove Bite Size* Party),
5 bars 39.0
raspberry cordial *(Schwan's)* 22.0
root beer float *(Schwan's)* 16.0
(Schwan's) 17.0
(Schwan's Gold 'N' Nugit) 23.0
(Schwan's Healthy Creation Creme Bar) 18.0
(Schwan's Krispie Krunch Bar) 12.0
(Schwan's Rainbow Stick) 18.0
(Schwan's Silver Mint) 14.0
(Snickers Singles) 19.0
(Snickers Snack Size), 4 bars 37.0
strawberry shake *(Schwan's Push-Ems)* 14.0
strawberry shortcake:
   (Col. Crunch) 22.0
   (Good Humor), 3 oz. 23.0
   (Good Humor), 3.75 oz. 26.0
toffee, English *(Schwan's)* 18.0
toffee crunch, English *(Weight Watchers)* 12.0
vanilla:
   (Ben & Jerry's) 29.0
   (Breyers), 4 oz. 27.0
   (Dove Bite Size Classic), 5 bars ... 31.0
   (Good Humor), 2.75 oz. 11.0
   (Good Humor Premium), 3 oz. ... 11.0
   (Good Humor Premium), 3.75 oz. ... 14.0
   (Klondike Original) 24.0
   (Klondike Reduced Fat–No Sugar Added) ... 19.0
   (Nestlé Crunch) 16.0
   (Popsicle) 15.0
   (3 Musketeers), 1.6 oz. 16.0
   (3 Musketeers Singles), 2.2 oz. ... 21.0
   French *(Dove Bite Size)*, 5 bars ... 33.0
   brownie *(Ben & Jerry's)* 43.0
   white coated *(DoveBar)* 26.0
vanilla with almonds:
   (Edy's/Dreyer's) 23.0
   (Häagen-Dazs), 3 oz. 21.0
   (Häagen-Dazs Single), 3.7 oz. ... 26.0
vanilla, dark chocolate coated:
   (DoveBar), 2.8 oz. 26.0

(DoveBar Single), 3.5 oz. 32.0
(Häagen-Dazs), 3.2 oz. 27.0
(Häagen-Dazs Single), 4 oz. 33.0
(Klondike) 24.0
(Milky Way) 23.0
(Milky Way Reduced Fat) 19.0
vanilla, ice coated:
   (Creamsicle Bar), 2.5 oz. 19.0
   (Creamsicle Bar), 2.7 oz. 20.0
   (Creamsicle Orange Pop), 1.75 oz. 13.0
   (Creamsicle Variety Pop), 1.75 oz. 14.0
   (Creamsicle Pop No Sugar Added) 5.0
vanilla, milk chocolate coated:
   (DoveBar), 2.8 oz. 25.0
   (DoveBar Single), 3.5 oz. 31.0
   (Edy's/Dreyer's) 22.0
   (Häagen-Dazs), 3 oz. 20.0
   (Häagen-Dazs Single), 3.5 oz. 24.0
vanilla and chocolate *(Good Humor* Number 1) 22.0
vanilla and chocolate *(Snoopy)* 18.0
vanilla with toffee crunch *(Ben & Jerry's Heath)* 33.0
(Weight Watchers Orange Vanilla Treat) 10.0
Ice cream cone, plain, unfilled, 1 piece:
(Oreo) 10.0
cinnamon *(Teddy Grahams)* 13.0
sugar *(Comet)* 11.0
waffle *(Comet)* 14.0
Ice cream cone, filled, 1 cone:
butter pecan *(Breyers)*, 5 oz. 31.0
chocolate *(Drumstick)* 36.0
chocolate dipped *(Drumstick)* 40.0
chocolate dipped *(Good Humor* Premium Sundae), 4.6 oz. 33.0
chocolate dipped *(Good Humor* Sundae), 4 oz. 36.0
chocolate dipped, with peanuts:
   (Good Humor American Glory) 36.0
   (Good Humor King) 48.0
   (Klondike Sundae) 34.0
cookies 'n cream *(Edy's/Dreyer's* Sundae) 31.0
pecan praline *(Schwan's Sundae Cone)* 36.0
(Schwan's Sundae Cone) 28.0
(Snickers) 34.0
vanilla *(Drumstick)* 35.0

Ice cream cone, filled *(cont.)*

vanilla caramel *(Drumstick)* 38.0

vanilla fudge:

    (Drumstick) 39.0

    (Edy's/Dreyer's Sundae) 31.0

    chocolate *(Schwan's Sundae Cone)* 37.0

    ripple *(Good Humor* Choco Taco) 37.0

Ice cream cup, filled, 1 piece:

chocolate:

    (Carnation), 3 fl. oz. 16.0

    (Sealtest) 19.0

    malt *(Carnation)*, 12 fl. oz. 48.0

    malt *(Milky Way)* 44.0

    sundae *(Carnation)*, 5 fl. oz. 30.0

    sundae *(Schwan's)* 17.0

fudge swirl *(Schwan's* Fat Free) 26.0

(Good Humor Sundae Twist) 33.0

peanut butter *(Good Humor Reese's)*, 2 oz. 14.0

peanut butter *(Good Humor Reese's)*, 3 oz. 20.0

strawberry:

    (Carnation), 3 fl. oz. 12.0

    (Sealtest) 19.0

    sundae *(Carnation)*, 5 fl. oz. 29.0

    sundae *(Schwan's)* 16.0

vanilla:

    (Carnation), 3 fl. oz. 11.0

    (Carnation), 5 fl. oz. 19.0

    (Schwan's) 13.0

    (Schwan's Nonfat) 20.0

    (Sealtest) 16.0

    (Sealtest Fat Free) 22.0

    (Sealtest No Sugar Added) 12.0

    malt *(Carnation)*, 12 fl. oz. 48.0

vanilla and chocolate *(Breyers)*, 6 oz. 26.0

Ice cream loaf, 2.4-oz. slice:

all flavors, except chocolate *(Vienetta)* 19.0

chocolate *(Vienetta)* 18.0

Ice cream nuggets, chocolate coated:

(Nestlé Crunch), 8 pieces 25.0

dark *(Bon-Bons)*, 5 pieces 16.0

dark *(Bon-Bons)*, 8 pieces 26.0

dark *(Bon-Bons)*, 9 pieces 30.0

milk *(Bon-Bons)*, 5 pieces 17.0
milk *(Bon-Bons)*, 8 pieces 27.0
milk *(Bon-Bons)*, 9 pieces 30.0
Ice cream pie, ⅛ pie:
grasshopper *(Schwan's)* 45.0
strawberry cheesecake *(Schwan's)* 49.0
Ice cream sandwich, 1 piece:
chocolate chip cookie:
    (Chipwich Jr.) 35.0
    (Good Humor Premium), 4 oz. 43.0
    (Good Humor Premium), 4.5 oz. 44.0
cookies and cream *(Cool Creations)* 34.0
(Good Humor), 3 oz. 27.0
(Good Humor American Glory), 3.5 oz. 28.0
(Good Humor Giant), 5 oz. 35.0
(Klondike Big Bear), 5 oz. 31.0
(Klondike Big Bear), 7 oz. 46.0
(Klondike Big Bear Fat Free) 33.0
mini *(Cool Creations)* 16.0
Neapolitan *(Good Humor* Giant), 5 oz. 39.0
(Popsicle) 28.0
(Schwan's) 24.0
vanilla *(Häagen-Dazs)*, 2.8 oz. 32.0
vanilla and chocolate *(Häagen-Dazs)*, 2.8 oz. 31.0
Ice cream and sorbet, see "Sorbet"
Icing, see "Frosting"
Italian cut beans, see "Green beans"
Italian sausage, see "Sausage"
Italian seasoning, 1 tsp. 6

J

FOOD AND MEASURE   **CARBOHYDRATE GRAMS**

Jack-in-the-Box, 1 serving:
breakfast items:
   Breakfast Jack 30.0
   Country Crock Spread, .2 oz. 0
   croissant, sausage 39.0
   croissant, supreme 39.0
   hash browns 14.0
   jelly, grape, .5 oz. 9.0
   pancake platter 59.0
   pancake syrup, 1.5 oz. 30.0
   sandwich, breakfast, sourdough 31.0
   sandwich, breakfast, ultimate 39.0
   scrambled egg pocket 31.0
sandwiches:
   cheeseburger, regular 32.0
   cheeseburger, double 35.0
   cheeseburger, ultimate 30.0
   chicken 38.0
   chicken, Caesar 44.0
   chicken, spicy crispy 55.0
   chicken, supreme 48.0
   chicken fajita pita 29.0
   chicken fillet, grilled 36.0
   hamburger, regular 31.0
   hamburger, quarter-pound 39.0
   hamburger, sourdough, grilled 39.0
   Jumbo Jack 41.0
   Jumbo Jack with cheese 42.0
entrees:
   chicken teriyaki bowl 115.0
   taco 15.0
   taco, monster 22.0
salads:
   chicken, garden 8.0
   side 3.0

finger foods:
    chicken strips, 4 pieces 18.0
    chicken strips, 6 pieces 28.0
    egg rolls, 3 rolls 54.0
    egg rolls, 5 rolls 92.0
    jalapeños, stuffed, 7 pieces 29.0
    jalapeños, stuffed, 10 pieces 41.0
    potato wedges with bacon and cheddar 49.0
fries:
    small 28.0
    regular 45.0
    jumbo 51.0
    super scoop 76.0
    seasoned, curly 39.0
onion rings 38.0
sauces:
    barbeque, 1 oz. 11.0
    buttermilk, .9 oz. 3.0
    soy, .3 oz. .... <1.0
    sweet and sour, 1 oz. 11.0
    tartar, 1 oz. 2.0
dressings, 2 oz.:
    blue cheese 11.0
    buttermilk, house 6.0
    Italian, low calorie 2.0
    Thousand Island 10.0
condiments:
    cheese, American or Swiss style, 1 slice 0
    croutons, .4 oz. 8.0
    hot sauce, 1 pkt. 1.0
    ketchup, 1 pkt. 3.0
    mayonnaise, 1 pkt. 0
    mustard, 1 pkt. 0
    salsa, 1 oz. 2.0
desserts:
    apple turnover 48.0
    carrot cake 58.0
    cheesecake 29.0
    cheesecake, chocolate chip cookie dough 44.0
shakes:
    cappuccino 80.0
    chocolate 85.0

Jack-in-the-Box, shakes *(cont.)*
  strawberry 85.0
  vanilla 73.0
Jackfruit:
(Frieda's), ⅓ cup 30.0
untrimmed, 1 lb. 30.5
trimmed, 1 oz. 6.8
Jackson wonder beans, dried *(Frieda's)*, ½ cup 22.0
Jalapeño, see "Pepper, jalapeño"
Jalapeño dip, 2 tbsp.:
(Kraft) 3.0
(Old El Paso) 4.0
and cheddar *(Breakstone's)* 2.0
and cheddar *(Frito-Lay)* 3.0
cheese *(Kraft* Premium) 1.0
Jalapeño relish *(Old El Paso)*, 1 tbsp. 1.0
Jam and preserves (see also "Fruit spreads" and "Jelly"),
  1 tbsp., except as noted:
all varieties:
  (Knott's Berry Farm), 1 tsp. 4.0
  (Smucker's) 13.0
  (Smucker's Light) 5.0
  (Smucker's Reduced Sugar) 6.0
apricot *(Kraft)* 13.0
blackberry *(Kraft)* 13.0
grape *(Kraft)* 14.0
mango *(Goya)* 11.0
orange marmalade *(Crosse & Blackwell)* 16.0
papaya *(Goya)* 11.0
passion fruit *(Goya)* 12.0
peach *(Kraft)* 14.0
pineapple *(Goya)* 11.0
pineapple *(Kraft)* 14.0
plum, red *(Kraft)* 13.0
raspberry *(Kraft)* 13.0
strawberry *(Goya)* 11.0
strawberry *(Kraft)* 13.0
Jambalaya dinner mix *(Luzianne)*, ¼ pkg. 43.0
Japanese burdock, see "Burdock root"
Java plum:
with seeds, 1 lb. 57.2
3 medium, .4 oz. 1.4

seeded, ½ cup 10.5
Jelly, 1 tbsp., except as noted:
all fruit flavors:
    (Knott's Berry Farm), 1 tsp. 4.0
    (Smucker's) 13.0
    except apple, grape, and strawberry *(Kraft)* 13.0
apple *(Kraft)* 14.0
apple mint *(Crosse & Blackwell)* 13.0
currant, red *(Crosse & Blackwell)* 14.0
grape *(Goya)* 11.0
grape *(Kraft)* 14.0
guava *(Goya)* 12.0
pepper, mild *(Tabasco)* 14.0
pepper, spicy *(Tabasco)* 12.0
strawberry *(Kraft)* 14.0
Jerk sauce *(World Harbors* Blue Mountain), 2 tbsp. 18.0
Jerusalem artichoke:
(Frieda's Sun Choke), ½ cup 14.0
untrimmed, 1 lb. 54.6
sliced, ½ cup 13.1
Jicama, see "Yam bean tuber"
Jujube:
raw, with seeds, 1 lb. 85.3
raw, seeded, 1 oz. 5.7
dried, 1 oz. 20.1
Jute, potherb:
raw, untrimmed, 1 lb. 16.3
raw, ½ cup 8
boiled, drained, ½ cup 3.1

K

FOOD AND MEASURE	CARBOHYDRATE GRAMS

Kabocha squash (Frieda's), ¾ cup, 3 oz. 7.0
Kale, ½ cup, except as noted:
fresh:
    raw, untrimmed, 1 lb. 27.7
    raw, chopped 3.4
    raw, chopped (Dole). 3.0
    boiled, drained, chopped 3.7
canned (Allens/Sunshine). 3.0
canned (Stubb's Harvest). 3.0
frozen (Seabrook), 3 oz. 2.0
Kale, Chinese (Frieda's Gai Lan), 1 cup 1.0
Kale, Scotch:
raw, untrimmed, 1 lb. 23.0
raw, chopped, ½ cup 2.8
boiled, drained, chopped, ½ cup 3.7
Kamranga, see "Carambola"
Kamut flakes, see "Cereal"
Kamut flour (Arrowhead Mills), ¼ cup 25.0
Kanpyo:
1 oz. 18.4
½ cup 17.6
Kasha, see "Buckwheat groats"
Kelp, see "Seaweed"
Ketchup, 1 tbsp.:
(Del Monte). 4.0
(Healthy Choice). 2.0
(Heinz) 4.0
(Hunt's/Hunt's No Salt Added) 3.0
(Smucker's) 7.0
KFC, 1 serving:
chicken, Original Recipe:
    breast 16.0
    drumstick. 4.0
    thigh 6.0
    wing, whole 5.0

chicken, *Extra Tasty Crispy:*
    breast 25.0
    drumstick 8.0
    thigh 18.0
    wing, whole 10.0
chicken, Hot & Spicy:
    breast 23.0
    drumstick 10.0
    thigh 13.0
    wing, whole 9.0
chicken, *Tender Roast:*
    breast, with or without skin 1.0
    drumstick, with or without skin . . . . <1.0
    thigh, with skin . . . . <2.0
    thigh, without skin . . . . <1.0
    wing, with skin 1.0
chicken potpie 69.0
Crispy Strips, 3 pieces 10.0
Hot Wings, 6 pieces 18.0
Kentucky Nuggets, 6 pieces 15.0
sandwiches, chicken:
    BBQ flavored 28.0
    Original Recipe 45.5
sides and specials:
    BBQ baked beans 33.0
    biscuit, 2-oz. piece 20.0
    coleslaw 21.0
    corn on the cob 34.0
    corn bread, 2-oz. piece 25.0
    garden rice 23.0
    green beans 7.0
    macaroni and cheese 21.0
    mashed potatoes with gravy 17.0
    Mean Greens 11.0
    potato salad 23.0
    potato wedges 28.0
    red beans and rice 21.0
Kidney beans:
dried, red:
    uncooked *(Arrowhead Mills),* ¼ cup 29.0
    uncooked, ¼ cup 27.6
    boiled, ½ cup 20.1

Kidney beans *(cont.)*
canned, red, ½ cup:
   (Eden Organic) 18.0
   (Hunt's) 19.5
   (Seneca) 20.0
   (Van Camp's New Orleans Style) 20.0
   with liquid 20.0
   baked *(B&M/Friends)* 32.0
   dark *(Allens/East Texas Fair/Trappey's)* 22.0
   dark *(Goya)* 18.0
   dark or light *(Green Giant/Joan of Arc)* 20.0
   dark or light *(Progresso)* 20.0
   dark or light *(Stokely)* 21.0
   dark or light *(Stokely* No Sugar) 19.0
   dark or light *(Van Camp's)* 20.0
   light *(Allens/Trappey's)* 22.0
   with bacon, light *(Trappey's* New Orleans) 20.0
   with chili gravy *(Trappey's)* 20.0
   with jalapeños, light *(Trappey's)* 19.0
canned, white *(Progresso* Cannellini), ½ cup 18.0
Kidney beans, sprouted:
raw, 1 lb. 18.6
raw, ½ cup 3.8
Kidneys, braised, 4 oz.:
beef 1.1
lamb 1.1
pork 0
veal 0
Kielbasa (see also "Polish sausage"):
(Boar's Head), 2 oz. 0
(Jones Dairy Farm Dinner), 1 link 1.0
Kimchee *(Frieda's),* ¼ cup 2.0
Kishka *(Hebrew National),* 2 oz. 10.0
Kiwi:
fresh:
   (Dole), 2 fruits, 5.3 oz. 25.0
   (Frieda's), 5 oz. 21.0
   with skin, 1 lb. 58.1
   1 large, 3.7 oz. 13.5
   1 medium, 3.1 oz. 11.3
dried *(Sonoma),* 7–8 pieces, 1 oz. 19.0
Kiwi punch *(After the Fall* Bear), 8 fl. oz. 24.0

Kiwi-strawberry drink, 8 fl. oz.:
(Snapple) 29.0
(Snapple Diet) 5.0
Knockwurst, beef:
(Boar's Head), 4 oz. 1.0
(Hebrew National), 3-oz. link 1.0
Kohlrabi:
(Frieda's), ⅔ cup, 3 oz. 5.0
raw, untrimmed, 1 lb. 12.9
raw, sliced, ½ cup 4.3
boiled, drained, sliced, ½ cup 5.5
Kumquat:
(Frieda's), 5 oz. 23.0
with seeds, 1 lb. 69.3
1 medium, .7 oz. 3.1
seeded, 1 oz. 4.7
Kun choy, see "Celery, Chinese"

FOOD AND MEASURE   **CARBOHYDRATE GRAMS**

Lamb, without added ingredients 0
Lamb curry entree, frozen *(Curry Classics)*, 10 oz. 16.0
Lamb's-quarter:
raw, untrimmed, 1 lb. 33.1
boiled, drained, chopped, ½ cup 4.5
Lard, pork 0
Lasagna entree, canned:
(Hormel), 7½ oz. 24.0
(Hormel Micro Cup), 7½ oz. 24.0
(Libby's Diner), 7¾ oz. 25.0
(Nalley), 1 cup 33.0
(Nalley), 7½ oz. 26.0
and beef *(Hormel* Micro Cup), 10½ oz. 34.0
cheese, three, with beef *(Nalley)*, 7½-oz. can 21.0
Italian *(Top Shelf)*, 10 oz. 28.0
Lasagna entree, freeze-dried *(Mountain House)*, 1 cup . . . 24.0
Lasagna entree, frozen:
(Celentano), 10 oz. 51.0
(Celentano), ½ of 14-oz. pkg. 33.0
(Celentano 25 oz.), 1 cup 31.0
(Celentano Great Choice), 10 oz. 42.0
(Celentano Value Pack), 1 cup 41.0
(Healthy Choice Roma)*, 13.5 oz. 60.0
Alfredo *(Weight Watchers)*, 9 oz. 45.0
Alfredo, with broccoli *(The Budget Gourmet* Special
   Selections)*, 9 oz. 47.0
bake *(Stouffer's)*, 10¼ oz. 47.0
cheese:
   (Lean Cuisine Classic)*, 11.5 oz. 38.0
   casserole *(Lean Cuisine* Lunch Classics)*, 10 oz. 40.0
   with chicken scaloppine *(Lean Cuisine* Cafe Classics)*,
      10 oz. 34.0
   extra *(Marie Callender's)*, 1 cup 32.0
   five *(Lean Cuisine* 96 oz.)*, approx. 1 cup 28.0
   five *(Stouffer's)*, 10¾ oz. 40.0

four *(Wolfgang Puck's)*, 12 oz. 15.0
Italian *(Weight Watchers)*, 11 oz. 38.0
three *(The Budget Gourmet)*, 10.5 oz. 40.0
chicken *(Lean Cuisine)*, 10 oz. 40.0
chicken *(Lean Cuisine 96 oz.)*, 8 oz. 30.0
Florentine *(Smart Ones)*, 10 oz. 34.0
garden *(Weight Watchers)*, 11 oz. 36.0
with meat sauce:
   (Banquet), 10.5 oz. 39.0
   (Banquet Bake at Home), 1 cup, 8 oz. 32.0
   (Banquet Family), 1 cup, 7 oz. 29.0
   (The Budget Gourmet Light), 9.4 oz. 38.0
   (Freezer Queen Deluxe Family), 1 cup, 8.3 oz. 39.9
   (Freezer Queen Homestyle), 10.5 oz. 41.0
   (Lean Cuisine), 10.5 oz. 35.0
   (Marie Callender's), 1 cup, 7 oz. 34.0
   (Marie Callender's Multi-Serve), 1 cup, 8.9 oz. 32.0
   (Schwan's), 1 cup 30.0
   (Smart Ones), 9 oz. 43.0
   (Stouffer's), 10½ oz. 39.0
   (Stouffer's 21 oz.), approx. 1 cup, 7 oz. 24.0
   (Stouffer's 40 oz.), approx. 1 cup, 8 oz. 28.0
   (Stouffer's 96 oz.), approx. 1 cup, 7.4 oz. 26.0
   (Swanson), 10 oz. 45.0
   (Weight Watchers), 10¼ oz. 38.0
   Bolognese *(The Budget Gourmet Special Selections)*,
     9 oz. 44.0
   Bolognese *(Weight Watchers)*, 9 oz. 45.0
   casserole *(Swanson)*, 1 pkg. 41.0
mozzarella *(The Budget Gourmet Special Selections)*, 9 oz. 52.0
primavera *(Celentano Great Choice)*, 10 oz. 32.0
primavera *(Celentano Selects)*, 10 oz. 33.0
sausage, Italian *(The Budget Gourmet)*, 10.5 oz. 43.0
vegetable:
   (Amy's Family), 7 oz. 27.0
   (Banquet), 10.5 oz. 41.0
   (Lean Cuisine), 10.5 oz. 35.0
   (Schwan's), 1 cup 31.0
   (Stouffer's), 10½ oz. 43.0
   (Stouffer's 96 oz.), 1 cup 34.0
   with cheese *(Amy's)*, 9.5 oz. 39.0
   cheesy *(Swanson)*, 1 pkg. 40.0

Lasagna entree, frozen, vegetable *(cont.)*
tofu *(Amy's)*, 9.5 oz. 41.0
zucchini *(Healthy Choice)*, 13.5 oz. 58.0
Lasagna entree mix:
(Master-A-Meal), ⅕ pkg. 30.0
tomato and vegetable *(Pasta Roni)*, approx. 1 cup* 36.0
Leek, fresh:
raw:
    untrimmed, 1 lb. 28.2
    1 medium, 9.9 oz. 17.6
    trimmed, chopped, ½ cup 7.4
boiled, drained, chopped, ½ cup 4.0
Leek, freeze-dried, 1 tbsp. 2
Lemon:
(Dole), 1 fruit 6.0
with peel, 2⅛″-diam. lemon, 3.9 oz. 11.6
1 wedge, ¼ medium 2.9
peeled, 2⅛″-diam. lemon 5.4
Lemon herb sauce mix *(Knorr)*, 1 tbsp. 4.0
Lemon juice:
fresh, 1 tbsp. 1.3
bottled *(ReaLemon)*, 1 tsp. 0
bottled *(Seneca)*, 1 tsp. 0
Lemon peel, fresh, 1 tbsp. 1.0
Lemon peel, candied:
(S&W), 1.1 oz. 23.0
diced *(Paradise/White Swan)*, 2 tbsp., 1 oz. 21.0
Lemon pepper:
(Lawry's), ¼ tsp. 0
(Tone's), ¼ tsp. 0
1 tsp. 1.5
Lemon sauce *(House of Tsang)*, 2 tbsp. 17.0
Lemonade, 8 fl. oz., except as noted:
(After the Fall) 23.0
(Heinke's Old Fashion) 29.0
(R.W. Knudsen) 29.0
(R.W. Knudsen Aseptic) 27.0
(Minute Maid) 31.0
(Santa Cruz) 29.0
(Snapple) 29.0
(Tropicana) 29.0
(Tropicana), 11.5 fl. oz. 39.0

(Veryfine Chillers), 11.5 fl. oz. 45.0
pink:
   (Minute Maid) 29.0
   (Snapple) 29.0
   (Snapple Diet) 4.0
   (Veryfine Chillers), 11.5 fl. oz. 45.0
frozen*:
   (R.W. Knudsen Natural/Organic) 29.0
   (Minute Maid/Minute Maid Pink) 30.0
   (Schwan's) 35.0
   (Schwan's Lite) 12.0
Lemonade fruit blends, 8 fl. oz.:
all fruit flavors:
   (R.W. Knudsen) 29.0
   (Minute Maid) 32.0
   (Santa Cruz) 29.0
cherry *(Snapple)* 31.0
cherry *(Veryfine* Chillers) 29.0
cranberry *(Heinke's)* 29.0
ginger *(R.W. Knudsen* Echinacea) 25.0
lime *(Veryfine* Chillers) 29.0
peach *(Snapple)* 31.0
peach *(Veryfine* Chillers) 31.0
strawberry *(Snapple)* 29.0
strawberry *(Veryfine* Chillers) 30.0
tangerine *(Veryfine* Chillers) 31.0
tropical *(Minute Maid)* 32.0
frozen*:
   cranberry *(Minute Maid)* 30.0
   raspberry *(Minute Maid)* 30.0
   tropical *(Minute Maid)* 32.0
Lemonade mix*, 8 fl. oz.:
(Country Time) 17.0
(Country Time Punch) 16.0
(Country Time/Kool-Aid Sugar Free) 0
(Crystal Light) 0
(Hi-C Pink) 26.0
(Kool-Aid Presweetened) 17.0
with sugar *(Kool-Aid* With Sugar) 25.0
Lentil:
dry, ¼ cup 27.4
dry, green or red *(Arrowhead Mills)*, ¼ cup 27.0

Lentil *(cont.)*
boiled, ½ cup 19.9
Lentil, canned *(Eden* Organic), ½ cup 13.0
Lentil, sprouted:
raw, 1 lb. 100.4
raw, ½ cup 8.4
stir-fried, ½ cup 24.1
Lentil dishes, canned *(Patak's* Moong Dhal), ½ cup 20.0
Lentil dishes, mix:
burgoo, spicy *(Buckeye Beans)*, 2½ tbsp. 21.0
cassoulet, sausage *(Buckeye Beans)*, 2½ tbsp. 18.0
hearty, and wild rice *(Spice Islands* Quick Meal), 1 pkg. . . . 37.0
and herb *(Eastern Traditions)*, 2 oz. 35.0
honey baked *(Buckeye Beans)*, 4 tbsp. 30.0
pilaf:
    (Casbah), 1 oz. 19.0
    (Near East), 1 cup* 37.0
    almond *(Spice Islands* Quick Meal), 1 pkg. 37.0
Lentil rice loaf, frozen *(Natural Touch)*, 1″ slice 14.0
Lentil salad, garden *(Cedar's)*, 2 tbsp. 4.0
Lettuce (see also "Salad blend mix"):
Bibb or Boston:
    untrimmed, 1 lb. 7.8
    1 head, 5″ diam. 3.8
    2 inner leaves 4
butter *(Dole)*, 1 head 4.0
cos or romaine:
    untrimmed, 1 lb. 10.1
    1 inner leaf 2
    shredded, ½ cup 7
    shredded *(Dole)*, 1½ cups 2.0
iceberg:
    (Dole), ⅙ head 4.0
    1 head, 6″ diam., approx. 1¼ lb. 11.3
    1 leaf, .7 oz. 4
    precut *(Dole)*, 3 oz. 3.0
leaf, shredded *(Dole)*, 1½ cups 1.0
looseleaf:
    untrimmed, 1 lb. 10.2
    1 leaf, approx. .4 oz. 4
    shredded, ½ cup 1.0

Lima beans, ½ cup, except as noted:
(Frieda's), ⅓ cup, 3 oz. 20.0
fresh:
   raw, untrimmed, 1 lb. 40.2
   raw, trimmed 15.7
   boiled, drained 20.1
mature, baby, boiled 21.2
mature, large, boiled 19.6
canned:
   (Goya) 18.0
   (Green Giant/Joan of Arc Butterbeans) 16.0
   (S&W Butterbeans) 18.0
   (Seneca) 15.0
   (Stokely/Stokely No Salt) 15.0
   (Stubb's Harvest Butter Beans) 22.0
   (Van Camp's Butter Beans) 22.0
   baby *(Allens* Butterbeans) 22.0
   green *(Allens/East Texas Fair/Sunshine* Limas/
      Butterbeans) 23.0
   green *(Del Monte)* 15.0
   green *(Goya)* 15.0
   green and white *(Allens)* 20.0
   large *(Allens* Butterbeans) 20.0
   mature, baby, green or butterbeans *(Stokely)* 19.0
   with bacon, baby green *(Trappey's* Limas) 22.0
   with bacon, baby white *(Trappey's* Limas) 21.0
   with ham and sauce *(Nalley),* 1 cup 34.0
   with sausage, large white *(Trappey's* Butterbeans) 21.0
dried, Christmas *(Frieda's)* 22.0
frozen:
   baby *(Birds Eye)* 24.0
   baby *(Green Giant Harvest Fresh)* 15.0
   baby *(Seabrook)* 22.0
   baby *(Stilwell)* 22.0
   baby, in butter sauce *(Green Giant),* ⅔ cup 18.0
   Fordhook *(Birds Eye)* 19.0
   Fordhook *(Stilwell)* 17.0
   plain or speckled *(Stilwell* Butterbeans) 20.0
Lime:
(Dole), 1 medium, 2.4 oz. 7.0
2″-diam. lime, 2.8 oz. 7.1
peeled, seeded, 1 oz. 3.0

Lime drink, 8 fl. oz.:
(After the Fall Key West) 25.0
(R.W. Knudsen Cactus Cooler) 29.0
frozen* *(Minute Maid* Limeade) 26.0
Lime juice, 1 tsp., except as noted:
fresh, 1 tbsp. 1.4
bottled or chilled *(ReaLime)* 0
sweetened *(Rose's)* 2.0
Ling, without added ingredients 0
Lingcod, without added ingredients 0
Linguine, plain:
dry, see "Pasta"
refrigerated *(Contadina),* 1¼ cups 46.0
refrigerated, plain or herb *(Di Giorno),* 2.5 oz. 39.0
Linguine dish, mix, garlic and butter *(Lipton* Pasta &
   Sauce), ⅓ cup mix or 1 cup* 40.0
Linguine entree, frozen:
with shrimp and clams *(The Budget Gourmet* Light), 9.5 oz. 38.0
with shrimp and clams marinara *(The Budget Gourmet),*
   9 oz. 36.0
with tomato sauce and sausage *(The Budget Gourmet*
   Special Selections), 10¼ oz. 48.0
Linguine entree, mix, approx. 1 cup*
chicken and broccoli *(Pasta Roni)* 49.0
chicken Parmesan, creamy *(Pasta Roni)* 51.0
Liquor[1], all proofs, 1 fl. oz. . . . . <.1
Litchee, see "Lychee"
Little Caesars, 1 serving:
Baby Pan!Pan!, 2 squares 67.3
Crazy Bread, 1 piece 15.9
Crazy Sauce, 6 oz. 13.7
Pan!Pan!, cheese only, 1 medium slice 22.1
Pan!Pan!, pepperoni, 1 medium slice 22.2
Pizza!Pizza!, cheese only, 1 medium slice 23.8
Pizza!Pizza!, pepperoni, 1 medium slice 23.9
salads, individual:
   antipasto 7.4
   Caesar 13.6
   Greek 12.3

[1]*Includes all pure distilled liquors: bourbon, brandy, gin, rum, Scotch, tequila,
vodka, etc.*

tossed 19.3
dressings, 1.5 oz.:
  blue cheese 7.9
  Caesar 2.6
  French 6.0
  Greek 4
  Italian, regular or fat free 3.0
  ranch 4.7
  Thousand Island 6.4
sandwiches, cold:
  ham and cheese 71.0
  Italian 71.3
  veggie 74.2
sandwiches, hot:
  Cheeser 75.2
  Meatsa 75.3
  pepperoni 73.6
  supreme 77.1
  veggie 78.7
Liver:
beef, pan-fried, 4 oz. 8.9
chicken, raw *(Tyson)*, 4 oz. 2.0
chicken, simmered, 4 oz. 1.0
chicken, chopped, 1 cup 1.2
duck, raw, 1 oz. 1.0
goose, raw, 1 oz. 1.8
lamb, pan-fried, 4 oz. 4.3
pork, braised, 4 oz. 4.3
turkey, simmered, 4 oz. 3.9
turkey, simmered, chopped, 1 cup 4.8
veal (calve's), braised, 4 oz. 3.1
Liver cheese *(Oscar Mayer)*, 1.3-oz. slice 1.0
Liver pâté, see "Pâté"
Liverwurst (see also "Braunschweiger"), 2 oz.:
(Boar's Head Strassburger/Smoked) 0
(Underwood) 3.0
pâté *(Boar's Head)* 0
spread *(Hormel)* 2.0
Lo bok, see "Radish, Oriental"
Lo mein entree mix, see "Entree mix, frozen"
Lobster, northern, meat only:
raw, 4 oz. 6

Lobster *(cont.)*
boiled or steamed, 4 oz. 1.5
boiled or steamed, 1 cup, 5.1 oz. 1.9
frozen, chunks *(Tyson* Delight), 3 oz. 11.0
"Lobster," imitation, frozen or refrigerated:
chunks *(Captain Jac Lobster Tasties),* ½ cup, 3 oz. 12.0
chunks *(Louis Kemp Lobster Delights),* ½ cup, 3 oz. 11.0
salad style *(Louis Kemp Lobster Delights),* ½ cup, 3 oz. . . . 11.0
tail style *(Captain Jac Lobster Tasties),* 4-oz. tail 17.0
Lobster sauce, rock *(Progresso),* ½ cup 6.0
Loganberry:
fresh, untrimmed, 1 lb. 64.2
fresh, 1 cup 21.5
frozen, ½ cup 9.6
Long beans, see "Yard-long beans"
Long John Silver's, 1 serving:
chicken, fish, and seafood:
   chicken, batter-dipped, 1 piece 11.0
   chicken, *Flavorbaked,* 1 piece . . . . <1.0
   chicken, popcorn, 3.3 oz. 17.0
   clams, 3 oz. 31.0
   fish, batter-dipped, 1 piece 12.0
   fish, *Flavorbaked,* 1 piece 1.0
   fish, popcorn, 3.6 oz. 27.0
   shrimp, batter-dipped, 1 piece 2.0
   shrimp, popcorn, 3.3 oz. 27.0
sandwiches, 1 piece:
   chicken, *Flavorbaked* 27.0
   fish, batter-dipped, without sauce 40.0
   fish, *Flavorbaked* 28.0
   Ultimate Fish 44.0
sides:
   cheese sticks, 1.6 oz. 12.0
   coleslaw 20.0
   corn cobbette, with or without butter, 1 piece 19.0
   french fries, 3 oz. 28.0
   green beans 5.0
   hush puppy, 1 piece 9.0
   potato, baked 49.0
   rice pilaf 26.0
   side salad 4.0

dressings:
    French, fat free, 1½ oz. 14.0
    Italian, 1 oz. 2.0
    ranch, 1 oz. 1.0
    ranch, fat free, 1½ oz. 13.0
    Thousand Island, 1 oz. 5.0
sauces/condiments:
    honey mustard, .4 oz. 5.0
    malt vinegar, .3 oz. 0
    margarine, .2 oz. 0
    shrimp sauce, .4 oz. 3.0
    sour cream, 1 oz. 1.0
    sweet 'n' sour, .4 oz. 5.0
    tartar sauce, .4 oz. 5.0
Longan:
fresh:
    untrimmed, 1 lb. 36.4
    1 medium, approx. .2 oz. 5
    shelled and seeded, 1 oz. 4.3
dried, 1 oz. 21.0
Loquat:
(Frieda's), 5 oz. 17.0
untrimmed, 1 lb. 34.1
1 medium, .6 oz. 1.2
peeled and seeded, 1 oz. 3.4
Lotus root:
(Frieda's), 1 cup, 3 oz. 15.0
raw, untrimmed, 1 lb. 61.8
raw, trimmed, 1 oz. 4.9
boiled, drained, 4 oz. 18.3
boiled, drained, 10 slices, 3.1 oz. 14.3
Lotus seed:
raw, in shell, 1 lb. 41.5
raw, 1 oz. 4.9
dried, 1 oz., 47 small or 36 large 18.3
fried, 1 cup 20.6
Lox, see "Salmon, smoked"
Lunch combinations *(Lunchables),* 1 pkg.:
bologna/American 22.0
bologna/wild cherry 60.0
chicken/turkey deluxe 25.0
ham/cheddar 21.0

Lunch combinations *(cont.)*

ham/fruit punch	54.0
ham/fruit punch, low fat	50.0
ham/*Surfer Cooler,* low fat	58.0
ham/Swiss	20.0
pizza, mozzarella/fruit punch	61.0
pizza/pepperoni/mozzarella	32.0
pizza/pepperoni/orange	62.0
pizza, two cheese	29.0
salami/American	21.0
turkey/cheddar	22.0
turkey/ham deluxe	25.0
turkey/Monterey Jack	20.0
turkey/*Pacific Cooler*	54.0
turkey/*Pacific Cooler,* low fat	55.0
turkey/*Surfer Cooler*	61.0

Lunch meat (see also specific listings), spiced loaf *(Oscar Mayer)*, 1-oz. slice 2.0
Lunch meat, canned, 2 oz.:
(Spam/Spam Less Salt/Lite) 0
spread *(Spam)* 1.0
Lunch "meat," vegetarian, canned *(Loma Linda Nuteena),* 3/8" slice 6.0
Lupin:
raw, 1/2 cup 36.3
boiled, 1/2 cup 8.2
Lupin beans, in jars *(Canto Lupini),* 1/4 cup 3.0
Lychee:
raw:
   in shell, 1 lb. 45.0
   shelled and seeded, 1 oz. 4.7
   shelled and seeded, 1/2 cup 15.7
dried, 1 oz. 20.0
Lychee, canned, in syrup *(Ka•Me),* 5 oz. 32.0
Lychee juice *(Ceres* Litchi), 8 fl. oz. 31.0

M

FOOD AND MEASURE   **CARBOHYDRATE GRAMS**

Macadamia nut, shelled:
(Frieda's), 5 pieces, 1.1 oz. 4.0
dried, 1 oz. 3.9
dried, 1 cup 18.4
oil-roasted, 1 oz. 3.7
Macaroni, uncooked (see also "Pasta, dry, uncooked"),
   2 oz., except as noted:
(Creamette) 42.0
elbow:
   (Eden) 39.0
   (Goya Coditos) 45.0
   1 cup 78.4
   whole wheat *(Eden)* 39.0
Macaroni, cooked (see also "Pasta, dry, cooked"):
4 oz. 32.1
elbow, 1 cup 39.7
small shells, 1 cup 32.6
spirals, 1 cup 38.0
vegetable (tri-color), 4 oz. 30.2
whole-wheat, 4 oz. 30.1
Macaroni dinner, and cheese, frozen *(Swanson* Budget),
   1 pkg. 43.0
Macaroni entree, canned, 7½ oz., except as noted:
and beef:
   (Kid's Kitchen Beefy) 23.0
   (Kid's Kitchen Cheezy Mac & Beef) 34.0
   (Libby's Diner), 7¾ oz. 31.0
   (Nalley), 1 cup 34.0
and cheese:
   (Chef Boyardee Bowl) 31.0
   (Franco-American), 1 cup 29.0
   (Hormel Micro Cup) 30.0
   (Kid's Kitchen) 30.0
   (Libby's Diner), 7¾ oz. 25.0
   (Nalley) 22.0

Macaroni entree, canned *(cont.)*
chili, see "Chili"
Macaroni entree, frozen:
and beef:

(Banquet Bake at Home), 1 cup, 8 oz.	31.0
(Freezer Queen Homestyle), 9 oz.	32.0
(Kid Cuisine Rip-Roaring), 9.6 oz.	58.0
(Lean Cuisine), 10 oz.	40.0
(Marie Callender's), 1 cup, 7 oz.	40.0
(Stouffer's), 11½ oz.	40.0
casserole *(Swanson)*, 1 pkg.	39.0

broccoli *(Swanson Mac & More)*, 1 pkg. 28.0
and cheese:

(Amy's), 9 oz.	58.0
(Banquet), 10.5 oz.	47.0
(Banquet Bake at Home), 1 cup, 8 oz.	39.0
(Banquet Family), 1 cup, 7 oz.	33.0
(The Budget Gourmet Value Classics Homestyle), 9 oz.	47.0
(Freezer Queen Family Side Dish), 1 cup, 8.6 oz.	40.0
(Healthy Choice), 9 oz.	45.0
(Kid Cuisine Magical), 10.6 oz.	68.0
(Lean Cuisine), 10 oz.	42.0
(Marie Callender's), 1 cup. 6.5 oz.	47.0
(Morton), 6.5 oz.	35.0
(Morton 16/28 oz.), 1 cup	40.0
(Schwan's), 1 cup	28.0
(Smart Ones), 9 oz.	42.0
(Stouffer's 12 oz.), approx. 1 cup, 6 oz.	31.0
(Stouffer's 20 oz.), approx. 1 cup, 8 oz.	32.0
(Stouffer's 40 oz.), approx. 1 cup, 8 oz.	40.0
(Stouffer's 76 oz.), approx. 1 cup. 8.4 oz.	38.0
(Swanson Entree), 1 pkg.	36.0
(Swanson Entree), 1 cup	34.0
(Swanson Mac & More Classic), 1 pkg.	30.0
(Tabatchnik Side Dish), 7.5 oz.	30.0
(Weight Watchers), 9 oz.	49.0
bake casserole, 3-cheese *(Swanson)*, 1 pkg.	53.0
and broccoli *(Lean Cuisine* Lunch Classics), 9¾ oz.	34.0
with broccoli *(Stouffer's)*, 10.5 oz.	37.0
with cheddar and Romano *(The Budget Gourmet* Special Selections), 9 oz.	50.0
cheddar, white *(Swanson Mac & More)*, 1 pkg.	27.0

pie *(Banquet)*, 6.5 oz. 36.0
salsa *(Swanson Mac & More)*, 1 pkg. 27.0
Italiano *(Swanson Mac & More)*, 1 pkg. 25.0
soy cheeze *(Amy's)*, 9 oz. 42.0
Macaroni entree mix, dry, except as noted:
and cheese:
   (Creamette), 1/3 pkg. 48.0
   (Kraft Original Dinner), 2½ oz. 47.0
   (Kraft Original Deluxe Dinner), 3½ oz. 44.0
   (Kraft Thick'n Creamy), 2½ oz. 48.0
   (Land O Lakes Deluxe Plus), approx. 1 cup* 45.0
   (Land O Lakes Original), approx. 1 cup* 49.0
   Alfredo *(Annie's)*, ½ cup 33.0
   all varieties *(Kraft* Dinner), 2½ oz. 47.0
   cheddar *(Fantastic)*, 3/8 cup 40.0
   cheddar *(Golden Grain)*, 1 cup* 40.0
   Parmesan *(Fantastic)*, 3/8 cup 40.0
   rotini, with broccoli *(Velveeta)*, 4½ oz. 46.0
   shells *(Land O Lakes)*, approx. 1 cup* 42.0
   shells *(Velveeta* Original), 4 oz. or approx. 1 cup* 44.0
   shells, with bacon *(Velveeta)*, 4 oz. or approx. 1 cup* . . 43.0
   shells, with salsa *(Velveeta* Original), 4 oz. or approx.
     1 cup* 47.0
   three cheese *(Knorr* Cup), 1 pkg. 40.0
Macaroni and cheese, see "Macaroni dinner" and
  "Macaroni entree"
Mace:
(McCormick), 1/4 tsp. 2
ground, 1 tbsp. 2.7
ground, 1 tsp. 9
Mackerel, fresh, canned, or smoked, meat only 0
Madras sauce, see "Curry sauce"
Mahimahi:
fresh, without added ingredients 0
frozen, fillet *(Peter Pan)*, 4 oz. 0
Mai tai drink mixer, bottled *(Mr & Mrs T)*, 4.5 fl. oz. 33.0
Malanga *(Frieda's)*, 2/3 cup, 3 oz. 23.0
Malt beverage *(Goya)*, 12 fl. oz. 39.0
Malt cooler, 12-oz. bottle:
(Bartles & Jaymes Original) 29.0
berry *(Bartles & Jaymes)* 33.0
black cherry *(Bartles & Jaymes)* 32.0

Malt cooler *(cont.)*

Fuzzy Navel *(Bartles & Jaymes)* 39.0
iced tea, Long Island *(Bartles & Jaymes)* 43.0
mai tai *(Bartles & Jaymes)* 40.0
Margarita *(Bartles & Jaymes)* 46.0
peach *(Bartles & Jaymes)* 33.0
piña colada *(Bartles & Jaymes)* 48.0
sangria *(Bartles & Jaymes)* 31.0
strawberry *(Bartles & Jaymes)* 33.0
strawberry daiquiri *(Bartles & Jaymes)* 36.0
tropical *(Bartles & Jaymes)* 37.0

Malted milk powder, 3 tbsp.:

natural *(Kraft)* 17.0
natural *(Nestlé Original)* 15.0
chocolate *(Kraft)* 15.0
chocolate *(Nestlé)* 18.0

Mammy apple:

fresh, untrimmed, 1 lb. 34.0
fresh, peeled, seeded, 1 oz. 3.5
frozen, chunks *(Goya)*, ⅓ pkg. 32.0

Mandarin orange, see "Tangerine, canned"

Mandioca, see "Yuca"

Mango:

fresh:

    untrimmed, 1 lb. 53.2
    10.6-oz. fruit 35.2
    peeled:
        (Frieda's), 5 oz. 23.0
        sliced *(Dole)*, ½ cup 14.0
        sliced, ½ cup 14.0
dried *(Frieda's)*, 4 pieces, 1.4 oz. 32.0
dried *(Sonoma)*, 2 oz. 44.0
in jars, in light syrup *(Sunfresh)*, ½ cup 25.0

Mango drink, 8 fl. oz.:

(Snapple Madness) 29.0
(Snapple Madness Diet) 5.0
(Tree Top More Mango) 30.0
tangerine *(Veryfine)* 27.0

Mango juice, 8 fl. oz.:

(After the Fall Montage) 27.0
(Ceres) 30.0
peach *(R.W. Knudsen)* 30.0

Mango nectar, 8 fl. oz., except as noted:
(Goya), 12 fl. oz. 56.0
(Libby's/Kern's) 36.0
orange *(Kern's)* 35.0
Manhattan mixer, bottled *(Holland House/Mr & Mrs T)*,
  2 fl. oz. 15.0
Manicotti, frozen, 2 pieces:
(Celentano), 7 oz. 40.0
mini *(Celentano)*, 4.8 oz. 32.0
Manicotti entree, frozen:
cheese:
    (Celentano), 10 oz. 41.0
    (Celentano), ½ of 14-oz. pkg. 27.0
    (Celentano Great Choice), 10 oz. 41.0
    (Celentano Value Pack), 2 pieces, 8 oz. 28.0
    (Stouffer's), 9 oz. 38.0
    (Weight Watchers), 9¼ oz. 31.0
    with meat sauce *(The Budget Gourmet)*, 10 oz. 38.0
    three cheese *(Healthy Choice)*, 11 oz. 40.0
Florentine *(Celentano)*, 10 oz. 28.0
Florentine *(Celentano Great Choice)*, 10 oz. 29.0
Maple syrup *(Cary's/Maple Orchard's/MacDonald's* Pure),
  ¼ cup 52.0
Margarine, all varieties and blends, 1 tbsp. 0
Margarita mixer:
bottled *(Holland House/Mr & Mrs T)*, 4 fl. oz. 29.0
bottled, strawberry *(Holland House/Mr & Mrs T)*, 3.5 fl. oz. 34.0
frozen* *(Bacardi)*, 8 fl. oz. 25.0
mix *(Bar-Tenders)*, 2 pkt., .9 oz. 21.0
Marinade (see also "Stir-fry sauce" and specific listings),
  1 tbsp., except as noted:
(House of Tsang Classic), ½ tbsp. 4.0
(House of Tsang Mandarin) 6.0
(Stubb's Legendary Moppin' Sauce) 1.0
Hawaiian *(Lawry's)* 4.0
hickory grill *(Adolph's Marinade in Minutes)* 4.0
lemon butter dill, seafood *(Ken's Steak House)* 3.0
lemon garlic *(Adolph's Marinade in Minutes)* 2.0
lemon pepper *(Lawry's)* 1.0
mesquite *(Adolph's Marinade in Minutes)* 5.0
red wine *(Lawry's)* 1.0
and stir-fry sauce *(Mary Rose* Sari) 1.0

Marinade _(cont.)_
teriyaki _(Adolph's Marinade in Minutes)_ 4.0
Marinade seasoning mix, 1 tbsp.*, except as noted:
lemon herb _(Adolph's Marinade in Minutes)_ 2.0
lemon pepper _(Adolph's Marinade in Minutes)_ 2.0
meat _(Lawry's Carne Asada)_, 1 tsp. 1.0
mesquite _(Adolph's Marinade in Minutes)_ 2.0
Parmesan herb _(Adolph's Marinade in Minutes)_ 1.0
scampi _(Adolph's Marinade in Minutes)_ 2.0
teriyaki _(Adolph's Marinade in Minutes)_ 3.0
Marjoram, dried:
(McCormick), ¼ tsp. 2
1 tbsp. 1.0
1 tsp. 4
Marmalade, see "Jam and preserves"
Marrow beans, dried _(Frieda's)_, ½ cup 22.0
Marrow squash, raw, trimmed, 1 oz. 1.0
Marshmallow topping, 2 tbsp.:
(Smucker's) 29.0
all varieties _(Marshmallow Fluff)_ 5.0
creme _(Kraft)_ 10.0
Masa, see "Corn flour" and Cornmeal"
Matzo, see "Cracker"
Mayonnaise, 1 tbsp.:
(Best Foods Real) 0
(Blue Plate) 0
(Hellmann's Real) 0
(Hellmann's/Best Foods Light) 1.0
(Hellmann's/Best Foods Low Fat) 4.0
(Kraft Real) 0
(Master Choice) 0
(Nalley Cholesterol Free) 2.0
(Nalley Real) 0
(Nalley Light) 1.0
(Smart Beat Super Light Reduced Fat) 2.0
(Weight Watchers Light/Light Low Sodium) 1.0
canola _(Smart Beat Reduced Fat)_ 2.0
dressing:
(Kraft Free) 2.0
(Kraft Light) 1.0
(Miracle Whip Salad) 2.0
(Miracle Whip Free/Miracle Whip Light) 3.0

   (Nalley Whip) 3.0
   (Smart Beat Nonfat) 3.0
   (Spin Blend/Spin Blend Nonfat) 3.0
   (Weight Watchers Fat Free/Weight Watchers Whipped) . . . 3.0
tofu (Nayonaise) 1.0

McDonald's, 1 serving:
breakfast biscuits:
   plain 32.0
   bacon, egg, and cheese 33.0
   sausage 32.0
   sausage and egg 33.0
breakfast dishes:
   burrito 23.0
   eggs, scrambled, 2 . . . . 1.0
   hash browns 14.0
   hotcakes, plain . : 53.0
   hotcakes, with syrup and margarine 100.0
   sausage 0
breakfast muffins:
   Egg McMuffin 27.0
   English 25.0
   Sausage McMuffin 26.0
   Sausage McMuffin, with egg 27.0
Danish and muffin:
   apple bran muffin 61.0
   apple Danish 51.0
   cheese Danish 47.0
   cinnamon roll 47.0
sandwiches:
   Arch Deluxe or Arch Deluxe with bacon 39.0
   Big Mac 45.0
   cheeseburger 35.0
   Crispy Chicken Deluxe 43.0
   Fish Filet Deluxe 54.0
   Grilled Chicken Deluxe 38.0
   hamburger 34.0
   Quarter Pounder 37.0
   Quarter Pounder, with cheese 38.0
Chicken McNuggets:
   4 pieces 10.0
   6 pieces 15.0
   9 pieces 23.0

McDonald's (cont.)

McNuggets sauce pkt.:

barbeque	10.0
honey	12.0
honey mustard	3.0
hot mustard	7.0
light mayonnaise	0
sweet and sour	11.0

french fries:

small	26.0
large	57.0
Super Size	68.0

salad, garden	7.0
salad, grilled chicken deluxe	7.0
salad croutons, 1 pkg.	7.0

salad dressing, 1 pkg.:

Caesar	7.0
ranch	10.0
red French, reduced calorie	23.0
vinaigrette, herb, fat free	11.0

desserts and shakes:

baked apple pie	34.0
chocolate chip cookie	22.0
ice cream cone, vanilla, reduced fat	23.0
McDonaldland Cookies, 1 pkg.	32.0
shake, chocolate or strawberry, small	60.0
shake, vanilla, small	59.0
sundae, hot caramel	61.0
sundae, hot fudge	52.0
sundae, strawberry	50.0
sundae nuts, 1/4 oz.	2.0

Meat, canned (see also "Meat spread"):

potted *(Goya),* 1/4 cup	0
potted *(Hormel),* 2 oz.	1.0
potted or deviled *(Libby's),* 3 oz.	0

"Meat," ground (see also " 'Hamburger,' ground"), frozen:

(Morningstar Farms Ground Meatless), 1/2 cup	4.0

Meat, lunch, see "Lunch meat" and specific listings

Meat, potted, see "Meat, canned"

Meat loaf dinner, frozen:

(Banquet Extra Helping), 19 oz.	49.0
(Freezer Queen Meal), 9.5 oz.	23.0

(Healthy Choice), 12 oz. 52.0
(Marie Callender's), 14 oz. 44.0
(Schwan's), 1 pkg. 52.0
(Swanson), 1 pkg. 44.0
(Swanson Budget), 1 pkg. 29.0
(Swanson Hungry Man), 1 pkg. 65.0
Meat loaf entree, frozen:
(Banquet Homestyle), 9.5 oz. 23.0
with whipped potato *(Lean Cuisine)*, 9⅜ oz. 24.0
with whipped potato *(Stouffer's Homestyle)*, 9⅞ oz. 26.0
with sauce and vegetables *(Swanson)*, 1 pkg. 20.0
tomato sauce and *(Freezer Queen Family)*, ⅙ of 28-oz. pkg. 10.0
tomato sauce with *(Morton)*, 9 oz. 24.0
"Meat" loaf mix, vegetarian *(Natural Touch)*, ¼ cup 10.0
Meat loaf seasoning mix:
(Adolph's Meal Makers), 1 tbsp. 7.0
(Durkee Pouch), ⅑ pkt. 3.0
(Durkee/French's Roasting Bag), ⅛ pkg. 2.0
(Lawry's), 1 tbsp. 7.0
Meat seasoning *(Aromat)*, ¼ tsp. 0
Meat spread (see also specific listings):
(Oscar Mayer Sandwich Spread), 2 oz. 8.0
Meat tenderizer, unseasoned *(Tone's)*, 1 tsp. 1.2
"Meatball," vegetarian, with gravy, canned
   (Loma Linda Tender Rounds), 6 pieces 5.0
Meatball entree, frozen:
Italian *(Schwan's)*, 6 pieces, 3 oz. 7.0
Italian style, with vegetables, in wine *(The Budget Gourmet*
   Italian Originals), 10 oz. 27.0
and spaghetti, see "Spaghetti entree"
Swedish:
   (The Budget Gourmet), 10 oz. 40.0
   (Healthy Choice), 9.1 oz. 35.0
   (Stouffer's), 10¼ oz. 43.0
   (Weight Watchers), 9 oz. 33.0
   with pasta *(Lean Cuisine)*, 9⅛ oz. 38.0
Meatball seasoning mix, Italian *(Durkee Pouch)*, ⅕ pkt. . . . 3.0
Meatball stew, canned:
(Dinty Moore), 1 cup 18.0
(Dinty Moore Cup), 7.5 oz. 16.0
Melon, see specific melon listings

Melon, mixed:
balls, frozen *(Stilwell)*, 1 cup 14.0
balls, frozen, cantaloupe and honeydew, ½ cup 6.9
salad, in jars, in extra light syrup *(Sunfresh* Lite), ½ cup . . 20.0
salad, in jars, in light syrup *(Sunfresh)*, ½ cup 20.0
Melonberry juice cocktail *(Snapple)*, 8 fl. oz. 29.0
Menudo, canned *(Goya)*, 1 cup 12.0
Menudo seasoning mix *(Gebhardt)*, ¼ tsp. 0
Mesquite sauce *(S&W)*, 1 tbsp. 3.0
Mesquite seasoning *(Tone's)*, ¼ tsp. 0
Mexican beans (see also "Chili beans"), canned or in jars,
   ½ cup:
(Allens/Brown Beauty) 21.0
(Chi-Chi's Ranchero) 18.0
(Old El Paso Mexe Beans) 19.0
(Stokely Red) 21.0
with bacon and jalapeños *(Rosarita Fiesta/3-Bean Recipe)* . . 22.0
with chicken and chilies *(Rosarita Fiesta/3-Bean Recipe)* . . 22.0
with chilies and chorizo *(Rosarita Fiesta/3-Bean Recipe)* . . 19.5
with jalapeños *(Brown Beauty)* 21.0
with jalapeños *(Trappey's* Mexi-Beans) 22.0
with onions and peppers *(Rosarita Fiesta/3-Bean Recipe)* . . 20.0
Mexican dinner (see also specific listings), frozen:
(Patio), 13¼ oz. 59.0
(Patio Fiesta), 12 oz. 51.0
(Patio Ranchera), 13 oz. 55.0
style:
   (Banquet Extra Helping), 22 oz. 100.0
   (Swanson Budget), 1 pkg. 52.0
   (Swanson Hungry Man), 1 pkg. 86.0
   combination *(Swanson)*, 1 pkg. 57.0
Mexican entree (see also specific listings), frozen:
(Banquet), 11 oz. 56.0
combination *(Banquet)*, 11 oz. 55.0
Mexican seasoning:
(Chi-Chi's Mix), 1 tsp. 1.0
(Tone's), 1 tsp. 1.3
with coriander or saffron *(Goya)*, ¼ tsp. 0
Milk, dairy pack or packaged, 1 cup:
buttermilk *(Friendship)* 12.0
buttermilk, cultured 11.7
(Lactaid 100) 13.0

(Lactaid Calcium Fortified/Nonfat) 13.0
low-fat:
   2% 11.7
   2% *(Lactaid* 100) 13.0
   2% *(Parmalat)* 13.0
   2%, protein fortified 13.5
   1% 11.7
   1% *(Lactaid)*................................ 13.0
   1% *(Parmalat)* 13.0
   1%, protein fortified 13.6
   skim 11.9
   skim *(Parmalat)*............................ 13.0
   skim *(Weight Watchers)* 13.0
whole:
   (America's Choice).......................... 11.0
   (Juniper Valley Organic/Lactose Free Organic) 12.0
   (Parmalat) 13.0
   3.3% fat 11.4
Milk, canned, 2 tbsp.:
condensed, sweetened:
   (Borden) 23.0
   (Carnation) 22.0
   (Eagle/Magnolia Brand/Meadow Gold/Star) 23.0
   (Goya) 22.0
   low-fat *(Borden)* 23.0
   low-fat *(Eagle)* 23.0
   skim *(Borden* Fat Free) 24.0
   skim *(Eagle* Fat Free) 24.0
evaporated:
   (Carnation)................................. 3.0
   (Pet/Pet Skimmed)........................... 3.0
   low-fat *(Carnation)*......................... 3.0
   skim *(Carnation)* 4.0
Milk, chocolate, see "Chocolate milk"
Milk, dry:
buttermilk, sweet cream, 1 cup 58.8
buttermilk, sweet cream, 1 tbsp. 3.2
whole, 1 oz. 10.9
whole, 1 cup 49.2
nonfat:
   (Carnation), ⅓ cup 12.0
   regular, 1 cup 62.4

Milk, dry, nonfat *(cont.)*

instant, 3.2-oz. pkt. 35.5

Milk, goat's:

(Meyenberg), 1 cup 11.0

1 cup 10.9

powdered *(Meyenberg),* 1 cup* 11.0

"Milk," nondairy (see also "Soy beverage"), 8 fl. oz.:

(EdenBlend) 16.0

(EdenRice) 21.0

(Rice Dream Original/*Rice Dream* Original Enriched) . . 25.0

carob *(Rice Dream)* 32.0

chocolate *(Rice Dream/Rice Dream* Enriched) 36.0

vanilla *(Rice Dream/Rice Dream* Enriched) 28.0

Milk, sheep's, 1 cup 13.1

Milk beverage, flavored (see also specific flavors):

Butterfinger (Nestlé Quik), 8 fl. oz. 30.0

shake, root beer *(Nestlé Killer),* 14 oz. 67.0

Milk shake, see "Milk beverage, flavored" and specific
flavors

Milkfish, without added ingredients 0

Millet:

raw, 1 oz. 20.7

cooked, 4 oz. 26.8

hulled *(Arrowhead Mills),* ¼ cup 34.0

Millet flour *(Arrowhead Mills),* ¼ cup 26.0

Mincemeat, see "Pie filling"

Mint baking chips *(Hershey's),* 1 tbsp. 10.0

Mint sauce *(Crosse & Blackwell),* 1 tsp. 1.0

Miso, soy, 1 tbsp., except as noted:

(Eden Hacho) 2.0

1 oz. 7.9

½ cup 38.6

with barley *(Eden Organic Mugi)* 3.0

with brown rice *(Eden Genmai)* 3.0

with white rice *(Eden Shiro)* 5.0

Mocha drink:

chilled *(Nestlé Mocha Cooler),* 1 cup 25.0

canned, cafe *(Carnation Instant Breakfast),* 10 fl. oz. . . . 35.0

mix, see "Coffee, flavored, mix"

Molasses, 1 tbsp.:

(Grandma's 4-Star/Gold/Green) 14.0

bead *(La Choy)* 12.0

blackstrap *(New Morning)* 13.0
dark or light *(Brer Rabbit)* 14.0
Monkfish, without added ingredients 0
Monosodium glutamate *(Tone's)*, 1 tsp. 0
Mortadella, 2 oz., except as noted:
(Boar's Head Cinghiale) 0
beef and pork, 1 oz. 9
with pistachios *(Boar's Head Cinghiale)* 3.0
Moth beans, boiled, 4 oz. 23.8
Mother's loaf, pork, 1 oz. 2.1
Mousse, frozen, 2.75 oz.:
chocolate *(Weight Watchers)* 31.0
triple chocolate caramel *(Weight Watchers)* 34.0
Mousse pudding, see "Pudding mix"
Muffin, 1 piece, except as noted:
(Arnold Bran'nola) 29.0
(Arnold Extra Crisp) 25.0
apple *(Awrey's)*, 1½ oz. 18.0
apple *(Awrey's)*, 2½ oz. 28.0
banana nut:
   (Awrey's Grande) 46.0
   (Tastykake), ½ piece, 2 oz. 26.0
   (Tastykake Family) 33.0
   mini *(Awrey's)*, 2 pieces 22.0
   mini *(Hostess)*, 3 pieces 16.0
blueberry:
   (Awrey's), 1½ oz. 19.0
   (Awrey's), 2½ oz. 30.0
   (Awrey's Grande) 43.0
   (Entenmann's) 24.0
   (Entenmann's Fat Free) 26.0
   (Tastykake), ½ piece, 2 oz. 30.0
   (Tastykake Family) 27.0
   (Tastykake Low Fat), ½ piece, 2 oz. 32.0
   loaf *(Hostess)*, 3.8 oz. 62.0
   mini *(Awrey's)*, 2 pieces 22.0
   mini *(Hostess)*, 3 pieces 18.0
   top *(Awrey's)*, 2½ oz. 31.0
carrot raisin *(Awrey's* Grande) 59.0
cheese streusel *(Awrey's* Grande) 48.0
chocolate chip, mini *(Hostess)*, 5 pieces 17.0
chocolate chocolate chip *(Awrey's* Grande) 51.0

Muffin *(cont.)*

cinnamon apple, mini *(Hostess)*, 5 pieces 16.0
corn:

    (Awrey's), 1½ oz. 20.0
    (Awrey's), 2½ oz. 33.0
    (Sara Lee) 30.0
    (Tastykake), ½ piece, 2 oz. 30.0
    (Tastykake Golden Family) 31.0
cranberry nut *(Awrey's)* 20.0
cranberry orange *(Tastykake* Low Fat), ½ piece, 2 oz. 33.0
English:

    (Awrey's) 28.0
    (Pepperidge Farm) 26.0
    (Roman Meal) 27.0
    (Tastykake) 26.0
    (Thomas') 25.0
    (Wonder) 25.0
    blueberry *(Thomas')* 31.0
    cinnamon raisin *(Pepperidge Farm)* 28.0
    cinnamon raisin *(Tastykake)* 20.0
    cranberry *(Thomas')* 31.0
    honey wheat *(Thomas')* 24.0
    oat bran *(Thomas')* 26.0
    raisin *(Thomas')* 31.0
    sandwich size *(Thomas'* 4 Pack/Twin) 38.0
    seven grain *(Pepperidge Farm)* 26.0
    sourdough *(Pepperidge Farm)* 26/0
    sourdough *(Tastykake)* 25.0
    sourdough *(Thomas')* 25.0
    sourdough, sandwich size *(Thomas' Em's)* 41.0
    wheat, sandwich size *(Thomas' Em's)* 39.0
lemon poppyseed *(Awrey's)* 19.0
lemon poppyseed *(Awrey's* Grande) 41.0
oat bran *(Hostess)* 22.0
onion, sandwich size *(Thomas' Em's)* 40.0
raisin *(Arnold)* 32.0
raisin bran:

    (Awrey's), 1½ oz. 18.0
    (Awrey's), 2½ oz. 30.0
    (Awrey's Grande) 47.0
    (Tastykake Low Fat), ½ piece, 2 oz. 38.0
    top *(Awrey's)* 30.0

raspberry, loaf *(Hostess)*, 3.8 oz. 62.0
sourdough *(Arnold)* 25.0
Muffin, frozen or refrigerated, 1 piece:
apple oatmeal *(Pepperidge Farm Wholesome Choice)* 28.0
banana nut *(Weight Watchers Fat Free)* 41.0
blueberry *(Pepperidge Farm Wholesome Choice)* 27.0
blueberry *(Weight Watchers Fat Free)* 38.0
bran, with raisins *(Pepperidge Farm Wholesome Choice)* . . . 30.0
chocolate chocolate chip *(Weight Watchers)* 39.0
corn *(Pepperidge Farm Wholesome Choice)* 27.0
English *(Thomas')* 25.0
English, honey wheat *(Thomas')* 24.0
honey bran *(Weight Watchers Fat Free)* 36.0
Muffin mix, 1 muffin*, except as noted:
apple cinnamon:
   (Betty Crocker) 24.0
   (Betty Crocker Fat Free) 26.0
   (Martha White) 31.0
   (Martha White), 1/4 cup 30.0
   (Martha White Low Fat) 34.0
   (Pillsbury) 31.0
   (Pillsbury), 1/3 cup 30.0
   (Robin Hood) 23.0
   (Robin Hood), 1/6 pkg. 22.0
   (Sweet Rewards Fat Free) 28.0
banana nut:
   (Betty Crocker) 24.0
   (Gold Medal/Robin Hood) 22.0
   (Gold Medal/Robin Hood), 1/6 pkg. 21.0
   (Martha White) 26.0
   (Martha White), 1/3 cup 25.0
blackberry *(Martha White)* 31.0
blackberry *(Martha White)*, 1/4 cup 30.0
blueberry:
   (Betty Crocker) 25.0
   (Betty Crocker Fat Free) 27.0
   (Duncan Hines) 28.0
   (Duncan Hines Bakery Style) 32.0
   (Duncan Hines Bakery Style), 1/12 pkg. 30.0
   (Martha White) 31.0
   (Martha White), 1/4 cup 30.0
   (Martha White Low Fat), 1/4 cup 34.0

Muffin mix, blueberry *(cont.)*
    (Pillsbury) 31.0
    (Pillsbury), 1/3 cup 30.0
    (Pillsbury Low Fat), 1/4 cup 34.0
    (Robin Hood) 25.0
    (Robin Hood), 1/6 pkg. 24.0
    (SnackWell's) 28.0
    (Sweet Rewards Fat Free) 27.0
    double *(Martha White)* 30.0
    double *(Martha White)*, 1/4 cup 31.0
    wild *(Betty Crocker)* 29.0
bran:
    (Martha White) 29.0
    multi *(Buckeye)*, 1/12 pkg. 25.0
    oat *(Arrowhead Mills)*, 1/3 cup 23.0
    oat *(Martha White)* 28.0
    oat *(Martha White)*, 1/3 cup 30.0
    wheat *(Arrowhead Mills)*, 1/3 cup 26.0
caramel nut *(Gold Medal/Robin Hood)* 11.0
caramel nut *(Gold Medal/Robin Hood)*, 1/6 pkg. 10.0
chocolate chip *(Duncan Hines)* 30.0
chocolate chocolate chip:
    (Martha White) 24.0
    (Pillsbury) 31.0
    (Pillsbury), 1/3 cup 30.0
cinnamon streusel *(Betty Crocker)* 22.0
cinnamon streusel *(Betty Crocker)*, 1/4 cup 21.0
cinnamon swirl *(Duncan Hines)* 33.0
corn:
    (Flako), 1/3 cup 23.0
    (Gladiola) 25.0
    (Gladiola), 1/4 cup 26.0
    (Gold Medal) 25.0
    (Gold Medal), 1/6 pkg. 24.0
    white *(Martha White)* 31.0
    white *(Martha White)*, 1/3 cup 32.0
honey pecan *(Martha White)* 21.0
honey pecan *(Martha White)*, 1/3 cup 22.0
lemon poppyseed:
    (Betty Crocker) 30.0
    (Martha White) 29.0
    (Martha White), 1/3 cup 30.0

oatmeal raisin *(Martha White)* 29.0
oatmeal raisin *(Martha White)*, ¼ cup 30.0
raspberry *(Martha White)* 30.0
raspberry *(Martha White)*, ¼ cup 31.0
raspberry swirl *(Duncan Hines)* 27.0
strawberry:
    (Martha White) 30.0
    (Martha White), ¼ cup 31.0
    (Martha White Low Fat) 34.0
    (Pillsbury) 31.0
    (Pillsbury), ⅓ cup 30.0
Muffin sandwich, see "Egg breakfast sandwich"
Mulberry:
untrimmed, 1 lb. 44.5
10 berries, .5 oz. 1.5
½ cup 6.9
Mullet, without added ingredients 0
Mung beans:
dry *(Arrowhead Mills)*, ¼ cup 28.0
boiled, ½ cup 19.3
Mung beans, sprouted, fresh:
raw:
    (Jonathan's), 1 cup 4.0
    1 lb. 26.9
    1 oz. 1.7
    ½ cup 3.1
boiled, drained, ½ cup 2.6
Mungo beans:
dry, ¼ cup 31.8
boiled, ½ cup 16.5
Mushroom:
fresh:
    (Dole), 5 medium, 3 oz. 3.0
    raw, pieces, ½ cup 1.6
    boiled, drained, pieces, ½ cup 4.0
    enoki, trimmed, 1 oz. 2.2
    enoki, 1 large, 4⅛" long 4
    oyster *(Frieda's)*, 3 oz. 4.0
    portobello *(Frieda's)*, 1 oz. 1.2
    shiitake *(Frieda's)*, 3 oz. 4.0
    shiitake, cooked, 4 medium or ½ cup pieces 10.4
    wood ear *(Frieda's)*, 3 oz. 4.0

Mushroom, fresh *(cont.)*
  yamabiko honshimeji *(Frieda's)*, 1.1 oz. 1.0
Mushroom, canned, ½ cup, except as noted:
(Seneca/Seneca No Salt) 5.0
(Seneca Jars) 4.0
all varieties *(BinB)*, 4¼-oz. can 4.0
all varieties *(Green Giant)* 4.0
shiitake *(Seneca)* 5.0
straw *(Roland)* 3.0
teriyaki, sliced *(Seneca)* 15.0
Mushroom, breaded, frozen:
(Empire Kosher), 7 pieces, 2.9 oz. 16.0
(Schwan's), 1 cup 22.0
Mushroom, dried:
chanterelle *(Frieda's)*, 2 pieces, .14 oz. 2.0
freeze-dried *(Tone's)*, ⅓ cup 2.0
morel *(Frieda's)*, 3 pieces, .14 oz. 2.0
padi straw *(Frieda's)*, 6 pieces, .14 oz. 2.0
porcini *(Frieda's)*, 5 pieces, .14 oz. 2.0
portobello *(Frieda's)*, 7 pieces, .14 oz. 1.0
shiitake, 4 medium, ½ oz. 11.3
stir-fry *(Frieda's)*, 4 pieces, .14 oz. 2.0
Mushroom, marinated *(Seneca)*, 1 oz. 2.0
Mushroom, pickled *(Seneca)*, 1 oz. 1.0
Mushroom blends:
pasta, soup, or steak *(Frieda's)*, 6 pieces, .14 oz. 2.0
poultry or sauce *(Frieda's)*, 4 pieces, .14 oz. 2.0
Mushroom entree mix, see "Entree mix, frozen"
Mushroom gravy, ¼ cup:
(Franco-American) 3.0
(Heinz Homestyle Fat Free) 3.0
country or with wine *(Pepperidge Farm)* 4.0
creamy *(Franco-American)* 4.0
Mushroom gravy mix:
(Durkee), ¼ cup* 3.0
(French's), ¼ cup* 3.0
(Loma Linda Gravy Quik), 1 tbsp. 3.0
brown *(Durkee)*, ¼ cup* 3.0
hunter *(Knorr)*, 1 tbsp. 4.0
Mushroom salad, all varieties *(Seneca)*, 1 tbsp. . . . . . . <1.0
Mushroom sauce:
(House of Tsang), 1 tbsp. 2.0

mix *(Knorr)*, 1/5 pkg. 2.0
Mussel, blue, meat only:
raw, 4 oz. 4.2
raw, 1 cup 5.5
boiled or steamed, 4 oz. 8.4
Mustard, in jars, 1 tsp., except as noted:
(Boar's Head Deli) 0
(Grey Poupon Deli) 0
(Grey Poupon Spicy) . . . . <1.0
(Gulden's Spicy) 0
(Hunt's) 0
(Kraft Pure) 0
(Nance's Sharp & Creamy/Hot) 2.0
all varieties *(French's)* 0
all varieties *(Hebrew National* Deli) 0
Chinese *(House of Tsang)*, 1 pkt. . . . . <1.0
Dijon *(Grey Poupon)* . . . . <1.0
Dijon *(Roland* Extra Strong) 0
horseradish *(Kraft)* 0
hot *(Eden* Organic) . . . . <1.0
honey *(Nance's)* 3.0
Mustard blend *(Best Foods/Hellmann's Dijonnaise)*, 1 tsp. . . . 1.0
Mustard greens:
fresh:
    raw, untrimmed, 1 lb. 20.7
    raw, chopped, 1 oz. or 1/2 cup 1.4
    boiled, drained, chopped, 1/2 cup 1.5
canned *(Allens/Sunshine)*, 1/2 cup 5.0
canned *(Stubb's Harvest)*, 1/2 cup 5.0
frozen, chopped *(Seabrook)*, 3 oz. 2.0
Mustard powder *(Spice Islands)*, 1 tsp. 3
Mustard sauce mix, herb *(Knorr)*, 1 tbsp. 5.0
Mustard seed, yellow:
(McCormick), 1/4 tsp. 2
1 tbsp. 3.9
1 tsp. 1.2
Mustard spinach, see "Spinach, mustard"
Mustard tallow, 1 tbsp. 0

N

FOOD AND MEASURE	CARBOHYDRATE GRAMS

Nacho dip (see also "Cheese dip"), mild *(Guiltless Gourmet)*, 2 tbsp. 5.0
Nacho dip mix *(Knorr)*, ½ tsp. 1.0
Natto, ½ cup 12.6
Navy beans:
dry, ¼ cup 31.5
boiled, ½ cup 24.0
canned, ½ cup:
   (Allens) 19.0
   (Eden Organic) 20.0
   (Stokely) 19.0
   with liquid 26.8
   bacon or bacon and jalapeño *(Trappey's)* 17.0
Navy beans, sprouted:
raw, 1 lb. 59.2
raw, ½ cup 6.8
boiled, drained, 4 oz. 17.0
Nectarine, fresh:
(Dole), 1 fruit, 5 oz. 16.0
untrimmed, 1 lb. 48.6
1 medium, 2½" diam., 5.3 oz. 16.0
sliced, ½ cup 8.1
New England sausage *(Oscar Mayer)*, 1.6 oz. 1.0
New Zealand spinach, see "Spinach, New Zealand"
Newburg sauce mix *(Knorr)*, ⅓ pkg. 5.0
Noodle, Chinese:
(Nasoya), 1 cup, 2¾ oz. 43.0
cellophane or long rice, dry, 2 oz. 48.0
chow mein:
   (Chun King), ½ cup 18.5
   (Frieda's), 4 oz. 40.0
   (La Choy), ½ cup 18.5
   (Mee Tu), ⅔ cup 19.0
   ½ cup 13.0
crispy, wide *(La Choy)*, ½ cup 16.0

egg, dried *(House of Tsang)*, 2 oz. 43.0
rice *(La Choy)*, ½ cup 21.0
Noodle, egg:
uncooked, 2 oz.:
    (Creamette/Penn Dutch) 39.0
    (Kluski) 40.0
    (Manischewitz) 42.0
    all varieties *(Creamette/Goodman's)* 40.0
    all varieties *(Eden* Organic) 42.0
    bow ties *(Mueller's)* 38.0
    and spinach *(Prince* Paglia E Fieno) 41.0
    yolk-free *(Borden)* 41.0
cooked, 1 cup 39.7
cooked, spinach, 1 cup 38.8
Noodle, egg-free, frozen *(Morningstar Farms* Homestyle),
  ½ cup 33.0
Noodle, Japanese, dry, except as noted:
(Nasoya), 1 cup, 2¾ oz. 43.0
soba, dry, 2 oz., except as noted:
    (Eden Organic Traditional), ½ cup 38.0
    (Eden Traditional) 37.0
    2 oz. 42.5
    buckwheat *(Eden* 100%) 41.0
    buckwheat *(Eden* 40%) 37.0
    lotus root *(Eden)* 37.0
    mugwort *(Eden)* 37.0
    wild yam *(Eden)* 37.0
soba, cooked, 1 cup 24.4
somen:
    (Eden Organic Traditional), ½ cup 38.0
    2 oz. 42.2
    cooked, 1 cup 48.5
spinach *(Nasoya)*, 1 cup, 2¾ oz. 42.0
udon:
    (Eden), 2 oz. 37.0
    (Eden Organic Traditional), ½ cup 38.0
    2 oz. 32.3
    brown rice *(Eden* Organic Traditional), ½ cup 38.0
    cooked, 4 oz. 23.0
Noodle dishes, canned or frozen, see "Noodle entree"
Noodle dishes, mix:
Alfredo *(Lipton* Noodles & Sauce), ½ pkg. 39.0

Noodle dishes, mix *(cont.)*
Alfredo *(Lipton* Noodles & Sauce), 1 cup* 42.0
Alfredo, broccoli *(Lipton* Noodles & Sauce), ½ pkg. 40.0
Alfredo, broccoli *(Lipton* Noodles & Sauce), 1 cup* 43.0
beef *(Lipton* Noodles & Sauce), ½ pkg. or 1 cup* 43.0
butter *(Lipton* Noodles & Sauce), ½ pkg. or 1 cup* 41.0
butter and herb *(Lipton* Noodles & Sauce), ½ pkg.
    or 1 cup* 42.0
cheddar *(Kraft* Dinner), 2.5 oz. 45.0
cheddar *(Master-A-Meal),* ⅕ pkg. 30.0
cheddar *(Nissin* Noodles and Sauce), 2.5 oz. 43.0
chicken/chicken flavor:
    (Kraft Dinner), 2.5 oz. 45.0
    (Lipton Noodles & Sauce), ½ pkg. or 1 cup* 42.0
    (Nissin Noodles and Sauce), 2.4 oz. 41.0
    broccoli *(Lipton* Noodles & Sauce), ½ pkg. 41.0
    broccoli *(Lipton* Noodles & Sauce), 1 cup* 44.0
    creamy *(Lipton* Noodles & Sauce), ½ pkg. 39.0
    creamy *(Lipton* Noodles & Sauce), 1 cup* 42.0
    tetrazzini *(Lipton* Noodles & Sauce), ½ pkg. 38.0
    tetrazzini *(Lipton* Noodles & Sauce), 1 cup* 41.0
Oriental *(Knorr* Cup), 1 pkg. 39.0
Oriental *(Pasta Roni),* approx. 1 cup* 38.0
Parmesan *(Lipton* Noodles & Sauce), ½ pkg. 37.0
Parmesan *(Lipton* Noodles & Sauce), 1 cup* 40.0
sour cream and chive *(Lipton* Noodles & Sauce), ½ pkg.
    or 1 cup* 41.0
Stroganoff *(Lipton* Noodles & Sauce), ½ pkg. 37.0
Stroganoff *(Lipton* Noodles & Sauce), 1 cup* 40.0
tomato, Italian *(Nissin* Noodles & Sauce), 2.4 oz. 42.0
Noodle entree, canned, 1 cup, except as noted:
with beef *(Hunt's* Homestyle) 22.0
with beef *(La Choy* Bi-Pack) 24.0
with chicken:
    (Dinty Moore), 7½ oz. 21.0
    (Hormel Micro Cup), 7½ oz. 21.0
    (Hormel Micro Cup), 10½ oz. 31.0
    (Hunt's Homestyle) 21.0
    (La Choy Bi-Pack) 23.0
    (Nalley Dinner) 21.0
    cacciatore *(Hunt's* Homestyle) 21.0
    and mushrooms *(Hunt's* Homestyle) 32.0

and vegetables *(Nalley)* 19.0
and vegetables *(Nalley)*, 7½ oz. 19.0
with franks *(Van Camp's Noodle Weenee)*, 1 can 34.0
rings *(Kid's Kitchen)*, 7.5 oz. 16.0
sweet and sour, with chicken *(La Choy* Entree) 49.0
with vegetables:
    (La Choy Entree) 27.0
    and beef *(La Choy* Entree) 27.0
    and chicken *(La Choy* Entree) 24.0
Noodle entree, frozen:
and beef *(Banquet* Family), 1 cup, 7 oz. 16.0
and chicken *(Banquet* Bake at Home), 1 cup, 8 oz. 24.0
and chicken, escalloped *(Marie Callender's/Marie Callender's*
    Multi-Serve), 1 cup 22.0
escalloped, and turkey *(The Budget Gourmet* Special
    Selections), 10¾ oz. 44.0
kung pao, and vegetables *(Weight Watchers* International
    Selections), 10 oz. 35.0
Romanoff *(Stouffer's)*, 12 oz. 48.0
Nut topping (see also specific listings), *(Planters)*, 2 tbsp.   . 3.0
Nutmeg, ground:
(McCormick), ¼ tsp. 3
1 tbsp. 3.5
1 tsp. 1.1
Nuts, see specific listings
Nuts, mixed, 1 oz., except as noted:
dry-roasted *(Planters)* 7.0
dry-roasted, with peanuts, salted or unsalted 7.2
honey-roasted *(Planters)* 9.0
oil-roasted:
    (Paradise/White Swan), ¼ cup, 1.2 oz. 6.0
    (Planters) 5.0
    (Planters Deluxe/Lightly Salted/Unsalted) 6.0
    with peanuts, salted or unsalted 6.1
    no Brazils *(Planters* 3½ oz./Lightly Salted) 6.0
    no peanuts *(Paradise/White Swan* Deluxe), ¼ cup,
       1.2 oz. 7.0
cashews, with almonds and macadamias *(Planters* Select) . . . 6.0
cashews, with almonds and pecans *(Planters* Select) 7.0
sesame, oil-roasted *(Planters)* 9.0
tamari-roasted *(Eden)* 9.0

O

FOOD AND MEASURE   **CARBOHYDRATE GRAMS**

Oat (see also "Cereal, ready-to-eat"):
whole-grain, 1 oz. 18.8
flakes, rolled *(Arrowhead Mills)*, ⅓ cup 23.0
rolled or oatmeal:
    dry, 1 oz. 19.0
    dry, ½ cup 27.0
    cooked, 1 cup 25.2
steel cut *(Arrowhead Mills)*, ¼ cup 29.0
Oat bran (see also "Cereal, ready-to-eat" and "Cereal,
   cooking/hot"):
dry:
    (Arrowhead Mills), ⅓ cup 23.0
    1 oz. 18.8
    ½ cup 31.1
cooked, 1 cup 25.1
Oat flour *(Arrowhead Mills)*, ⅓ cup 20.0
Oat groats *(Arrowhead Mills)*, ¼ cup 29.0
Oatmeal, see "Oat" and "Cereal"
Oaxacan chili, See "Pepper, chili"
Ocean perch:
fresh, without added ingredients 0
frozen *(Schwan's)*, 4 oz. .... <1.0
Ocean perch entree, battered, frozen *(Van de Kamp's)*,
   2 fillets 19.0
Octopus, meat only:
raw, 4 oz. 2.5
boiled or steamed, 4 oz. 5.0
Octopus, canned, 2 oz.:
(Goya) 3.0
in garlic sauce *(Goya)* 3.0
à la marinara *(Goya)* 4.0
in olive oil *(Goya)* 3.0
spiced, in red sauce *(Reese)* 4.0
Oheloberry:
1 lb. 31.0

½ cup 4.8
10 berries, .4 oz. 8
Oil, all varieties 0
Oil substitute (Baking Healthy), 1 tbsp. 7.0
Okra:
fresh:
    raw, untrimmed, 1 lb. 29.8
    raw, 8 pods, 3″ × ⅝″, 3.9 oz. 7.3
    raw, sliced, ½ cup 3.8
    boiled, drained, 8 pods, 3″ × ⅝″ 6.1
    boiled, drained, sliced, ½ cup 5.8
canned, ½ cup:
    cut (Allens/Trappey's) 6.0
    cut (Stubb's Harvest) 6.0
    with tomatoes (Allens/Trappey's) 5.0
    with tomatoes and corn (Allens/Trappey's) 6.0
    Creole gumbo (Trappey's) 6.0
frozen:
    boiled, drained, sliced, ½ cup 7.5
    whole (Seabrook), 9 pods, 3 oz. 5.0
    whole (Stilwell), 9 pods, 3 oz. 6.0
    cut (Stilwell), ¾ cup 4.0
    and tomatoes (Stilwell), ⅔ cup 5.0
Old-fashioned drink mixer, bottled (Holland House),
    2 fl. oz. 20.0
Old-fashioned loaf (Oscar Mayer), 1 oz. 2.0
Olive, pickled:
black, see "ripe," below
Calamata (Krinos), 3 pieces 2.0
Calamata (Zorba), 5 pieces 2.0
green, all varieties (B&G), 1 oz. . . . . <1.0
green, with pits:
    10 small 4
    10 large 5
    10 giant 9
green, pitted, 1 oz. 4
green, cracked (Krinos), ½ oz. 2.0
green, queen/Spanish (S&W), 2 pieces 1.0
green, queen/Spanish (Zorba), 2 pieces 1.0
ripe, with pits (Lindsay), 5 medium or 4 large 0
ripe, with pits (S&W), 1 super colossal 1.0

Olive *(cont.)*
ripe, pitted:
  (Lindsay), 6 small, 5 medium, 4 large, or 1⅓ tbsp.
    chopped 1.0
  (S&W), 3 extra large or jumbo 1.0
  (Vlasic), 4 large or 6 small 1.0
  California *(Vlasic),* 1 tsp. chopped or 4–6 pieces 1.0
  Spanish *(Vlasic),* 8 small 1.0
ripe, Greek:
  (Krinos), ½ oz. 2.0
  (Krinos Alfonso), ½ oz. 1.0
  (Krinos Nafplion), ½ oz. 2.0
  (Zorba), 1.7-oz. piece 6.0
  10 medium 1.7
  10 extra large 2.3
  pitted, 1 oz. 2.5
ripe, oil-cured *(Krinos),* ½ oz. 3.0
ripe, oil-cured *(Progresso),* 3 pieces 3.0
royal *(Krinos),* ½ oz. 1.0
salad *(Goya),* ¼ cup 0
stuffed, Manzanilla:
  (Goya), 4 pieces 0
  (Lindsay), 5 pieces 1.0
  (S&W), 3 pieces 1.0
stuffed, queen:
  (Goya), 2 pieces 0
  (Lindsay), 2 pieces 1.0
  (S&W 4¾ oz.), 2 pieces 1.0
  (S&W 7 oz.), 2 pieces 1.0
  (S&W 10 oz.), 1 piece 1.0
  queen *(Vlasic),* ½ oz. 1.0
  stuffed, with tuna *(Goya),* 4 pieces 1.0
Olive loaf:
(Boar's Head), 2 oz. . . . . <1.0
(Oscar Mayer), 1-oz. slice 2.0
Olive oil 0
Olive salad, drained *(Progresso),* 2 tbsp. 1.0
Omelet, see "Egg breakfast"
Ong choy, see "Spinach, water"
Onion, mature:
fresh or stored, raw:
  (Frieda's Boiler/Cipolline), 3 onions, 3 oz. 7.0

(Frieda's Maui), 1/3 cup, 3 oz. 3.0
(Frieda's Pearl), 2/3 cup, 3 oz. 7.0
raw, untrimmed, 1 lb. 35.2
raw, trimmed, 1 oz. 2.4
raw, chopped, 1/2 cup 6.9
raw, chopped, 1 tbsp. 9
boiled, drained, chopped, 1/2 cup 10.7
boiled, drained, chopped, 1 tbsp. 1.5
canned or in jars:
  whole (Green Giant), 1/2 cup 8.0
  whole (S&W), 1/2 cup 8.0
  cocktail (Crosse & Blackwell), 1 tbsp. 1.0
  cocktail (S&W 4 oz.), 12 pieces, 1.1 oz. 1.0
  cocktail (S&W 16 oz.), 8 pieces, 1.1 oz. 1.0
  sweet, in sauce (Boar's Head Vidalia), 1 tbsp. 2.0
  wild, marinated (Krinos Volvi), 1 oz. 2.0
frozen:
  whole, small (Birds Eye), 17 pieces 7.0
  boiled, drained, 1 tbsp. 1.0
  chopped (Ore-Ida), 3/4 cup 6.0
  in cream sauce (Birds Eye), 1/2 cup 10.0
  rings, see "Onion rings"
Onion, cocktail, see "Onion"
Onion, dried:
flakes, 1/4 cup 11.7
flakes, 1 tbsp. 4.2
minced, 1 tsp. 1.9
Onion, green (scallion), raw:
untrimmed, 1 lb. 32.0
chopped, trimmed, with tops:
  1 oz. 2.1
  1/2 cup 3.7
  1 tbsp. 4
freeze-dried (McCormick), 1/4 tsp. 2
Onion, Welsh:
untrimmed, 1 lb. 19.2
trimmed, 1 oz. 1.8
Onion dip, 2 tbsp.:
creamy (Kraft Premium) 2.0
French:
  (Breakstone's) 2.0
  (Frito-Lay) 4.0

Onion dip, French *(cont.)*
   (Heluva Good) 2.0
   (Heluva Good Free) 3.0
   (Knudsen Premium) 2.0
   (Kraft) 4.0
   (Kraft Premium) 2.0
   (Nalley) 3.0
   (Old Dutch) 3.0
   (Ruffles) 4.0
   (Ruffles Low Fat) 6.0
   (Sealtest) 2.0
green *(Kraft)* 4.0
toasted *(Breakstone's)* 2.0
sour cream and *(Lay's* Low Fat) 6.0
Onion dip mix, and chive *(Knorr)*, ½ tsp. 1.0
Onion gravy, ¼ cup:
roasted, and garlic *(Pepperidge Farm)* 4.0
zesty *(Heinz* Homestyle) 3.0
mix*:
   (Durkee) 3.0
   (French's) 4.0
   (Loma Linda Gravy Quik) 3.0
   brown *(Durkee)* 4.0
   brown, Lyonnaise *(Knorr)* 4.0
Onion powder:
(McCormick), ¼ tsp. 0.6
(Tone's), ¼ tsp. 1.0
1 tsp. 2.4
Onion rings, canned *(French's French Fried Real Onions)*,
   2 tbsp. 3.0
Onion rings, frozen:
(Mrs. Paul's Old Fashioned), 7 rings, 3 oz. 29.0
(Ore-Ida Classic/Gourmet), 4 rings 26.0
(Ore-Ida Onion Ringers), 6 rings 26.0
(Schwan's), 3 oz. 18.0
Onion salt:
(Durkee California), ½ tsp. 0
(Tone's), 1 tsp. 4
Onion sprouts:
(Jonathan's), 1 cup 5.0
(Shaw's Premium Salad), 2 oz. 0
Opo squash *(Frieda's)*, ⅔ cup, 3 oz. 3.0

Opossum, without added ingredients . . . . : 0
Orange:
(Dole), 1 fruit 21.0
all varieties, untrimmed, 1 lb. 38.9
blood *(Frieda's)*, 5 oz. 16.0
California:
    navel, $2^7/_8$"-diam. orange 16.3
    navel, sections without membrane, ½ cup 9.6
    Valencia, $2^5/_8$"-diam. orange 14.4
    Valencia, sections without membrane, ½ cup 10.7
Florida, $2^{11}/_{16}$"-diam. orange 17.4
Florida, sections without membrane, ½ cup 10.7
Orange, in jars, in light syrup *(Sunfresh)*, ½ cup 18.0
Orange, mandarin, see "Tangerine"
Orange drink, 8 fl. oz., except as noted:
(Capri Sun), 6.75 fl. oz. 26.0
(Hi-C) . . . . : 32.0
(Hi-C Box) 34.0
(Lincoln) 33.0
orangeade *(Snapple)* 29.0
punch *(Kool-Aid Bursts)*, 6.75 fl. oz. 24.0
tropical *(Farmers Market)* 29.0
chilled or frozen* *(Bright & Early)* 30.0
frozen* *(Schwan's Vita-Sun)* 23.0
Orange drink blends, 8 fl. oz.:
cranberry *(Tropicana Twister)* 32.0
cranberry *(Tropicana Twister* Light) 7.0
guava nectar *(Kern's)* 36.0
peach *(Tropicana Twister)* 31.0
pineapple *(Lincoln)* 32.0
raspberry *(Tropicana Twister)* 31.0
raspberry *(Tropicana Twister* Light) 9.0
strawberry-banana *(Tropicana Twister)* 29.0
strawberry-banana *(Tropicana Twister* Light) 9.0
strawberry-guava *(Tropicana Twister)* 29.0
Orange drink mix*, 8 fl. oz.:
(Kool-Aid with Sugar) 16.0
(Tang) 24.0
(Tang Sugar Free) 1.0
Orange juice:
fresh, 8 fl. oz. 25.6
fresh, juice from $2^5/_8$"-diam. orange 8.9

Orange juice *(cont.)*
(Apple & Eve), 10 fl. oz. 32.0
(Dole), 10 fl. oz. 33.0
(Minute Maid Box), 8.45 fl. oz. 28.0
(S&W), 6-fl.-oz. can 22.0
(Seneca), 8 fl. oz. 28.0
(Tree Top), 8 fl. oz. 28.0
(Tree Top), 5.5 fl. oz. 19.0
(Tree Top), 10 fl. oz. 35.0
(Tree Top), 11.5 fl. oz. 40.0
(Tropicana Pure Premium), 8 fl. oz. 27.0
(Tropicana Pure Premium + Fiber), 8 fl. oz. 30.0
(Tropicana Ruby Red Pure Premium), 8 fl. oz. 28.0
(Veryfine), 8 fl. oz. 24.0
(Veryfine), 11.5 fl. oz. 34.0
chilled or frozen*, all varieties *(Minute Maid)*, 8 fl. oz. 27.0
frozen* *(Schwan's)*, 8 fl. oz. 28.0
frozen *(Seneca TreeSweet)*, 2 oz. 26.0
Orange juice blends, 8 fl. oz., except as noted:
grapefruit, 6 fl. oz. 19.1
kiwi–passion fruit *(Tropicana* Tropics) 26.0
mango *(R.W. Knudsen)* 30.0
peach-mango *(Tropicana* Tropics) 28.0
pineapple *(Tropicana* Tropics) 27.0
punch *(Juicy Juice)* 30.0
punch *(Veryfine* Juice-Ups) 35.0
Orange juice float *(R.W. Knudsen)*, 8 fl. oz. 33.0
Orange peel:
1 tbsp. 1.5
candied *(S&W)*, 58 pieces, 1.1 oz. 23.0
candied, diced *(Paradise/White Swan)*, 2 tbsp., 1.1 oz. 23.0
Orange roughy, see "Roughy, orange"
Orange sauce, mandarin *(Ka•Me)*, 1 tbsp. 11.0
Oregano, dried:
(McCormick), 1/4 tsp. 3
1 tsp. 5
Mexican *(McCormick)*, 1/4 tsp. 2
Oriental five spice *(Tone's)*, 1 tsp. 1.9
Oriental sauce (see also "Stir-fry sauce" and specific
  listings), 1 tsp., except as noted:
(House of Tsang Chow Chow) 0
(House of Tsang Imperial), 1 tbsp. 5.0

(House of Tsang Namasu) 2.0
brown, spicy *(House of Tsang)* 3.0
hot and spicy *(House of Tsang* Hunan) 0
Oyster, meat only:
Eastern, wild:
    raw, 1 lb. 17.7
    raw, 6 medium, 3 oz. 3.3
    baked, broiled, or microwaved, 4 oz. 5.4
    steamed or poached, 4 oz. 8.9
Eastern, farmed, raw, 4 oz. 6.3
Eastern, farmed, baked, broiled, or microwaved, 4 oz. 8.3
Pacific:
    raw, 4 oz. 5.6
    raw, boiled, or steamed, 1 medium, 1.75 oz. 2.5
    boiled or steamed, 4 oz. 11.2
Oyster, canned:
Eastern, wild, with liquid, 4 oz. 4.4
Eastern, wild, with liquid, 1 cup 9.7
whole *(S&W),* 2 oz. 2.0
smoked *(Reese* Petite), 2 oz. 6.0
smoked *(S&W),* 2 oz. 6.0
Oyster plant, see "Salsify"
Oyster and shrimp sauce *(TryMe* Caribbean Clipper), 1 tsp. . 2.0
Oyster stew, see "Soup"

P

Palm, hearts of:

(Goya), ½ cup	3.0
(Haddon House), 4.5 oz.	4.0

Pancake, frozen, 3 pieces, except as noted:

(Aunt Jemima Lowfat)	33.0
(Aunt Jemima Original)	40.0
(Downyflake)	47.0
(Hungry Jack Microwave Original)	45.0
blueberry (Aunt Jemima)	40.0
blueberry (Hungry Jack Microwave)	45.0
buttermilk:	
(Aunt Jemima)	38.0
(Hungry Jack Microwave)	46.0
(Schwan's)	49.0
mini (Hungry Jack Microwave), 11 pieces	44.0

Pancake batter, frozen, ½ cup:

(Aunt Jemima Original)	50.0
blueberry (Aunt Jemima)	55.0
buttermilk (Aunt Jemima)	51.0

Pancake breakfast, frozen, 1 pkg.:

(Swanson Kids Breakfast Blast Mini)	54.0
with bacon (Swanson Great Starts)	42.0
with sausage (Swanson Great Starts)	52.0
silver dollar, eggs and (Swanson Great Starts)	22.0
silver dollar, and sausage (Swanson Great Starts)	36.0

Pancake mix, dry:

(Aunt Jemima Complete), ⅓ cup	39.0
(Aunt Jemima Original), ⅓ cup	34.0
(Betty Crocker Complete), ⅓ cup	39.0
(Bisquick Shake 'N Pour), ½ cup	39.0
(Gladiola), ½ cup	41.0
(Hungry Jack Original), ⅓ cup	32.0
(Hungry Jack Premeasured), ½ pkt.	38.0
(Hungry Jack Extra Lights), ⅓ cup	33.0
(Hungry Jack Hungry Lights Complete), ⅓ cup	30.0

(Martha White Flapstax), ½ cup 45.0
blueberry *(Bisquick Shake 'N Pour)*, ½ cup 40.0
buckwheat *(Arrowhead Mills)*, ⅓ cup 25.0
buckwheat *(Aunt Jemima)*, ¼ cup 28.0
buttermilk:
    (Arrowhead Mills), ¼ cup 25.0
    (Aunt Jemima Complete), ⅓ cup 38.0
    (Aunt Jemima Complete Reduced Calorie), ⅓ cup 30.0
    (Betty Crocker Complete), ⅓ cup 39.0
    (Bisquick Shake 'N Pour), ½ cup 38.0
    (Hungry Jack), ⅓ cup 33.0
    (Hungry Jack Complete), ⅓ cup 32.0
    (Robin Hood), ⅓ cup 31.0
corn, blue *(Arrowhead Mills)*, ⅓ cup 28.0
gluten-free *(Arrowhead Mills)*, ¼ cup 24.0
kamut *(Arrowhead Mills)*, ¼ cup 26.0
multigrain *(Arrowhead Mills)*, ¼ cup 24.0
oat bran *(Arrowhead Mills)*, ⅓ cup 25.0
whole grain *(Arrowhead Mills)*, ¼ cup 24.0
whole wheat *(Aunt Jemima)*, ¼ cup 28.0
wild rice *(Arrowhead Mills)*, ⅓ cup 30.0
Pancake syrup (see also "Maple syrup"), ¼ cup:
(Aunt Jemima)........................ 53.0
(Aunt Jemima Lite) 27.0
(Country Kitchen)...................... 53.0
(Country Kitchen Lite).................... 26.0
(Golden Griddle)....................... 57.0
(Hungry Jack) 17.0
(Hungry Jack Lite) 8.0
(Karo) 60.0
(Log Cabin)......................... 52.0
(Log Cabin Lite)....................... 26.0
(Mrs. Richardson's) 52.0
(Mrs. Richardson's Lite) 26.0
butter flavor:
    (Aunt Jemima Butterlite) 26.0
    (Aunt Jemima Rich) 52.0
    (Country Kitchen) 53.0
    maple *(Hungry Jack)* 17.0
    maple *(Hungry Jack* Lite) 8.0
butter or maple flavor *(S&W* Reduced Calorie) 15.0
Pancreas, without added ingredients 0

Papaya:
fresh:
    1-lb. papaya, 3½″ × 5⅛″ 29.8
    peeled, cubed, ½ cup 6.9
    peeled *(Frieda's)*, 1 oz. 2.8
    peeled and cubed *(Dole)*, ½ cup 7.0
dried *(Frieda's)*, ⅓ cup, 1.4 oz. 29.0
dried *(Sonoma)*, 2 pieces, 2 oz. 41.0
frozen, slices *(Goya)*, ⅓ pkg. 11.0
canned, in light syrup *(Ka•Me)*, ¾ cup 29.0
in jars, slices, in light syrup *(Sunfresh)*, ½ cup 17.0
Papaya, creamed *(R.W. Knudsen)*, 2 fl. oz. 10.0
Papaya drink, 8 fl. oz., except as noted:
(Farmer's Market) 32.0
colada *(Snapple)* 29.0
juice *(After the Fall* Pele's) 25.0
nectar:
    (Goya), 12 fl. oz. 56.0
    (R.W. Knudsen) 34.0
    (Libby's/Kern's), 11.5 fl. oz. 51.0
    (Santa Cruz) 28.0
punch *(Lincoln)* 32.0
Pappadum:
(Patak's), 3 pieces, 1 oz. 13.0
snack crisps *(Tamarind Tree)*, 30 pieces, 1 oz. 16.0
Paprika:
(McCormick), ¼ tsp. 3
1 tbsp. 3.9
1 tsp. 1.2
Parfait, frozen *(Weight Watchers)*, 1 piece:
double fudge brownie 39.0
praline toffee crunch 40.0
strawberry 35.0
Parsley:
fresh:
    untrimmed, 1 lb. 27.3
    1 oz. 1.8
    10 sprigs, approx. .4 oz. 6
    chopped, ½ cup 1.9
    chopped *(Dole)*, 1 tbsp. 7
dried:
    (McCormick), ¼ tsp. 0

1 tbsp. 7
1 tsp. 2
freeze-dried, ¼ cup 6
freeze-dried, 1 tbsp. 2
Parsley root, raw:
(Frieda's), ⅔ cup, 3 oz. 2.0
1 lb. 10.4
1 oz. 7
Parsnip:
raw, untrimmed, 1 lb. 69.4
raw, sliced, ½ cup 12.1
boiled, drained, 1 medium, 9″ × 2¼″ diam. 31.3
boiled, drained, sliced, ½ cup 15.2
Passion fruit:
fresh, purple:
    (Frieda's), 5 oz. 33.0
    untrimmed, 1 lb. 55.1
    1 medium, approx. 1.2 oz. 4.2
    trimmed, 1 oz. 6.6
frozen, chunks *(Goya),* ⅓ pkg. 15.0
Passion fruit juice:
fresh, purple, 8 fl. oz. 33.6
fresh, yellow, 8 fl. oz. 36.0
bottled *(Snapple),* 10 fl. oz. 39.0
Passion fruit–mango drink *(Heinke's),* 8 fl. oz. 33.0
Pasta, dry, uncooked (see also "Macaroni" and "Noodle"),
    2 oz., except as noted:
plain 42.6
all varieties:
    (Creamette/Prince) 42.0
    (Delverde) 41.0
    (Goya Estrellas) 45.0
    (Mueller's) 42.0
    with egg *(Herb's)* 42.0
    kamut *(Eden* Organic) 33.0
    except angel-hair, egg pastina, fettuccine, and light and
        fluffy noodles *(San Giorgio)* 42.0
angel-hair *(San Giorgio)* 40.0
egg pastina *(San Giorgio)* 40.0
elbows, regular or hot pepper *(Eden* Organic), ½ cup 41.0
extra fine *(Eden* Organic), ½ cup 40.0

Pasta, dry, uncooked *(cont.)*
fettuccine:
    (Prince) 40.0
    (San Giorgio) 39.0
    Florentine *(San Giorgio)* 39.0
    garlic and herb *(San Giorgio)*............... 41.0
finbows *(Eden* Organic), ½ cup 41.0
kamut and quinoa *(Eden* Organic) 40.0
kuzu and sweet potato *(Eden* Organic) 47.0
linguine, tomato-basil *(Prince)* 41.0
mung bean *(Eden* Organic) 47.0
noodles, light and fluffy, all varieties *(San Giorgio)*....... 40.0
noodle-style, yolk free *(Mueller's)* 42.0
penne, tomato-pepper-basil *(Prince)* 41.0
pesto twists *(Eden* Organic), ½ cup 40.0
ribbons, all varieties except spinach *(Eden* Organic) 40.0
ribbons, spinach *(Eden* Organic) 41.0
rice *(Eden* Organic)......................... 44.0
shells *(Goya* Conchas)....................... 45.0
spaghetti:
    (Eden Organic) 40.0
    (Prince Square/Thin) 40.0
    parsley-garlic 41.0
    whole wheat *(Eden* Organic) 40.0
spirals:
    sesame rice *(Eden* Organic), ½ cup 37.0
    spinach *(Eden* Organic), ½ cup 41.0
    vegetable *(Eden* Organic), ½ cup 40.0
tri-color *(Mueller's)*......................... 42.0
tubes *(Eden* Organic), ½ cup 41.0
vegetable alphabets, rotini, spirals, or shells *(Eden/Herb's)*,
    ½ cup 40.0
Pasta, dry, cooked, 1 cup:
plain 39.7
corn 39.1
spinach 36.6
whole wheat 37.2
Pasta, refrigerated (see also specific pasta listings), plain:
uncooked, with egg, 2 oz. 31.0
uncooked, spinach, with egg, 2 oz. 31.6
cooked, with egg, 4 oz. 28.3
cooked, spinach, with egg, 4 oz. 28.4

Pasta dinner, see specific listings
Pasta dishes, frozen (see also "Pasta entree, frozen"):
Alfredo *(Green Giant Pasta Accents),* 2 cups 25.0
cheddar, creamy *(Green Giant Pasta Accents),* 2⅓ cups . . . 36.0
cheddar, white *(Green Giant Pasta Accents),* 1¾ cups 38.0
Florentine *(Green Giant Pasta Accents),* 2 cups 44.0
garden blend, early *(Schwan's),* ½ cup 8.0
garden blend, summer *(Schwan's),* 1 cup 18.0
garden herb *(Green Giant Pasta Accents),* 2 cups 32.0
garlic *(Green Giant Pasta Accents),* 2 cups 36.0
Italian blend *(Schwan's),* 1 cup 12.0
primavera *(Green Giant Pasta Accents),* 2¼ cups 40.0
rotini *(Schwan's),* 1 cup 28.0
Pasta dishes, mix (see also specific pasta listings):
broccoli, and mushroom *(Pasta Roni),* approx. 1 cup* 49.0
butter and herb *(Lipton* Pasta & Sauce), ½ pkg. or 1 cup* 40.0
cheese:
   cheddar, mild *(Lipton* Pasta & Sauce), ½ pkg. 38.0
   cheddar, mild *(Lipton* Pasta & Sauce), 1 cup* 41.0
   cheddar broccoli *(Lipton* Pasta & Sauce), ½ pkg. 26.0
   cheddar broccoli *(Lipton* Pasta & Sauce), 1 cup* 49.0
   four, corkscrews *(Pasta Roni),* 1 cup* 49.0
chicken:
   herb Parmesan *(Lipton* Pasta & Sauce), ½ pkg.
     or 1 cup* 43.0
   roasted garlic *(Lipton* Pasta & Sauce), ½ pkg. 40.0
   roasted garlic *(Lipton* Pasta & Sauce), 1 cup* 43.0
   stir-fry *(Lipton* Pasta & Sauce), ½ pkg. or 1 cup* 43.0
fagioli, with white beans *(Fantastic* One Pot Meals), ½ cup 30.0
garlic:
   creamy *(Lipton* Pasta & Sauce), ½ pkg. 47.0
   creamy *(Lipton* Pasta & Sauce), 1 cup* 50.0
   creamy, corkscrews *(Pasta Roni),* approx. 1 cup* 41.0
   and herb *(Spice Islands* Quick Meal), 1 pkg. 32.0
   and olive oil *(Pasta Roni),* approx. 1 cup* 48.0
   roasted, and olive oil, with tomatoes *(Lipton* Pasta &
     Sauce), ½ pkg. or 1 cup* 42.0
   herb, savory, with garlic *(Lipton* Pasta & Sauce), ½ pkg.
     or 1 cup* 52.0
Mediterranean gemelli and red lentils *(Fantastic* One Pot
   Meals), ⅜ cup 31.0
mixed *(Buckeye* Oceans of), 2 oz. 42.0

Pasta dishes, mix *(cont.)*

mushroom, creamy *(Lipton* Pasta & Sauce), ½ pkg. 43.0

mushroom, creamy *(Lipton* Pasta & Sauce), 1 cup* 46.0

Parmesan *(Pasta Roni* Parmesano), approx. 1 cup* 49.0

primavera *(Knorr* Cup), 1 pkg. 36.0

primavera *(Spice Islands* Quick Meal), 1 pkg. 32.0

salad:

    (Buckeye Sunny Day), ¹/₁₀ pkg. 23.0

    Caesar *(Kraft),* 2.5 oz. 30.0

    garden primavera *(Kraft),* 2.5 oz. 34.0

    hearty *(Buckeye),* ⅛ pkg. 27.0

    Italian, light *(Kraft),* 2.5 oz. 34.0

    Italian herb *(Fantastic),* ⅔ cup 34.0

    Parmesan peppercorn *(Kraft),* 2.5 oz. 28.0

    ranch, classic, with bacon *(Kraft),* 2.5 oz. 30.0

    seasoned *(Buckeye* Sunny), ¹/₉ pkg. 26.0

    spicy Oriental *(Fantastic),* ⅔ cup 37.0

spinach and mushroom *(Spice Islands* Quick Meal), 1 pkg. 29.0

tomato, creamy, basil *(Spice Islands* Quick Meal), 1 pkg. . . 40.0

tomato, creamy, twists *(Knorr* Cup), 1 pkg. 41.0

Pasta entree, canned (see also specific listings):

spirals, and chicken *(Libby's Diner),* 7¾ oz. 16.0

twists *(Franco-American),* 1 cup 41.0

Pasta entree, freeze-dried:

primavera *(Mountain House),* 1 cup 32.0

Roma *(AlpineAire),* 1⅓ cups 47.0

Pasta entree, frozen (see also "Pasta dishes, frozen" and

    specific pasta listings):

cheddar bake with *(Lean Cuisine),* 9 oz. 36.0

cheddar and broccoli *(Banquet),* 10.5 oz. 48.0

cheddar, with beef and tomatoes *(Stouffer's),* 11 oz. 45.0

primavera:

    (Schwan's), 1 cup 21.0

    Alfredo *(Lean Cuisine Lunch Classics),* 10 oz. 46.0

    with chicken *(Marie Callender's),* 1 cup, 6.5 oz. 22.0

rings *(Swanson Fun Feast* Razzlin'), 1 pkg. 57.0

and sausage in cream suace *(The Budget Gourmet* Italian

    Originals), 10.5 oz. 43.0

sausage and peppers *(Banquet),* 10.5 oz. 43.0

and spinach Romano *(Weight Watchers* International

    Selections), 10.4 oz. 32.0

with tomato basil sauce *(Weight Watchers* International
    Selections), 9.6 oz. 33.0
vegetable Italiano *(Healthy Choice),* 10 oz. 48.0
wheels and cheese *(Swanson Fun Feast),* 1 pkg. 60.0
wide ribbon with ricotta *(The Budget Gourmet* Special
    Selections), 10¼ oz. 41.0
wine and mushroom sauce, with chicken *(The Budget*
    Gourmet Italian Originals), 10 oz. 37.0
Pasta flour, see "Semolina flour"
Pasta salad, see "Pasta dishes, mix"
Pasta sauce, tomato (see also "Pasta sauce, refrigerated,"
    "Tomato sauce," and specific sauce listings), ½ cup,
    except as noted:
(Del Monte). 14.0
(Eden Organic/Organic No Salt). 12.0
(Healthy Choice Traditional) 10.0
(Hunt's Chunky) 8.0
(Hunt's Homestyle Traditional) 9.0
(Hunt's Light Traditional) 7.0
(Hunt's Original Traditional) 11.0
(Paesana Casalinga) 7.0
(Patsy's Fileto di Pomodoro) 7.0
(Pomodoro Fresca Solo) 6.0
(Porino's) 11.0
(Prego Traditional) 23.0
(Prego Low Sodium) 11.0
(Prego Extra Chunky Tomato Supreme) 20.0
(Pritikin Original) 7.0
(Progresso) 12.0
(Ragú Light No Sugar Added) 9.0
(Ragú Old World Traditional) 10.0
all varieties, except no sugar added *(Ragú* Light) 11.0
with basil:
    (Barilla) 10.0
    (Classico Di Napoli) 8.0
    (Del Monte) 11.0
    (Del Monte D'Italia) 9.0
    (Hunt's Classic) 9.0
    (Porino's) 14.0
    (Prego) 19.0
    summer tomato *(Five Brothers)* 8.0
    zesty *(Prego Extra Chunky)* 22.0

Pasta sauce *(cont.)*

beef or beef and pork *(Porino's)*	13.0
cheese, four *(Classico* Di Parma)	7.0
cheese, four *(Del Monte* D'Italia)	8.0
cheese, three *(Prego)*	18.0
cheese and garlic, Italian style *(Hunt's* Original)	10.0
cheese, wine, and herbs *(Porino's)*	19.0
fra diavolo *(Patsy's)*	11.0

garden:

(Porino's Chunky)	17.0
(Porino's Gardina Fresca)	11.0
(Pritikin Chunky)	6.0
combination *(Prego Extra* Chunky)	16.0
combination *(Ragú* Gardenstyle)	18.0
style *(Del Monte)*	11.0
vegetable primavera *(Five Brothers)*	9.0
garlic *(Prego Extra Chunky* Supreme)	23.0
garlic, roasted *(Healthy Choice* Garlic Lovers)	11.5
garlic, roasted, and sun-dried tomatoes *(Healthy Choice* Garlic Lovers)	11.0
garlic and cheese *(Prego Extra* Chunky)	22.0

garlic and herb:

(Del Monte)	11.0
(Healthy Choice)	10.0
(Hunt's Classic)	9.0
(Hunt's Light)	7.0
garlic and mushroom *(Healthy Choice* Garlic Lovers)	10.0

garlic and onion:

(Del Monte)	13.0
(Hunt's Chunky)	13.0
(Hunt's Classic)	10.0
(Ragú Gardenstyle)	19.0
green pepper and mushroom *(Del Monte)*	12.0
green and red pepper *(Ragú* Gardenstyle)	19.0
hot *(Pomodoro Fresca* Cayenne)	6.0
Italian, herb *(Del Monte)*	12.0
Italian, spice *(Aunt Millie's* Family Style)	16.0

marinara:

(Angelia Mia), ¼ cup	4.0
(Aunt Millie's)	9.0
(Barilla)	10.0
(Colavita)	11.0

(Del Monte D'Italia Classic) 9.0
(Hunt's Chunky) 12.0
(Paesana) 9.0
(Patsy's) 11.0
(Prego) 12.0
(Prince Chunky) 13.0
(Prince Traditional) 9.0
(Pritikin) 4.0
(Progresso) 8.0
(Progresso Authentic) 9.0
(Ragú Old World) 9.0
(Rao's Homemade) 4.0
with burgundy wine *(Five Brothers)* 9.0
with pizza paste *(Aunt Millie's)* 9.0
meat/meat flavor:
   (Aunt Millie's) 9.0
   (Aunt Millie's Family Style) 16.0
   (Del Monte) 13.0
   (Hunt's Homestyle) 9.0
   (Hunt's Light) 8.0
   (Hunt's Original) 12.0
   (Prego) 21.0
   (Progresso) 12.0
   (Ragú Old World) 9.0
mushroom:
   (Aunt Millie's) 10.0
   (Aunt Millie's Family Style) 16.0
   (Del Monte) 15.0
   (Five Brothers) 10.0
   (Healthy Choice) 10.0
   (Healthy Choice Chunky) 9.0
   (Hunt's Homestyle) 8.0
   (Hunt's Light) 8.0
   (Hunt's Original) 11.0
   (Prego) 23.0
   (Prego Extra Chunky Supreme) 21.0
   (Prince Chunky) 13.0
   (Progresso) 11.0
   (Ragú Old World) 10.0
   (Weight Watchers) 11.0
with spice, extra *(Prego* Extra Chunky) 19.0
super *(Ragú* Gardenstyle) 19.0

Pasta sauce *(cont.)*

mushroom and garlic *(Barilla)* 9.0
mushroom and garlic *(Healthy Choice Super Chunky)* 10.0
mushroom and green pepper *(Prego Extra Chunky)* 18.0
mushroom and green pepper *(Ragú Gardenstyle)* 18.0
mushroom and onion *(Prego Extra Chunky)* 18.0
mushroom and onion *(Ragú Gardenstyle)* 19.0
mushroom Parmesan *(Prego)* 19.0
mushroom and ripe olive *(Classico Di Sicilia)* 8.0
mushroom and sweet peppers *(Healthy Choice Super
  Chunky)* 9.0
mushroom and tomato *(Prego Extra Chunky)* 19.0
olive, black, and mushrooms *(Porino's)* 14.0
olive, green and black *(Barilla)* 9.0
with olives and mushrooms *(Classico Di Sicilia)* 8.0
onion and garlic:
  (Classico Di Sorrento) 9.0
  (Porino's) 14.0
  (Prego/Prego Extra Chunky) 19.0
oregano, zesty *(Prego Extra Chunky)* 25.0
with Parmesan *(Hunt's Classic)* 8.0
with Parmesan *(Prego)* 19.0
pepper, sweet or red:
  and garlic *(Barilla)* 8.0
  and onion *(Classico Di Salerno)* 8.0
  and onion *(Porino's)* 14.0
  red *(Del Monte D'Italia)* 9.0
  spicy *(Barilla)* 9.0
  spicy *(Classico Di Roma Arrabbiata)* 6.0
  with pesto *(Classico Di Genoa)* 10.0
sausage, Italian *(Hunt's Chunky)* 9.5
sausage, Italian, and fennel *(Classico D'Abruzzi)* 7.0
sausage and pepper *(Prego Extra Chunky)* 22.0
sausage, pepper, and mushroom *(Porino's)* 20.0
spinach and cheese *(Classico Di Firenze)* 8.0
sun-dried tomato *(Classico Di Capri)* 8.0
with tomato bits *(Angelia Mia)* 11.0
with vegetables:
  (Hunt's Chunky) 13.0
  (Prego Extra Chunky Supreme) 15.0
  Italian *(Healthy Choice Chunky)* 9.0
  primavera *(Healthy Choice Super Chunky)* 9.5

primavera *(Ragú* Gardenstyle) 17.0
zucchini and Parmesan *(Classico* Di Milano) 9.0
Pasta sauce, refrigerated, tomato, ½ cup, except as noted:
cheese, four *(Di Giorno),* ¼ cup 2.0
garden vegetable *(Contadina* Fat Free) 9.0
marinara *(Contadina)* 10.0
marinara *(Di Giorno)* 12.0
meat, traditional *(Di Giorno)* 12.0
olive oil and garlic, with grated cheese *(Di Giorno),* ¼ cup . 3.0
primavera *(Tutta Pasta)* 11.0
puttanesca *(Tutta Pasta)* 12.0
red bell pepper *(Contadina)* 10.0
roasted garlic and artichoke *(Monterey Pasta Company)* 8.0
tomato:
    basil *(Contadina* Fat Free) 9.0
    chunky, with basil *(Di Giorno* Light) 16.0
    plum, and basil *(Contadina)* 9.0
    plum, and mushroom *(Di Giorno)* 15.0
vodka *(Tutta Pasta)* 14.0
Pasta sauce mix (see also specific listings):
(Knorr Parma Rosa), 2 tbsp. 8.0
(Lawry's), 1 tbsp. 6.0
garlic and herb *(Knorr),* ⅓ pkg. 7.0
garlic and herb *(Spice Islands),* ¼ pkg. 3.0
primavera *(Spice Islands* Pouch), ⅕ pkg. 3.0
salad *(Durkee* Pouch), 2 tsp. 2.0
spaghetti:
    (Durkee), ½ cup* 5.0
    (Durkee Family), 2 tsp. 4.0
    American style *(Durkee),* ½ cup* 6.0
    with mushrooms *(Durkee),* ½ cup* 4.0
    zesty *(Durkee),* 2 tsp. 5.0
Pastrami, 2 oz.:
(Healthy Deli) 2.0
(Hebrew National) 0
brisket or Romanian *(Boar's Head)* 2.0
round *(Boar's Head)* . . . . <1.0
round *(Hebrew National)* 0
turkey, see "Turkey pastrami"
Pastry, see specific listings
Pastry filling (see also "Pie filling"), canned, 2 tbsp.:
almond *(Solo)* 23.0

Pastry filling *(cont.)*

apple, Dutch *(Solo)* 20.0
apricot *(Solo)* 17.0
blueberry, wild *(Solo)* 17.0
cherry *(Solo)* 20.0
date *(Solo)* 22.0
nut, fancy *(Solo)* 25.0
pecan *(Solo)* 24.0
pineapple *(Solo)* 19.0
poppy seed *(Solo)* 30.0
prune plum *(Solo)* 18.0
raspberry *(Solo)* 19.0
strawberry *(Solo)* 18.0
Pastry shell *(Stella D'Oro)*, 1-oz. shell 17.0
Pastry shell, frozen (see also "Pie crust"):
dough *(Goya* Discos), 1 piece 20.0
patty *(Pepperidge Farm)*, 1 shell 23.0
sheet, puff *(Pepperidge Farm)*, 1/6 sheet 23.0
tart:
  (Oronoque), 3″ shell 12.0
  (Pet-Ritz), 3″ shell 11.0
  (Pet-Ritz), 1/4 of 6″ shell 9.0
Pâté, liver (see also "Liverwurst"), canned:
1 oz. 4
1 tbsp. 2
chicken liver:
  1 oz. 1.9
  1 tbsp. 9
  canned *(Chef Giovanni's)*, 2 oz. 5.0
goose liver, smoked, 1 oz. 1.3
goose liver, smoked, 1 tbsp. 6
liver *(Sells)*, 1/4 cup 3.0
"Pâté," vegetarian *(Bonavita* Swiss), 1 oz. 3.0
Pea pod, Chinese, see "Peas, edible-podded"
Peach, fresh:
(Dole), 2 fruits 19.0
untrimmed, 1 lb. 38.2
2½″-diam. peach, approx. 4 per lb. 9.7
peeled and pitted, sliced, 1/2 cup 9.4
Peach, canned, halves or slices, 1/2 cup, except as noted:
(Hunt's) 24.0
(S&W Ready-Cut California Sun) 20.0

(S&W Ready-Cut Tropical Sun) 19.0
with cinnamon *(S&W Sweet Memory* Ready-Cut Sun) 19.0
in juice, cling:
    (Del Monte Naturals) 15.0
    (Del Monte Naturals Snack Cup), 4-oz. cup 13.0
    (Libby's Lite) 13.0
    (S&W Natural) 19.0
    ½ cup 14.3
in extra light syrup:
    cling 18.3
    cling *(Del Monte* Snack Cup), 4-oz. cup 13.0
    cling *(Del Monte* Lite) 15.0
    freestone *(Del Monte* Lite) 14.0
in heavy syrup:
    cling *(Del Monte* Snack Cup), 4-oz. cup 20.0
    cling *(Del Monte/Del Monte* Melba) 24.0
    cling *(S&W)* 24.0
    cling or freestone 25.5
    freestone *(Del Monte)* 24.0
    freestone *(S&W)* 23.0
raspberry flavor, cling, in heavy syrup *(Del Monte)* 20.0
spiced *(Del Monte* Natural Harvest) 21.0
spiced, in heavy syrup:
    (Del Monte) 24.0
    (S&W), 4.3-oz. piece 23.0
    1 peach and 2 tbsp. syrup 17.7
Peach, dried:
(Sonoma), 3–5 pieces, 1.4 oz. 31.0
sulfured, halves, ½ cup 49.1
sulfured, 10 halves, 4.6 oz. 79.7
sun-dried *(Del Monte)*, 1.4 oz., ⅓ cup 26.0
Peach, frozen, sliced:
(Big Valley), ⅔ cup 13.0
(Schwan's), 1⅓ cups 13.0
(Stilwell), 1 cup 14.0
sweetened, 10-oz. pkg. 68.1
Peach butter *(Smucker's)*, 1 tbsp. 11.0
Peach drink, 8 fl. oz.:
(After the Fall) 27.0
(Farmer's Market) 31.0
(Tree Top Quake) 30.0
Peach dumpling, frozen *(Pepperidge Farm)*, 1 piece 47.0

Peach juice *(Ceres)*, 8 fl. oz. 29.0
Peach juice blend:
(Dole Orchard), 8 fl. oz. 34.0
(Dole Orchard), 10 fl. oz. 42.0
Peach nectar:
(Goya), 8 fl. oz. 36.0
(Goya), 12 fl. oz. 54.0
(R.W. Knudsen), 8 fl. oz. 30.0
(Libby's), 8 fl. oz. 36.0
(Libby's/Kern's), 11.5 fl. oz. 52.0
6 fl. oz. 26.0
Peanut, shelled, except as noted:
all varieties, raw, in shell, 1 lb. 53.4
unroasted, 1 oz. 4.5
boiled, salted, 1 oz. 6.0
dry-roasted, 1 oz., except as noted:
    (Little Debbie) 5.0
    (Planters/Planters Unsalted) 6.0
    (Planters Lightly Salted) 5.0
    (Planters Lightly Salted), 1¾-oz. pkg. 9.0
    salted or unsalted 6.0
    salted or unsalted, ½ cup 15.7
honey-roasted:
    (Frito-Lay), ¼ cup 10.0
    (Planters), 1 oz. 8.0
    (Smart Snackers), .7 oz. 7.0
    dry-roasted *(Planters)*, 1.7-oz. pkg. 17.0
    oil-roasted *(Planters* Reduced Fat), 1 oz. 12.0
hot *(Frito-Lay)*, ¼ cup 6.0
hot and spicy:
    (Planters Heat), 1 oz. 5.0
    (Planters Heat), 1.7-oz. pkg. 9.0
    (Planters Heat), 2-oz. pkg. 10.0
    (Planters Heat Munch 'N Go Singles), 2.5-oz. pkg. 13.0
oil-roasted:
    (Pennant), 1 oz. 6.0
    (Planters), 2-oz. bag 11.0
    (Planters Fun Size), 2 bags, 1 oz. 6.0
    (Planters Lightly Salted), 1¾-oz. pkg. 8.0
    (Planters Munch 'N Go), 1 oz. 6.0
    cocktail *(Planters/Planters* Unsalted), 1 oz. 6.0
    cocktail *(Planters* Lightly Salted), 1 oz. 5.0

fancy *(Paradise/White Swan)*, ¼ cup, 1½ oz. 7.0
salted *(Planters)*, 1 oz. 5.0
salted *(Planters)*, 1.7-oz. pkg. 10.0
salted or unsalted, 1 oz. 5.3
salted or unsalted, ½ cup 13.6
salted *(Frito-Lay)*, 1 oz. 2.0
Spanish *(Planters)*, 1 oz. 5.0
Spanish, raw *(Planters)*, 1 oz. 6.0
sweet *(Planters Sweet N Crunchy)*, 1 oz. 16.0
Peanut butter, 2 tbsp.:
all varieties *(Jif Reduced Fat)* 15.0
chunky or crunchy:
   (Adams Natural/Unsalted) 5.0
   (Adams No-Stir) 4.0
   (Arrowhead Mills) 6.0
   (Knotts All Natural) 5.0
   (Peter Pan/Peter Pan Plus) 6.0
   (Peter Pan Very Low Sodium) 12.0
   (Peter Pan Whipped) 5.0
   (Real Brand) 5.0
   (Roasted Honey Nut Skippy Super Chunk) 7.0
   (Roaster Fresh/Roaster Fresh Unsalted) 5.0
   (Simply Jif) 7.0
   (Skippy Super Chunk) 6.0
   (Skippy Super Chunk Reduced Fat) 13.0
   (Smucker's Natural/Natural No Salt) 7.0
   (Teddie Super) 7.0
   extra *(Jif)* 7.0
   spread *(Peter Pan Smart Choice)* 14.5
creamy or smooth:
   (Adams Natural/No-Stir) 4.0
   (Adams Unsalted) 5.0
   (Arrowhead Mills) 6.0
   (Jif) 7.0
   (Peter Pan) 6.5
   (Peter Pan Very Low Sodium/Peter Pan Plus) 6.0
   (Peter Pan Whipped) 5.0
   (Real Brand) 5.0
   (Roasted Honey Nut Skippy/Skippy) 6.0
   (Roaster Fresh/Roaster Fresh Unsalted) 5.0
   (Simply Jif) 6.0
   (Skippy Reduced Fat) 14.0

Peanut butter, creamy or smooth *(cont.)*
  (*Smucker's* Natural/Natural No Salt) 7.0
  (*Teddie/Teddie* Unsalted) 7.0
  spread (*Peter Pan Smart Choice*) 14.5
Peanut butter bits, baking (*Reese's*), 1 tbsp. 7.0
Peanut butter caramel topping (*Smucker's*), 2 tbsp. 24.0
Peanut butter and jelly (*Smucker's Goober*), 3 tbsp. 24.0
Peanut butter snack, see "Cookie" and "Cracker"
Peanut flour, 1 cup:
defatted 20.8
low-fat 18.8
Peanut sauce, Oriental:
(*House of Tsang Bangkok Padang*), 1 tbsp. 4.0
cooking (*Kylin Singapore Satay*), ¼ cup 7.0
Pear (see also specific listings):
fresh, with peel:
  (*Dole*), 1 fruit 25.0
  untrimmed, 1 lb. 63.1
  Bartlett, 1 medium, 2½ per lb. 25.1
  sliced, ½ cup 12.5
dried:
  (*Sonoma*), 3–4 pieces, 1.4 oz. 33.0
  2 oz. 39.5
  halves, ½ cup 62.7
Pear, cactus, see "Prickly pear"
Pear, canned, halves or slices, ½ cup, except as noted:
(*S&W* Ready-Cut California Sun) 19.0
in water 9.0
in juice:
  (*Del Monte* Naturals/Lite) 15.0
  (*Libby's* Lite) 13.0
  1 half and 1⅔ tbsp. juice 10.0
in extra light syrup:
  (*Del Monte* Naturals/Lite) 15.0
  (*Del Monte* Snack Cup), 4-oz. cup 13.0
  1 half and 1⅔ tbsp. syrup 9.4
in light syrup 19.0
in light syrup, 1 half and 1¾ tbsp. syrup 12.0
in heavy syrup:
  (*Del Monte*) 24.0
  (*Del Monte* Snack Cup), 4-oz. cup 20.0
  1 half and 1¾ tbsp. syrup 15.1

Bartlett, in juice *(S&W* Natural) 21.0
Bartlett, in heavy syrup *(S&W)* 22.0
ginger flavor *(Del Monte* Natural) 22.0
Pear, Asian:
(Frieda's), 5 oz. 15.0
1 medium, 2¼″ × 2½″ diam. 13.0
Pear juice, 8 fl. oz.:
(After the Fall Harvest) 22.0
(After the Fall Rouge River) 24.0
(Heinke's Organic) 30.0
(R.W. Knudsen Organic) 30.0
Pear nectar:
(Libby's), 8 fl. oz. 38.0
(Libby's/Kern's), 11.5 fl. oz. 54.0
(Santa Cruz), 8 fl. oz. 30.0
canned, 6 fl. oz. 29.6
Peas, butter, frozen *(Stilwell),* ½ cup 20.0
Peas, cream, canned *(Allens/East Texas Fair),* ½ cup 17.0
Peas, crowder, ½ cup:
canned *(Allens/East Texas Fair/Homefolks)* 19.0
frozen *(Stilwell)* 22.0
Peas, edible-podded:
fresh:
    raw, untrimmed, 1 lb. 32.2
    raw, trimmed, ½ cup 5.4
    boiled, drained, ½ cup 5.6
    snow *(Frieda's),* 1 cup, 3 oz. 6.0
    sugar snap *(Frieda's),* ⅔ cup, 3 oz. 6.0
frozen:
    (Birds Eye), ½ cup 7.0
    (Schwan's), ⅔ cup 6.0
    10-oz. pkg. 20.5
    boiled, drained, ½ cup 7.2
    sugar snap *(Green Giant),* ¾ cup 7.0
    sugar snap *(Green Giant Harvest Fresh),* ⅔ cup 10.0
Peas, field, ½ cup:
canned, fresh shell:
    (Sunshine) 21.0
    with snaps *(Allens/East Texas Fair/Homefolks)* 21.0
    with snaps *(Goya)* 19.0
canned, dry, with bacon *(Trappey's)* 15.0
canned, dry, with snaps and bacon *(Trappey's)* 19.0

Peas, field *(cont.)*
frozen, with snaps *(Stilwell)* 20.0
Peas, green, fresh:
(Dole), 2.5 oz. 5.0
(Frieda's), 1/3 cup 22.0
raw, in pod, 1 lb. 24.9
raw, shelled, 1/2 cup 10.4
boiled, drained, 1/2 cup 12.5
Peas, green, canned, 1/2 cup:
(Del Monte/Del Monte No Salt) 11.0
(Goya) 16.0
(Goya Tender Sweet) 12.0
(S&W Petit Pois/Sweet) 12.0
(Seneca/Seneca No Salt) 12.0
(Stokely/Stokely No Salt) 10.0
early June *(Sun-Vista)* 18.0
early June, dry *(Crest Top)* 20.0
early or sweet:
   (Green Giant/Green Giant 50% Less Sodium) 11.0
   (LeSueur) 12.0
   (LeSueur 50% Less Sodium) 11.0
very young, small *(Del Monte)* 10.0
with liquid, regular or low-sodium 10.7
Peas, green, dried:
(Goya), 1/4 cup 24.0
freeze-dried *(AlpineAire)*, 1/2 cup 14.0
freeze-dried *(Mountain House)*, 1/2 cup 12.0
Peas, green, frozen, 2/3 cup, except as noted:
(Birds Eye), 1/2 cup 13.0
(Schwan's) 12.0
(Seabrook) 12.0
(Stilwell) 12.0
baby early *(LeSueur Harvest Fresh)* 13.0
early June *(LeSueur)* 11.0
sweet:
   (Green Giant) 13.0
   (Green Giant Harvest Fresh) 12.0
   baby *(LeSueur)* 11.0
tiny *(Birds Eye)* 11.0
in butter sauce, baby, early *(Green Giant LeSueur)*, 3/4 cup 16.0
in butter sauce, sweet *(Green Giant)*, 3/4 cup 16.0

Peas, green, combinations:
canned, ½ cup:
    with mushrooms and onions *(LeSueur)* 11.0
    with pearl onions *(Green Giant)* 11.0
    with pearl onions *(S&W)* 11.0
canned, and carrots, ½ cup:
    (Del Monte) 11.0
    (Goya) 9.0
    (Green Giant) 11.0
    (S&W) 10.0
    (Seneca) 11.0
    (Stokely) 10.0
    (Stokely No Salt/Sugar) 9.0
frozen:
    and carrots *(Stilwell)*, ½ cup 9.0
    and mushrooms *(LeSueur)*, ¾ cup 10.0
    and pearl onion *(Birds Eye)*, ⅔ cup 18.0
    and pearl onions *(Green Giant)*, ⅔ cup 12.0
    and pearl onions *(Green Giant Harvest Fresh)*, ½ cup . . 10.0
    and potatoes and carrots *(Green Giant American*
      Mixtures), ⅔ cup 12.0
Peas, lady, canned, ½ cup:
(Sunshine) 17.0
with snaps *(East Texas Fair)* 17.0
Peas, pepper, canned *(Allens/East Texas Fair/Homefolks)*,
  ½ cup 22.0
Peas, purple hull, ½ cup:
canned *(East Texas)* 21.0
canned *(Stubb's Harvest)* 21.0
frozen *(Stilwell)* 21.0
Peas, snow or Chinese, see "Peas, edible-podded"
Peas, split, see "Split peas"
Peas, sprouted, mature seeds:
raw, 1 lb. 128.2
raw, ½ cup 17.0
boiled, drained, 4 oz. 24.8
Peas, sugar snap, see "Peas, edible-podded"
Peas, sweet, see "Peas, green"
Peas, white acre, canned *(East Texas Fair)*, ½ cup 17.0
Peas and carrots or onions, see "Peas, green,
  combinations"

Pecan, shelled, except as noted:

chips *(Planters)*, 2-oz. pkg. 9.0

halves *(Paradise/White Swan)*, ¼ cup 5.0

halves *(Planters)*, 1 oz. 4.0

halves *(Planters Gold Measure)*, 2-oz. pkg. 9.0

pieces *(Planters)*, 2-oz. pkg. 9.0

dried:

   in shell, 1 lb. 43.8

   1 oz. 5.2

   halves, 1 cup 19.7

   chopped, 1 cup 21.7

dry-roasted, salted or unsalted, 1 oz. 6.3

honey-roasted *(Planters)*, 1 oz. 9.0

oil-roasted, salted or unsalted, 1 oz. 4.6

Pecan filling, see "Pastry filling"

Pecan flour, 1 oz. 14.4

Pecan topping, with syrup *(Smucker's)*, 2 tbsp. 22.0

Pectin, see "Fruit pectin"

Penne:

dry, plain, see "Pasta"

refrigerated *(Tutta Pasta)*, 1 cup 58.0

Penne dishes, mix, dry, except as noted:

Alfredo *(Knorr)*, ¾ cup 44.0

herb and butter *(Pasta Roni)*, approx. 1 cup* 43.0

with sun-dried tomato Parmesan *(Knorr)*, ½ cup 51.0

Penne entree, canned, in meat sauce *(Franco-American)*,

   1 cup 40.0

Penne entree, frozen:

(The Budget Gourmet Special Selections), 9 oz. 48.0

Bolognese *(Lean Cuisine)*, 9.5 oz. 40.0

spicy, and ricotta *(Weight Watchers* International

   Selections), 10.2 oz. 45.0

with sun-dried tomato *(Weight Watchers)*, 10 oz. 41.0

with tomato sauce *(Healthy Choice)*, 8 oz. 36.0

with tomato basil sauce *(Lean Cuisine Lunch Classics)*,

   10 oz. 55.0

Pepper, seasoning

black:

   whole, 1 tsp. 1.9

   ground, 1 tbsp. 4.2

   ground, 1 tsp. 1.7

chili, 1 tsp. 1.2

red or cayenne, 1 tbsp. 3.0
red or cayenne, 1 tsp. 1.0
white:
    (McCormick), ¼ tsp. 4
    (Tone's), ¼ tsp. 0
    1 tbsp. 4.9
    1 tsp. 1.7
Pepper, banana, 1 oz.
hot or mild *(Vlasic)* 1.0
mild *(Nalley)* 1.0
Pepper, bell, see "Pepper, sweet"
Pepper, cherry:
(Trappey's), 2 pieces 2.0
hot:
    (B&G), 1 oz. 2.0
    (Hebrew National), 1⅓ pieces 4.0
    (Progresso), 1 piece 2.0
    sliced, drained *(Progresso)*, 2 tbsp. 2.0
sweet *(Nalley)*, 1 oz. 2.0
Pepper, chili, raw:
all varieties *(Frieda's Chiles)*, 1 pepper, 1.1 oz. 3.0
green and red, without seeds:
    untrimmed, 1 lb. 31.3
    1 medium, 1.6 oz. 4.3
    chopped, ½ cup 7.1
Pepper, chili, in jars:
chopped, with liquid, ½ cup 4.2
green, whole:
    (Chi-Chi's), ¾ chili 1.0
    (Nalley), 1 oz. 2.0
    (Rosarita), 1.2 oz. 1.0
    peeled *(Old El Paso)*, 1 chili 1.0
green, chopped *(Old El Paso)*, 2 tbsp. 2.0
green, diced, 2 tbsp.:
    (Chi-Chi's) 1.0
    (Pancho Villa) 1.0
    (Rosarita) 1.5
yellow, hot *(Del Monte)*, 4 pieces, 1 oz. 3.0
Pepper, chili, relish, pickle *(Patak's)*, 1 tbsp. 1.0
Pepper, chilpotle, spice sauce *(Del Monte)*, 2 tbsp. 4.0
Pepper, jalapeño, canned or in jars, except as noted:
fresh, see "Pepper, chili"

Pepper, jalapeño *(cont.)*
whole:
    (Chi-Chi's), 1 oz. 1.0
    (Clemente Jacques), 1 oz. 2.0
    (Goya), 2 pieces 2.0
    (Nalley), 1 oz. 1.0
    (Rosarita), 1.2 oz. 1.5
    (Trappey's), 2 pieces 3.0
    peeled *(Old El Paso)*, 3 pieces, 1.1 oz. 3.0
diced *(La Victoria)*, 1.1 oz. 2.0
diced *(Rosarita)*, 1.1 oz. 1.0
hot *(Vlasic)*, 1 oz. 2.0
marinated *(La Victoria)*, 1.1 oz. 2.0
nacho, sliced *(La Victoria)*, 1.1 oz. .... <1.0
nacho, sliced *(Rosarita)*, 1.1 oz. 1.0
pickled:
    (Clemente Jacques), 1 oz. 1.0
    (La Victoria), 1.1 oz. 2.0
    (Old El Paso), 2 pieces 1.0
    sliced *(Clemente Jacques)*, 1 oz. 2.0
    sliced *(Old El Paso)*, 1.1 oz., 2 tbsp. 3.0
    nacho, sliced *(Del Monte)*, 1 oz., 2 tbsp. 1.0
sliced *(Nalley)*, 1 oz. 1.0
wheels *(Chi-Chi's)*, 1 oz. 1.0
Pepper, nacho, pickled *(Goya)*, 14 slices 2.0
Pepper, roasted, see "Pepper, sweet, in jars"
Pepper, serrano, canned *(Stubb's Legendary)*, 1 oz. 1.0
Pepper, stuffed, frozen:
(Stouffer's), 10 oz. 24.0
(Stouffer's), ½ of 15½-oz. pkg. 20.0
jalapeño *(Schwan's)*, 3 pieces 22.0
Pepper, sweet:
fresh, green *(Dole)*, 1 medium, 5.3 oz. 7.0
fresh, green and red:
    raw, untrimmed, 1 lb. 23.9
    raw, 1 medium, 3¾″ × 3″ diam. 4.8
    raw, chopped, ½ cup 3.2
    boiled, drained, 1 medium 4.9
    boiled, drained, chopped, ½ cup 4.6
fresh, yellow, raw, 1 large, 5″ × 3″ diam. 11.8
fresh, yellow, raw, 10 strips, 1.8 oz. 3.3
in jars, see "Pepper, sweet, in jars" and "Pimiento"

freeze-dried, 1 tbsp. 3
frozen, chopped, 1 oz. 1.3
Pepper, sweet, in jars:
(B&G), 1 oz. 2.0
(Hebrew National/Rosoff/Shorr's Filet), 1 oz. 2.0
fried, drained *(Progresso),* 2 tbsp. 3.0
red *(B&G),* 1 oz. 5.0
rings *(Vlasic),* 1 oz. 6.0
roasted *(Progresso),* 1 piece 3.0
roasted, fire, with garlic and oil *(Paesana),* 2 tbsp. 2.0
sun-dried, marinated *(Antica Italia),* 1 oz. 2.0
Pepper dip, red *(Victoria),* 2 tbsp. 12.0
Pepper salad:
(B&G), 1 oz. 3.0
drained *(Progresso),* 2 tbsp. 1.0
Pepper sauce, hot, 1 tsp., except as noted:
(Durkee RedHot) 0
(Frank's Original Red Hot) 0
(Gebhardt) 0
(Goya) 0
(Pickapeppa), 1 tbsp. 4.0
(Try Me Tiger) 2.0
(Try Me Cajun/Tennessee Sunshine) 0
all varieties *(Tabasco)* 0
hot or original *(Hunt's)* 0
in vinegar *(Goya)* 0
Pepper steak, see "Beef entree"
Pepper "steak" entree, vegetarian, frozen *(Hain),* 10 oz. . . 41.0
Pepper stir fry, frozen *(Birds Eye),* 3 oz., approx. 1 cup . . . 5.0
Peppercorn sauce mix *(Knorr),* 2 tsp. 3.0
Peppered loaf, pork and beef, 1 oz. 1.3
Pepperoncini:
(Krinos), ¼ cup 2.0
(Nalley), 1 oz. 1.0
(Progresso Tuscan), 3 peppers 2.0
(Zorba), 5 pieces, 1.1 oz. 2.0
salad *(Vlasic),* 1 oz. 1.0
Pepperoni:
(Boar's Head), 1 oz. 0
(Hormel/Leoni/Rosa Grande), 1 oz. 0
(Oscar Mayer), 15 slices, 1.1 oz. 0
(Patrick Cudahy 3 oz.), 16 slices, 1.1 oz. 0

Pepperoni *(cont.)*
(Patrick Cudahy 6 oz.), 15 slices, 1.1 oz. 0
(Patrick Cudahy Stick), 1 oz. 0
pork and beef, 1 sausage, 10¼" long, approx. 9 oz. 7.1
pork and beef, 1 oz. 8
"Pepperoni," vegetarian *(Yves Veggie Cuisine)*, 3½ slices . 5.0
Pepperoni sandwich (see also "Bread, stuffed"), frozen,
   1 piece:
(Schwan's), 4.4-oz. piece 33.0
bagel *(Hormel Quick Meal)* 41.0
Perch, without added ingredients 0
Perch entree, frozen, battered *(Van de Kamp's)*, 2 pieces . . 19.0
Persimmon:
fresh:
   hachiya, trimmed *(Frieda's)*, 1 oz. 10.1
   Japanese, untrimmed, 1 lb. 70.8
   Japanese, 1 medium, 2½" × 3½", 7.1 oz. 31.2
   native *(Dole)*, 1 medium 8.0
   native, untrimmed, 1 lb. 124.6
   native, 1 medium, 1.1 oz. 8.4
dried:
   (Sonoma), 6–8 pieces 35.0
   fuyu *(Frieda's)*, ⅓ cup, 1.4 oz. 35.0
   Japanese, 1 oz. 20.0
Pesto sauce, ¼ cup:
in jars *(Sonoma)* 6.0
refrigerated:
   (Contadina Reduced Fat) 11.0
   (Di Giorno) 3.0
   sun-dried tomato *(Contadina)* 10.0
   tomato, creamy *(Contadina)* 12.0
Pesto sauce mix:
(Knorr), ⅓ pkg. 2.0
(Spice Islands), ¼ pkg. 1.0
creamy *(Knorr)*, ⅕ pkg. 3.0
red bell pepper *(Knorr)*, ⅓ pkg. 6.0
tomato *(Spice Islands)*, ¼ pkg. 3.0
tomato, sun-dried *(Knorr)*, ⅓ pkg. 9.0
Pheasant, without added ingredients 0
Phyllo pastry, see "Fillo pastry"
Picante sauce (see also "Salsa"), 2 tbsp.:
(Pace) 2.0

all varieties:
  (Chi-Chi's) 2.0
  (Hunt's Homestyle) 2.0
  (Old El Paso Thick 'n Chunky) 2.0
  (Rosarita) 2.0
  (Sun-Vista) 2.0
black bean (Arthur's) 3.0
black-eye pea (Arthur's) 3.0
garlic, with corn and honey (Arthur's) 3.0
hot or mild (Arthur's) 2.0
medium (Nalley Superba) 2.0
mesquite (Arthur's) 2.0
mild (Nalley Superba) 1.0
Pickle, cucumber, 1 oz., except as noted:
(B&G Sandwich Toppers New York Deli Style) 1.0
bread and butter:
  (B&G Sandwich Toppers) 7.0
  (Mrs. Fanning's), 3 slices, 1 oz. 6.0
  (Shorr's) 3.0
  chips (B&G) 7.0
  chips (B&G Unsalted) 6.0
  chips (Claussen), 4 slices, 1 oz. 4.0
  chunks or slices (Nalley Banquet) 6.0
  sandwich (Claussen), 2 slices, 1.2 oz. 5.0
  sandwich stackers (Vlasic) 7.0
chips (Nalley Cucumber) 9.0
chips, with honey (Pickle Eater's) 6.0
dill:
  (Vlasic Milwaukee) 1.0
  all varieties (Nalley) 1.0
  whole, 3¾" long, 2.3 oz. 2.7
  whole or halves (Del Monte) .... <1.0
  baby (Pickle Eater's) 0
  hamburger chips (Del Monte) 0
  hamburger chips/slices (Claussen), 10 slices, 1.1 oz. 0
dill, kosher:
  (Claussen Halves/Whole) 1.0
  (Claussen Mini), .8-oz. piece 1.0
  (Hebrew National Barrel/Hot), 1 pickle 4.0
  (Nalley) 1.0
  (Pickle Eater's/Pickle Eater's No Salt) 0
  all varieties (B&G/B&G Sandwich Toppers) 0

Pickle, dill, kosher *(cont.)*
  all varieties *(Vlasic)* 1.0
  slices *(Claussen)*, 2 slices, 1.1 oz. 1.0
  spears *(Claussen)*, 1.2-oz. spear 1.0
  spears *(Pickle Eater's)* 1.0
  tiny *(Del Monte)* 1.0
dill, Polish or zesty, spears *(Vlasic)* 1.0
kosher:
  (Shorr's Deli) 1.0
  whole *(Rosoff/Shorr's)* 1.0
  halves *(Hebrew National/Rosoff/Shorr's)* 1.0
  spears *(Hebrew National/Shorr's)* 1.0
sour *(Claussen* New York Deli/New York Garlic Deli),
  ½ pickle 1.0
sour, kosher:
  (Hebrew National/Rosoff/Shorr's New Half Sours) 1.0
  garlic *(Hebrew National/Shorr's)* 1.0
  spears *(Rosoff/Shorr's* Half Sour) 1.0
sour slices *(Claussen* New York Garlic Deli), 2 slices,
  1.2 oz. 1.0
sweet:
  (B&G Mixed) 8.0
  (Nalley) 8.0
  all varieties *(Del Monte)* 10.0
  all varieties *(Vlasic)* 10.0
  gherkins *(B&G)* 9.0
  gherkins *(Nalley)* 7.0
  midgets *(Nalley)* 8.0
  nubbins *(Nalley)* 6.0
Pickle dip, dill *(Nalley)*, 2 tbsp. 5.0
Pickle and pepper loaf *(Boar's Head)*, 2 oz. 2.0
Pickle and pimiento loaf *(Oscar Mayer)*, 1-oz. slice 3.0
Pickle relish, cucumber (see also specific listings), 1 tbsp.,
  except as noted:
dill, chunky *(Nalley)* 0
emerald *(B&G)* 4.0
hamburger:
  (B&G) 4.0
  (Del Monte) 6.0
  (Nalley) 3.0
  ½ cup 42.0
  1 tbsp. 5.2

hot dog:

(B&G) 5.0
(Del Monte) 4.0
(Nalley) 3.0
½ cup 28.5
1 tbsp. 3.5
India (B&G) 4.0
India (Heinz) 5.0
piccalilli, tomato (B&G) 5.0
piccalilli, tomato (Pickle Eater's) 2.0
red hot (Ron's) 4.0
sweet:

(B&G) 4.0
(B&G Unsalted) 5.0
(Claussen) 3.0
(Del Monte) 5.0
(Hebrew National) 4.0
(Nalley) 4.0
½ cup 42.8
1 tbsp. 5.3
honey (Pickle Eater's) 4.0
Pickled vegetables, see "Vegetables, mixed, pickled" and
specific vegetable listings
Pickling spice (Tone's), 1 tsp. 1.2
Pico de gallo, see "Salsa"
Pie, ⅙ pie, except as noted:
apple (Entenmann's Homestyle) 42.0
coconut custard (Entenmann's) 35.0
lemon (Entenmann's) 45.0
lemon meringue (Entenmann's), ⅕ pie 51.0
Pie, frozen:
apple:

(Amy's), 8 oz. 42.0
(Banquet), ⅕ pie 41.0
(Mrs. Smith's 8"), ⅙ pie 41.0
(Mrs. Smith's 9"), ⅛ pie 44.0
(Mrs. Smith's 10"), ⅒ pie 43.0
(Mrs. Smith's Old Fashioned 9"), ⅛ pie 50.0
(Mrs. Smith's Reduced Fat), ⅙ pie 43.0
(Mrs. Smith's Reduced Fat No Sugar), ⅙ pie 32.0
(Sara Lee Homestyle), ⅛ pie 42.0
(Schwan's), ⅟₁₂ pie 37.0

Pie, frozen, apple *(cont.)*
    lattice *(Mrs. Smith's)*, 1/5 pie 46.0
apple, Dutch:
    (Mrs. Smith's 8"), 1/6 pie 48.0
    (Mrs. Smith's 9"), 1/8 pie 52.0
    (Mrs. Smith's 10"), 1/10 pie 50.0
    (Mrs. Smith's Old Fashioned), 1/8 pie 49.0
apple-cranberry *(Mrs. Smith's)*, 1/6 pie 43.0
banana cream:
    (Banquet), 1/3 pie 39.0
    (Mrs. Smith's), 1/4 pie 37.0
    (Pet-Ritz), 1/3 pie 44.0
berry *(Mrs. Smith's)*, 1/6 pie 44.0
blackberry *(Mrs. Smith's)*, 1/6 pie 43.0
blueberry *(Mrs. Smith's)*, 1/6 pie 39.0
Boston creme, see "Cake, frozen"
cherry:
    (Banquet), 1/5 pie 39.0
    (Mrs. Smith's 8"), 1/6 pie 41.0
    (Mrs. Smith's 9"), 1/8 pie 45.0
    (Mrs. Smith's 10"), 1/10 pie 44.0
    (Mrs. Smith's Old Fashioned 9"), 1/8 pie 48.0
    (Mrs. Smith's Reduced Fat 8"), 1/6 pie 44.0
    (Mrs. Smith's Reduced Fat No Sugar 8"), 1/6 pie 35.0
    (Schwan's), 1/10 pie 42.0
    lattice *(Mrs. Smith's)*, 1/5 pie 47.0
chocolate cream:
    (Banquet), 1/3 pie 43.0
    (Mrs. Smith's), 1/4 pie 42.0
    (Pet-Ritz), 1/3 pie 44.0
    French silk *(Mrs. Smith's)*, 1/5 pie 55.0
chocolate mocha *(Weight Watchers)*, 2.75-oz. pie 31.0
coconut cream:
    (Banquet), 1/3 pie 39.0
    (Mrs. Smith's), 1/4 pie 40.0
    (Pet-Ritz), 1/3 pie 44.0
coconut custard *(Mrs. Smith's)*, 1/5 pie 35.0
fudge vanilla cream *(Pet-Ritz)*, 1/3 pie 44.0
lemon:
    cream *(Banquet)*, 1/3 pie 43.0
    cream *(Mrs. Smith's)*, 1/4 pie 40.0
    cream *(Pet-Ritz)*, 1/3 pie 44.0

meringue *(Mrs. Smith's)*, 1/5 pie 55.0
meringue *(Sara Lee Homestyle)*, 1/6 pie 59.0
lime, key *(Pet-Ritz)*, 1/3 pie 44.0
mince/mincemeat *(Banquet)*, 1/5 pie 46.0
mince/mincemeat *(Mrs. Smith's)*, 1/6 pie 48.0
Mississippi mud *(Weight Watchers)*, 2.45-oz. pie 24.0
peach:
    (Banquet), 1/5 pie 36.0
    (Mrs. Smith's 8"), 1/6 pie 38.0
    (Mrs. Smith's 9"), 1/8 pie 46.0
(Schwan's), 1/10 pie 45.0
peanut butter chocolate cream *(Pet-Ritz)*, 1/3 pie 44.0
pecan *(Mrs. Smith's 8")*, 1/6 pie 73.0
pecan *(Mrs. Smith's 10")*, 1/8 pie 68.0
pumpkin:
    (Banquet), 1/5 pie 40.0
    (Schwan's), 1/10 pie 37.0
    hearty *(Mrs. Smith's 8")*, 1/5 pie 42.0
    hearty *(Mrs. Smith's 9")*, 1/8 pie 39.0
pumpkin cream *(Pet-Ritz)*, 1/3 pie 44.0
pumpkin custard:
    (Mrs. Smith's 8"), 1/5 pie 44.0
    (Mrs. Smith's 9"), 1/8 pie 39.0
    (Mrs. Smith's 10"), 1/10 pie 42.0
raspberry, red *(Mrs. Smith's)*, 1/6 pie 43.0
strawberry *(Mrs. Smith's)*, 1/5 pie 45.0
strawberry-rhubarb *(Mrs. Smith's)*, 1/6 pie 44.0
Pie, snack, 1 pie, except as noted:
(Tastykake Tastyklair) 53.0
apple:
    (Drake's), 2 pies, 4 oz. 60.0
    (Hostess), 4.4 oz. 60.0
    (Pet-Ritz) 58.0
    (Tastykake) 45.0
    French *(Tastykake)* 61.0
blueberry:
    (Hostess), 4.4 oz. 58.0
    (Pet-Ritz) 61.0
    (Tastykake) 54.0
Boston creme, see "Cake, snack"
cherry:
    (Drake's), 2 pies, 4 oz. 60.0

Pie, snack, cherry *(cont.)*

(Hostess), 4.4 oz. 61.0
(Pet-Ritz) 56.0
(Tastykake) 61.0
coconut creme (Tastykake) 47.0
lemon:
(Hostess), 4.4 oz. 59.0
(Pet-Ritz) 61.0
(Tastykake) 50.0
marshmallow, banana (Little Debbie) 54.0
marshmallow, chocolate (Little Debbie) 53.0
oatmeal creme (Little Debbie) 48.0
peach (Hostess), 4.4 oz. 58.0
peach (Tastykake) 47.0
pineapple (Tastykake) 45.0
pineapple, cheese (Tastykake) 50.0
pumpkin (Tastykake) 47.0
raisin creme (Little Debbie) 44.0
strawberry (Tastykake) 49.0
Pie crust:
chocolate cookie (Oreo), 1/6 crust 18.0
chocolate cookie (Ready Crust), 1/8 crust 14.0
cookie crumbs (Nilla), 2 tbsp. 13.0
cookie crumbs (Oreo), 2 tbsp. 13.0
graham:
(Honey Maid), 1/6 crust 18.0
(Ready Crust Mini), .8-oz. crust 15.0
crumbs (Honey Maid), 2 tbsp. 13.0
crumbs (Sunshine), 2 tbsp. 13.0
shortbread (Ready Crust 9"), 1/8 crust 15.0
vanilla cookie (Nilla), 1/6 crust 20.0
Pie crust, frozen or refrigerated (see also "Pastry shell"),
1/8 crust, except as noted:
(Oronoque Orchards 6"), 1/4 crust 10.0
(Oronoque Orchards 9") 7.0
(Pet-Ritz 9") 9.0
(Pet-Ritz 95/8") 14.0
(Pillsbury) 9.0
deep dish:
(Oronoque Orchards 9") 8.0
(Oronoque Orchards 10") 11.0
all varieties (Pet-Ritz) 11.0

graham *(Oronoque Orchards)* 13.0
vegetable shortening *(Pet-Ritz)* 10.0
Pie crust mix:
(Betty Crocker), ⅛ of 9″ crust* 9.0
(Flako), ¼ cup dry 13.0
(Pillsbury), ⅛ of 9″ crust* 10.0
Pie filling (see also "Pastry filling"), canned, ⅓ cup, except
  as noted:
apple:
  (Comstock) 25.0
  (Comstock More Fruit) 20.0
  (Lucky Leaf/Lucky Leaf Premium) 22.0
  (Lucky Leaf Lite) 15.0
  (Musselman's 21 oz.) 22.0
  (Musselman's 24 oz.) 25.0
  cinnamon 'n spice *(Comstock* More Fruit) 27.0
  cranberry *(Comstock)* 22.0
apricot *(Comstock)* 23.0
apricot *(Lucky Leaf)* 22.0
banana cream *(Comstock)* 21.0
blackberry *(Comstock)* 26.0
blackberry *(Lucky Leaf)* 26.0
blueberry:
  (Comstock) 25.0
  (Comstock More Fruit) 21.0
  (Lucky Leaf/Lucky Leaf Premium) 26.0
  (Lucky Leaf Lite) 14.0
  (Musselman's) 24.0
  cranberry *(Comstock)* 25.0
cherry:
  (Comstock/Comstock More Fruit) 23.0
  (Comstock Lite) 15.0
  (Comstock More Fruit Lite) 13.0
  (Lucky Leaf/Musselman's) 24.0
  (Lucky Leaf/Musselman's Lite) 14.0
  dark sweet *(Comstock)* 24.0
  dark sweet *(Lucky Leaf/Musselman's)* 26.0
cherry-cranberry *(Comstock)* 22.0
chocolate cream *(Comstock)* 22.0
coconut cream *(Comstock)* 19.0
coconut creme *(Lucky Leaf)* 25.0

Pie filling *(cont.)*
lemon:
   (Comstock) 28.0
   (Lucky Leaf/Musselman's 22 oz.) 31.0
   (Lucky Leaf/Musselman's 25 oz.) 32.0
lemon creme *(Lucky Leaf)* 31.0
mincemeat:
   (Comstock) 40.0
   (Lucky Leaf) 33.0
   (None Such) 45.0
   (S&W), ¼ cup 43.0
   with brandy and rum *(None Such)* 47.0
   condensed *(None Such)*, 4 tsp. 36.0
peach *(Comstock More Fruit)* 19.0
peach *(Lucky Leaf)* 21.0
pineapple *(Comstock)* 27.0
pineapple *(Lucky Leaf/Musselman's)* 26.0
pumpkin, mix:
   (Comstock) 24.0
   (Libby's), ½ cup 25.0
   (Stokely) 24.0
raisin *(Comstock)* 29.0
raisin *(Lucky Leaf)* 25.0
raspberry *(Comstock)* 25.0
strawberry *(Comstock)* 23.0
strawberry *(Lucky Leaf/Musselman's)* 21.0
strawberry-rhubarb *(Lucky Leaf)* 23.0
Pie filling mix, see "Pudding mix"
Pie glaze, see "Glaze, fruit"
Pie mix, ⅙ pie⁎:
chocolate silk *(Jell-O)* 38.0
coconut cream *(Jell-O)* 37.0
Pierogi, frozen or refrigerated:
(Schwan's), 3 pieces 34.0
potato cheese *(Empire Kosher)*, 4 oz. 38.0
potato onion *(Empire Kosher)*, 4 oz. 36.0
potato onion *(Giorgio)*, 3 pieces 42.0
Pigeon peas:
fresh:
   in pods, 1 lb. 52.0
   shelled, raw, ½ cup 18.4
   boiled, drained, ½ cup 15.0

mature, dried *(Goya)*, ¼ cup 24.0
mature, dried, boiled, ½ cup 19.5
Pigeon peas, canned, ½ cup:
dried *(El Jib)* 18.0
green *(Tupi)* 14.0
Pig's feet:
simmered, 4 oz. 0
pickled *(Hormel)*, 2 oz. 0
pickled, cured, 1 oz. . . . . <1.0
Pignolia nuts, see "Pine nuts"
Pike, without added ingredients 0
Pili nuts, dried:
shelled, 1 oz. 1.1
shelled, 1 cup 4.8
Pimiento, drained:
(Goya), ¼ pepper 1.0
(S&W), 2¼ oz. 3.0
Piña colada mixer:
bottled *(Holland House/Mr & Mrs T)*, 4.5 fl. oz. 43.0
canned *(Goya)*, ⅓ cup 20.0
frozen* *(Bacardi)*, 8 fl. oz. 35.0
mix *(Bar-Tenders)*, 1.2-oz. pkt. 31.0
Pine nuts, dried:
pignolia:
 (Frieda's), ¼ cup 4.0
 (Krinos), .5 oz. 0
 (Progresso), 1 oz. 2.0
 1 oz. 4.0
 1 tbsp. 1.4
pinyon, 1 oz. 5.5
pinyon, 10 kernels 2
Pineapple
fresh:
 untrimmed, 1 lb. 29.2
 baby, trimmed *(Frieda's Sugarloaf)*, 1 oz. 3.9
 diced, ½ cup 9.6
 sliced *(Dole)*, 2 slices 21.0
canned, in juice:
 4 oz. 17.8
 all varieties, except sliced *(Del Monte)*, ½ cup 17.0
 chunks or tidbits *(Dole)*, ½ cup 15.0
 crushed *(Dole)*, ½ cup 17.0

Pineapple, canned, in juice *(cont.)*
sliced *(Del Monte)*, 2 slices 16.0
sliced *(Dole)*, 2 slices, 4 oz. 15.0
tidbits *(Del Monte* Snack Cup), 4-oz. cup 15.0
canned, in light syrup:
all varieties, except sliced *(Dole)*, ½ cup 20.0
chunks, in jars *(Sunfresh)*, ½ cup 17.0
sliced *(Dole)*, 3½ slices, 4 oz. 16.0
with mandarin orange *(Dole)*, ½ cup 19.0
canned, in heavy syrup:
4 oz. 22.9
all varieties, except sliced *(Dole)*, ½ cup 24.0
chunks, tidbits, or crushed, ½ cup 25.8
crushed or chunks *(Del Monte)*, ½ cup 24.0
sliced *(Del Monte)*, 2 slices 23.0
sliced *(Dole)*, 2 slices, 4 oz. 23.0
sliced *(S&W)*, ½ cup 23.0
canned, in extra heavy syrup, crushed *(Dole)*, ½ cup 29.0
dried *(Sonoma)*, 1.4 oz. 30.0
frozen, sweetened, chunks, ½ cup 27.1
Pineapple, candied:
(Paradise/White Swan), 6 pieces, 1 oz. 22.0
assorted *(Paradise/White Swan)*, 2 tbsp., 1 oz. 22.0
green *(Paradise/White Swan)*, 7 pieces, 1 oz. 22.0
red *(Paradise/White Swan)*, 8 pieces, 1.1 oz. 24.0
slices, natural or colored *(S&W* Glace), 2.2 oz. 46.0
wedges, natural or colored *(S&W* Glace), 5 pieces, 1 oz. . . 21.0
Pineapple drink:
(Tropicana Punch 16 oz.), 8 fl. oz. 31.0
(Tropicana Punch), 10 fl. oz. 40.0
Pineapple drink blend, 8 fl. oz., except as noted:
coconut *(Farmer's Market)* 29.0
coconut nectar *(Kern's)* 36.0
coconut nectar *(Kern's)*, 11.5 fl. oz. 52.0
grapefruit, pink *(Dole)*, 6 fl. oz. 25.0
grapefruit, pink *(Dole)* 32.0
orange, frozen* *(Schwan's Vita-Sun)* 24.0
Pineapple juice:
(Del Monte), 6 fl. oz. 20.0
(Del Monte), 8 fl. oz. 29.0
(Del Monte Not From Concentrate), 8 fl. oz. 29.0
(Dole Canned/Chilled), 8 fl. oz. 29.0

(Dole Reconstituted), 6 oz. 22.0
(Dole Reconstituted), 8 fl. oz. 26.0
(Dole Single Strength), 6 oz. 22.0
(Dole Single Strength), 8 fl. oz. 29.0
(Goya), 12 fl. oz. 46.0
(S&W), 6 fl. oz. 23.0
(S&W), 8 fl. oz. 29.0
(S&W), 12 fl. oz. 45.0
frozen* *(Dole),* 8 fl. oz. 30.0
frozen* *(Minute Maid),* 8 fl. oz. 31.0
Pineapple juice blend, 8 fl. oz., except as noted:
coconut *(R.W. Knudsen)* 32.0
grapefruit *(Dole),* 6 fl. oz. 24.0
grapefruit, frozen* *(Dole)* 29.0
orange:
   (Dole Chilled) 27.0
   (Dole Glass), 10 fl. oz. 36.0
   frozen* *(Dole)* 29.0
   frozen* *(Minute Maid)* 31.0
orange-banana:
   (Dole Chilled) 29.0
   (Dole Glass), 10 fl. oz. 40.0
orange-berry *(Dole)* 32.0
orange-guava *(Dole)* 29.0
orange-strawberry *(Dole)* 32.0
passion fruit–banana *(Dole* Chilled) 29.0
passion fruit–banana *(Dole* Glass), 10 fl. oz. 39.0
Pineapple topping, 2 tbsp.:
(Kraft) 28.0
(Smucker's) 28.0
Pink beans:
dried, ¼ cup 33.7
dried, boiled, ½ cup 23.5
canned *(Goya),* ½ cup 20.0
canned, in tomato sauce *(Goya* Guisadas), ½ cup 17.0
Pinquito beans, canned *(S&W),* ½ cup 20.0
Pinto beans:
dried:
   (Arrowhead Mills), ¼ cup 27.0
   (Goya), ¼ cup 22.0
   ¼ cup 30.5
   boiled, ½ cup 21.8

Pinto beans *(cont.)*

canned, ½ cup:

(Allens/East Texas Fair/Brown Beauty)	20.0
(Eden Organic)	18.0
(Eden Organic Jars)	22.0
(Gebhardt)	17.5
(Goya)	18.0
(Green Giant/Joan of Arc)	20.0
(Las Palmas)	19.0
(Old El Paso)	19.0
(Progresso)	18.0
(Stokely)	19.0
(Sun-Vista)	12.0
with liquid	17.5
with bacon *(Trappey's/Trappey's* Jala-pinto)	20.0
spiced, see "Chili beans"	
spicy *(Eden* Organic)	24.0
in tomato sauce *(Goya* Guisadas)	18.0

Pinto beans, sprouted, boiled, drained, 4 oz. ... 4.6

Pistachio nut, shelled, except as noted:

dried:

(Dole), 1 oz.	7.0
(Sonoma), ¼ cup	9.0
in shell *(Dole),* 1 oz.	3.0
in shell, 1 lb.	56.3
1 oz.	7.1
dry-roasted, in shell, salted, 1 lb.	64.9
dry-roasted, in shell *(Planters),* ½ cup, 1 oz. edible	7.0

dry-roasted:

(Planters), 1 oz.	7.0
(Planters Munch 'N Go Singles), 2-oz. pkg.	6.0
salted or unsalted, 1 cup	35.2
salted or unsalted, 1 oz.	7.8

Pita, see "Bread, pita/pocket"

Pitanga:

untrimmed, 1 lb.	29.9
1 medium, .3 oz.	.5
½ cup	6.5

Pizza, frozen:

artichoke heart *(Wolfgang Puck's* 10"), ½ pie	34.0
bacon burger *(Totino's Party),* ½ pie, 5.25 oz.	33.0

Canadian bacon:
   (Jeno's Crisp 'n Tasty), 6.9-oz. pie 49.0
   (Schwan's Special Recipe), ⅓ pie, 5.6 oz. 37.0
   (Tombstone Original 12″), ¼ pie 36.0
   (Totino's Party), ½ pie, 5.2 oz. 33.0
cheese:
   (Amy's), 1 serving 39.0
   (Celentano Thick Crust), ½ pie 62.0
   (Celeste Large), ¼ pie 32.0
   (Celeste Large Premium), ¼ pie 33.0
   (Celeste for One), 1 pie 52.0
   (Empire Kosher 3 Pack), 3-oz. pie 23.0
   (Empire Kosher 10 oz.), ½ pie 38.0
   (Jeno's Microwave For One), 3.7-oz. pie 25.0
   (Jeno's Crisp 'n Tasty), 6.9-oz. pie 51.0
   (Kid Cuisine Pirate), 8 oz. 71.0
   (Schwan's Deep Dish Single), 6-oz. pie 48.0
   (Schwan's Special Recipe), ⅓ pie, 5.3 oz. 37.0
   (Swanson Fun Feast), 1 pkg. 57.0
   (Tombstone For One ½ Less Fat), 6.5-oz. pie 45.0
   (Totino's Microwave for One), 3.7-oz. pie 25.0
   (Totino's Party), ½ pie, 4.9 oz. 33.0
   (Totino's Party Family Size), ⅓ pie, 5.6 oz. 38.0
cheese, extra:
   (Marie Callender's), ½ pie, 4.5 oz. 30.0
   (Tombstone Original 9″), ½ pie 42.0
   (Tombstone Original 12″), ¼ pie 36.0
   (Tombstone For One), 7-oz. pie 41.0
   (Weight Watchers), 5.74 oz. 49.0
cheese, four:
   (Celeste for One Original), 1 pie 47.0
   (Schwan's Deep Dish), ¼ of 10½″ pie 38.0
   (Tombstone Special Order 12″), ⅕ pie 37.0
   (Wolfgang Puck's), ½ of 10.75-oz. pie 40.0
   hot and zesty or zesty *(Celeste* for One), 1 pie 50.0
cheese, three:
   (Pappalo's Deep Dish), ¼ pie, 5.3 oz. 46.0
   (Pappalo's Deep Dish for One), 7.2-oz. pie 61.0
   (Pappalo's for One), 7.7-oz. pie 50.0
   (Pappalo's Pizzaria Style 9″), ½ pie 45.0
   (Pappalo's Pizzaria Style 12″), ¼ pie 40.0
   (Totino's Select), ⅓ pie, 4.4 oz. 30.0

Pizza, frozen, cheese, three *(cont.)*

    Italian *(Tombstone* ThinCrust), ¼ pie, 4.9 oz. 25.0

cheese, two:

    with Canadian bacon *(Totino's* Select), ⅓ pie, 4.9 oz. . . . 30.0

    with pepperoni *(Totino's* Select), ⅓ pie, 4.8 oz. 30.0

    with sausage *(Totino's* Select), ⅓ pie, 5 oz. 31.0

chicken, spicy *(Wolfgang Puck's)*, ½ of 10.75-oz. pie 36.0

chicken and broccoli *(Marie Callender's)*, ½ pie, 4.5 oz. . . . 34.0

combination:

    (Jeno's Microwave for One), 4.2-oz. pie 25.0

    (Jeno's Crisp 'n Tasty), 7-oz. pie 49.0

    (Totino's Microwave for One), 4.2-oz. pie 25.0

    (Totino's Party), ½ pie, 3.4 oz. 34.0

    (Totino's Party Family), ¼ pie, 4.4 oz. 28.0

    (Weight Watchers Deluxe), 6.57 oz. 47.0

deluxe:

    (Celeste Large), ¼ pie 35.0

    (Celeste Large Premium), ¼ pie 34.0

    (Celeste for One), 1 pie 53.0

    (Marie Callender's), ½ pie, 4.5 oz. 30.0

    (Tombstone Original 9"), ⅓ pie 28.0

    (Tombstone Original 12"), ¼ pie 29.0

hamburger:

    (Jeno's Crisp 'n Tasty), 7.3-oz. pie 49.0

    (Kid Cuisine Big League), 8.3 oz. 61.0

    (Tombstone Original 9"), ⅓ pie 28.0

    (Tombstone Original 12"), ⅕ pie 29.0

    (Totino's Party), ½ pie, 5.5 oz. 33.0

Italiano, zesty *(Totino's Party)*, ½ pie, 5.4 oz. 35.0

meat:

    five *(Marie Callender's)*, ½ pie, 4.5 oz. 36.0

    four *(Pappalo's* Deep Dish), ⅕ pie, 4.5 oz. 37.0

    four *(Pappalo's* Pizzaria Style 12"), ¼ pie 40.0

    four *(Tombstone* Special Order 9"), ⅓ pie 35.0

    four *(Tombstone* Special Order 12"), ⅙ pie 31.0

    four, combo, Italian *(Tombstone* ThinCrust), ¼ pie,

        5.1 oz. 25.0

    three *(Jeno's* Crisp 'n Tasty), 7-oz. pie 48.0

    three *(Schwan's* Deep Dish), ¼ of 10½" pie 38.0

    three *(Totino's* Party), ½ pie, 5.25 oz. 33.0

Mexican style:

    (Schwan's Deep Dish Single), 5.4-oz. pie 40.0

supreme taco *(Tombstone* ThinCrust), ¼ pie, 5.1 oz. . . . 26.0
zesty *(Totino's* Microwave for One), 4.2-oz. pie 25.0
zesty *(Totino's Party),* ½ pie, 5.5 oz. 34.0

pepperoni:

(Celeste Large), ¼ pie 33.0
(Celeste Large Premium), ¼ pie 34.0
(Celeste Pizza for One), 1 pie 53.0
(Hormel Quick Meal), 5.9-oz. pie 47.0
(Jeno's Microwave for One), 4-oz. pie 25.0
(Jeno's Crisp 'n Tasty), 6.8-oz. pie 49.0
(Marie Callender's), ½ pie, 4.5 oz. 30.0
(Pappalo's Deep Dish), ⅕ pie, 4.4 oz. 37.0
(Pappalo's Deep Dish for One), 7-oz. pie 55.0
(Pappalo's for One), 7-oz. pie 48.0
(Pappalo's Pizzaria Style 9″), ½ pie 45.0
(Pappalo's Pizzaria Style 12″), ¼ pie 40.0
(Schwan's Deep Dish Single), 6-oz. pie 47.0
(Schwan's Special Recipe), ⅓ pie, 5.4 oz. 37.0
(Tombstone Original 9″), ⅓ pie 28.0
(Tombstone Original 12″), ⅕ pie 29.0
(Tombstone for One), 7-oz. pie 41.0
(Tombstone For One ½ Less Fat), 6.8-oz. pie 45.0
(Tombstone Special Order 9″), ⅓ pie 35.0
(Tombstone Special Order 12″), ⅙ pie 31.0
(Totino's Microwave for One), 4 oz. 25.0
(Totino's Party), ½ pie, 5.1 oz. 33.0
(Totino's Party Family), ⅓ pie, 5.6 oz. 37.0
(Weight Watchers), 5.56 oz. 46.0
double cheese *(Tombstone Double Top),* ⅙ pie, 4.6 oz.   25.0
Italian *(Tombstone* ThinCrust), ¼ pie, 5 oz. 25.0
super *(Schwan's* Deep Dish), ¼ of 10½″ pie 38.0

sausage:

(Celeste for One), 1 pie 52.0
(Jeno's Microwave for One), 4.1-oz. pie 25.0
(Jeno's Crisp 'n Tasty), 7-oz. pie 49.0
(Pappalo's Deep Dish), ⅕ pie, 4.6 oz. 37.0
(Pappalo's Pizzaria Style 9″), ½ pie 46.0
(Pappalo's Pizzaria Style 12″), ¼ pie 40.0
(Schwan's Deep Dish Single), 6-oz. pie 47.0
(Schwan's Special Recipe), ¼ pie, 4.5 oz. 28.0
(Tombstone Original 9″), ⅓ pie 28.0
(Tombstone Original 12″), ⅕ pie 29.0

Pizza, frozen, sausage *(cont.)*

(Totino's Microwave For One), 4.1-oz. pie 25.0

(Totino's Party), ½ pie, 5.4 oz. 34.0

(Totino's Party Family), ¼ pie, 4.5 oz. 28.0

double cheese *(Tombstone Double Top),* ⅙ pie, 4.8 oz. 25.0

and herb *(Wolfgang Puck's),* ½ of 10.75-oz. pie 36.0

Italian *(Tombstone* ThinCrust), ¼ pie, 5.1 oz. 25.0

Italian *(Tombstone For One),* 7-oz. pie 40.0

sausage, three *(Tombstone Special Order 9"),* ⅓ pie 35.0

sausage, three *(Tombstone Special Order 12"),* ⅙ pie 31.0

sausage and mushroom *(Tombstone Original 12"),* ⅕ pie . . 29.0

sausage and pepperoni:

(Celeste Large Premium), ¼ pie 33.0

(Marie Callender's), ½ pie, 4.5 oz. 29.0

(Pappalo's Deep Dish), ⅕ pie, 4.6 oz. 37.0

(Pappalo's Deep Dish for One), 7.26-oz. pie 56.0

(Pappalo's for One), 7.2-oz. pie 48.0

(Pappalo's Pizzaria Style 9"), ½ pie 45.0

(Pappalo's Pizzaria Style 12"), ¼ pie 40.0

(Schwan's Special Recipe), ¼ pie, 4.4 oz. 28.0

(Tombstone Original 9"), ⅓ pie 28.0

(Tombstone Original 12"), ⅕ pie 29.0

(Tombstone For One), 7-oz. pie 40.0

(Totino's Select), ⅓ pie, 5 oz. 30.0

double cheese *(Tombstone Double Top),* ⅙ pie, 4.8 oz. 25.0

spinach feta *(Amy's),* 1 serving 40.0

supreme:

(Celeste Suprema for One), 1 pie 56.0

(Celeste Suprema Large), ⅕ pie 27.0

(Jeno's Crisp 'n Tasty), 7.2-oz. pie 49.0

(Pappalo's Deep Dish), ⅕ pie, 4.9 oz. 38.0

(Pappalo's Deep Dish for One), 7.6-oz. pie 54.0

(Pappalo's for One), 7.6-oz. pie 48.0

(Pappalo's Pizzaria Style 9"), ½ pie 31.0

(Pappalo's Pizzaria Style 12"), ¼ pie 41.0

(Schwan's Deep Dish), ¼ of 10½" pie 39.0

(Schwan's Deep Dish Single), 6-oz. pie 44.0

(Schwan's Special Recipe), ¼ pie, 5.1 oz. 32.0

(Tombstone Original 12"), ⅕ pie 29.0

(Tombstone Light), ⅕ pie, 4.9 oz. 30.0

(Tombstone For One), 7.6-oz. pie 41.0

(Tombstone for One ½ Less Fat), 7.7-oz. pie 45.0

(*Totino's* Microwave for One), 4.3-oz. pie 25.0
(*Totino's* Select), 1/3 pie, 5.5 oz. 31.0
(*Totino's Party*), 1/2 pie, 5.5 oz. 34.0
Italian (*Tombstone* ThinCrust), 1/4 pie, 5.3 oz. 26.0
super (*Tombstone Special Order 9"*), 1/3 pie 36.0
super (*Tombstone Special Order 12"*), 1/6 pie 31.0
tomato and mozzarella (*Marie Callender's*), 1/2 pie, 4.5 oz. . . 40.0
vegetable:
  (*Celeste* for One), 1 pie 52.0
  (*Tombstone* Light), 1/5 pie, 4.6 oz. 31.0
  (*Tombstone For One* 1/2 Less Fat), 7.3-oz. pie 46.0
  grilled, cheeseless (*Wolfgang Puck's*), 1/2 of 10.75-oz.
    pie 42.0
  primavera (*Marie Callender's*), 1/2 pie, 4.5 oz. 40.0
  roasted (*Amy's*), 1 serving 43.0
Pizza, bagel, frozen (*Empire* Kosher), 2-oz. piece 15.0
Pizza, breakfast, frozen, 1 piece:
bacon (*Schwan's Bright Starts* Singles) 36.0
western (*Schwan's* Bright Starts Singles) 36.0
Pizza, croissant, frozen, 1 piece:
cheese (*Pepperidge Farm*) 39.0
deluxe (*Pepperidge Farm*) 40.0
pepperoni (*Pepperidge Farm*) 39.0
Pizza, English muffin, frozen (*Empire* Kosher), 2-oz. piece 15.0
Pizza, French bread, frozen:
bacon cheddar (*Stouffer's*), 1/2 of 11 3/8-oz. pkg. 46.0
cheese:
  (*Healthy Choice*), 6 oz. 51.0
  (*Lean Cuisine*), 6 oz. 49.0
  (*Stouffer's*), 1/2 of 10 3/8-oz. pkg. 40.0
  double (*Stouffer's*), 1/2 of 11 3/4-oz. pkg. 46.0
cheeseburger (*Stouffer's*), 1/2 of 11 7/8-oz. pkg. 44.0
deluxe (*Lean Cuisine*), 6 1/8 oz. 44.0
deluxe (*Stouffer's*), 1/2 of 12 3/8-oz. pkg. 45.0
meat, three (*Stouffer's*), 1/2 of 12 1/2-oz. pkg. 48.0
pepperoni:
  (*Healthy Choice*), 6 oz. 49.0
  (*Lean Cuisine*), 5 1/4 oz. 45.0
  (*Stouffer's*), 1/2 of 11 1/4-oz. pkg. 41.0
pepperoni and mushroom (*Stouffer's*), 1/2 of 12 1/4-oz. pkg. . . 47.0
sausage (*Healthy Choice*), 6 oz. 48.0
sausage (*Stouffer's*), 1/2 of 12-oz. pkg. 46.0

Pizza, French bread *(cont.)*
sausage and pepperoni *(Stouffer's)*, ½ of 12½-oz. pkg. 45.0
supreme *(Healthy Choice)*, 6 oz. 51.0
vegetable *(Healthy Choice)*, 6 oz. 45.0
vegetable, deluxe *(Stouffer's)*, ½ of 12¾-oz. pkg. 46.0
white *(Stouffer's)*, ½ of 10⅛-oz. pkg. 45.0
Pizza, Italian bread, frozen, 1 piece:
cheese, four *(Celeste)* 32.0
chicken, zesty *(Celeste)* 34.0
deluxe *(Celeste)* 36.0
pepperoni *(Celeste)* 37.0
Pizza crust, refrigerated, ¼ crust:
(Pillsbury) 33.0
(Totino's) 25.0
Pizza crust mix*:
(Martha White), ¼ crust 32.0
(Ragú Pizza Quick), ⅕ of 12″ crust 24.0
(Robin Hood), ¼ crust 33.0
deep pan *(Martha White)*, ⅕ crust 28.0
Pizza Hut, 1 slice of medium pie, except as noted:
Bigfoot, 1 slice:
    cheese 25.0
    pepperoni 25.0
    pepperoni, mushroom, and sausage 25.0
breadsticks, 5 pieces 129.0
hand-tossed:
    cheese 29.0
    beef 29.0
    ham 29.0
    Meat Lovers 29.0
    pepperoni 29.0
    Pepperoni Lovers 29.0
    pork topping 29.0
    sausage, Italian 29.0
    supreme 30.0
    supreme, super 30.0
    Veggie Lovers 30.0
pan pizza:
    cheese 28.0
    beef 28.0
    ham 28.0
    Meat Lovers 28.0

pepperoni 28.0
Pepperoni Lovers 28.0
pork topping 28.0
sausage, Italian 27.0
supreme 28.0
supreme, super 28.0
Veggie Lovers 29.0
Personal Pan Pizza:
pepperoni, 1 pie 69.0
supreme, 1 pie 70.0
Thin 'N Crispy:
cheese 21.0
beef 21.0
ham 21.0
Meat Lovers 21.0
pepperoni 21.0
Pepperoni Lovers 22.0
pork topping 21.0
sausage, Italian 21.0
supreme 21.0
supreme, super 22.0
Veggie Lovers 22.0
Pizza pepper *(Lawry's),* 1/4 tsp. 0
Pizza roll, see "Pizza snacks"
Pizza sandwich, frozen:
cheese *(Amy's Pocketfuls),* 4.5-oz. piece 38.0
deluxe *(Lean Pockets),* 4.5-oz. piece 37.0
meat, mega *(Totino's* Big & Hearty), 4.8-oz. piece 35.0
pepperoni:
    (Croissant Pockets), 4.5-oz. piece 38.0
    (Deli Stuffs), 4.5-oz. piece 42.0
    (Hot Pockets), 4.5-oz. piece 38.0
    (Totino's Big & Hearty), 4.8-oz. piece 34.0
pepperoni and sausage *(Hot Pockets),* 4.5-oz. piece 38.0
sausage *(Hot Pockets),* 4.5-oz. piece 37.0
vegetable *(Ken & Robert's Veggie Pockets),* 1 piece 41.0
vegetable, pepperoni style *(Amy's),* 4.5-oz. piece 28.0
Pizza sauce, 1/4 cup:
(Angelia Mia) 5.0
(Angelia Mia Fully Prepared) 4.0
(Angelia Mia Prima Choice Super Heavy) 6.0
(Contadina) 4.0

Pizza sauce *(cont.)*
(Contadina Chunky) 6.0
(Contadina Pizza Squeeze) 6.0
(Pastorelli Italian Chef) 6.0
(Prince Traditional) 4.0
(Progresso) 5.0
(Ragú Pizza Quick 100% Natural) 4.0
(Ragú Pizza Quick Traditional) 5.0
with cheese:
   Italian *(Contadina)* 4.0
   Italian *(Contadina Pizza Squeeze)* 6.0
   three *(Contadina* Chunky) 5.0
garlic and basil *(Ragú* Pizza Quick) 6.0
mushroom *(Contadina* Chunky) 5.0
mushroom *(Ragú* Pizza Quick) 6.0
pepperoni *(Contadina)* 4.0
pepperoni *(Ragú* Pizza Quick) 5.0
tomato, chunky *(Ragú* Pizza Quick) 7.0
Pizza seasoning *(Tone's/Presti's)*, ¾ tsp. 1.0
Pizza snacks, 6 pieces, except as noted:
(Schwan's Wonton Rolls), 5 pieces, 5 oz. 42.0
cheese, double *(Hot Pockets* Pizza Snacks), 3 oz. 29.0
cheese, three *(Totino's Pizza Rolls)* 24.0
combination *(Totino's Pizza Rolls)* 22.0
hamburger and cheese *(Totino's Pizza Rolls)* 22.0
meat, three *(Totino's Pizza Rolls)* 22.0
nuggets *(Hormel Quick Meal)*, 5 pieces, 2.8 oz. 25.0
pepperoni *(Hot Pockets* Pizza Snacks), 3 oz. 30.0
pepperoni and cheese *(Totino's Pizza Rolls)* 22.0
pepperoni and sausage *(Hot Pockets Pizza Snacks)*, 3 oz. ... 26.0
sausage *(Hot Pockets* Pizza Snacks), 3 oz. 27.0
sausage and cheese *(Totino's Pizza Rolls)* 22.0
sausage and mushroom *(Totino's Pizza Rolls)* 23.0
spicy Italian style *(Totino's Pizza Rolls)* 22.0
supreme *(Totino's Pizza Rolls)* 23.0
Plantain:
raw:
   (Frieda's), 3 oz. 27.0
   untrimmed, 1 lb. 94.0
   1 medium, 9.7 oz. 57.1
   sliced, ½ cup 23.6
cooked, sliced, ½ cup 24.0

fried *(Goya* Tostone), 3 pieces 37.0
Plum:
fresh:
    (Dole), 2 medium 17.0
    with pits, 1 lb. 55.5
    pitted, sliced, ½ cup 10.7
    Japanese or hybrid, 1 medium, 2⅛″ diam. 8.6
canned:
    in juice, ½ cup 19.1
    in juice, 3 plums and 2 tbsp. liquid 14.4
    in light syrup, ½ cup 20.5
    in light syrup, 3 plums and 2¾ tbsp. liquid 21.7
    in syrup *(Oregon)*, ½ cup 25.0
    in heavy syrup, ½ cup 30.0
    in heavy syrup *(Comstock)*, ½ cup 26.0
    in heavy syrup, 3 plums and 2¾ tbsp. liquid 30.9
    in heavy syrup, whole *(S&W)*, ½ cup 33.0
Plum sauce:
(Ka•Me), 2 tbsp. 19.0
(La Choy), 1 tbsp. 6.0
Poblano chili, see "Pepper, chili"
Poi:
1 oz. 7.7
½ cup 32.7
Pocket sandwich, see specific listings
Poke greens, canned *(Allens)*, ½ cup 5.0
Pokeberry shoots, ½ cup:
raw, trimmed 3.0
boiled, drained 2.5
Polenta, refrigerated:
(Frieda's), 4 oz. 21.0
(San Gennaro), 2 slices, ½″ 15.0
basil and garlic *(San Gennaro)*, 2 slices, ½″ 15.0
Italian herb *(Frieda's)*, 4 oz. 17.0
sun-dried tomato *(San Gennaro)*, 2 slices, ½″ 16.0
wild mushroom *(Frieda's)*, 4 oz. 17.0
Polenta mix *(Fantastic)*, 1 cup* 46.0
Polish sausage (see also "Kielbasa"):
(Schwan's), 2.7-oz. link 4.0
beef *(Hebrew National)*, 3-oz. link 1.0
beef *(Hebrew National)*, 4-oz. link 1.0
skinless *(John Morrell)*, 2 oz. 3.0

Pollock, without added ingredients 0
Pomegranate:
(Dole), 1 medium 26.0
(Frieda's), 5 oz. 24.0
untrimmed, 1 lb. 43.6
1 medium, 9.7 oz. 26.4
Pomegranate juice *(R.W. Knudsen),* 8 fl. oz. 37.0
Pompano, without added ingredients 0
Popcorn, unpopped:
(Arrowhead Mills), 1/4 cup, 1 3/4 oz. 36.0
(Orville Redenbacher Original/Hot Air/White), 2 tbsp. 22.0
microwave:
    (Redenbudders Movie Theater), 2 tbsp. 16.0
    (Redenbudders Movie Theater Light), 2 tbsp. 19.0
    (Smart Pop), 2 tbsp. 19.5
    butter *(Orville Redenbacher),* 2 tbsp. 15.0
    butter *(Orville Redenbacher* No Salt Added), 2 tbsp. . . . 19.0
    butter *(Orville Redenbacher* Snack Size), 1 bag 25.0
    butter *(Pop•Secret/Pop•Secret Movie Theater),* 3 tbsp. 17.0
    butter *(Pop•Secret* Jumbo Pop), 3 tbsp. 18.0
    butter *(Pop•Secret* Single Serving), 1/4 cup 24.0
    butter *(Pop•Secret Movie Theater* Jumbo Pop), 3 tbsp. 18.0
    butter *(Redenbudders* Movie Theater), 2 tbsp. 16.0
    butter *(Smart Pop* Movie Theater), 2 tbsp. 20.0
    butter *(Smart Pop* Snack Size), 1 bag 34.0
    butter, light *(Orville Redenbacher),* 2 tbsp. 20.0
    butter, light *(Orville Redenbacher* Snack Size), 1 bag . . . 30.0
    butter, light *(Pop•Secret),* 3 tbsp. 22.0
    butter, light *(Pop•Secret* Single Serving), 1/4 cup 25.0
    butter, light *(Pop•Secret Movie Theater),* 1/4 cup 22.0
    butter, light *(Redenbudders* Movie Theater), 2 tbsp. 19.0
    butter, 94% fat free *(Pop•Secret),* 3 tbsp. 26.0
    butter, real *(Pop•Secret),* 3 tbsp. 17.0
    caramel *(Orville Redenbacher),* 2 tbsp. 23.0
    cheddar, golden or white *(Orville Redenbacher),* 2 tbsp. 15.0
    cheese, cheddar or nacho *(Pop•Secret),* 3 tbsp. 19.0
    herb and garlic *(Redenbudders),* 2 tbsp. 16.0
    natural *(Orville Redenbacher),* 2 tbsp. 17.5
    natural *(Orville Redenbacher* Light/No Salt Added),
      2 tbsp. 19.0
    natural *(Pop•Secret),* 3 tbsp. 17.0
    natural, light *(Pop•Secret),* 3 tbsp. 22.0

natural, 94% fat free *(Pop•Secret)*, 3 tbsp. 26.0
zesty *(Redenbudders)*, 2 tbsp. 16.0
Popcorn, popped:
(Barrel O'Fun Canola), 3 cups 14.0
(Barrel O'Fun Light), 3 cups 22.0
(Chester's Triple Mix), 1½ cups 19.0
(Frieda's), 2 cups 23.0
(Wise Choice), 2½ cups 18.0
air popped:
    (Bachman), 2¾ cups 15.0
    (Bachman Lite), 5 cups 23.0
    white or yellow *(Jolly Time)*, 5 cups 24.0
butter/butter flavor:
    (Borden), 1-oz. bag 14.0
    (Chester's), 3 cups 15.0
    (Smart Snackers), .66-oz. bag 14.0
    (Smartfood), 3 cups 15.0
    (Smartfood Reduced Fat), 3⅓ cups 21.0
    (Wise Reduced Fat), 3 cups 19.0
caramel:
    (Barrel O'Fun Fat Free), ¾ cup 27.0
    (Chester's), ¾ cup 27.0
    (Cracker Jack Fat Free), 1 cup, 1 oz. 27.0
    (Smart Snackers), .9-oz. bag 22.0
    (Wise Fat Free), 1 cup 26.0
    air popped *(Greenfield)*, ⅔ cup 23.0
caramel with peanuts:
    (Barrel O'Fun), ⅔ cup 21.0
    (Cracker Jack), ⅔ cup 23.0
    (Cracker Jack), 1.25-oz. box 29.0
    (Old Dutch), 1 oz. 23.0
cheddar, white:
    (Barrel O'Fun), 3 cups 13.0
    (Chester's), 3 cups 17.0
    (Smart Snackers), .66-oz. bag 12.0
    (Smartfood), 2 cups 17.0
    (Smartfood Reduced Fat), 3 cups 19.0
cheese, 2½ cups, except as noted:
    (Barrel O'Fun) 14.0
    (Barrel O'Fun Low Fat) 20.0
    3 cups 14.0

Popcorn, popped *(cont.)*
microwave:

    (Jolly Time/Jolly Time Light), 4 cups 16.0

    cheese, cheddar or nacho *(Pop•Secret)*, 1 cup 3.0

    cheese, cheddar or nacho *(Pop•Secret)*, 5 cups 16.0

    natural *(Pop•Secret)*, 1 cup 4.0

    natural *(Pop•Secret)*, 4 cups 16.0

    natural, light or 94% fat free *(Pop•Secret)*, 1 cup 4.0

    natural, light *(Pop•Secret)*, 6 cups 20.0

    natural, 94% fat free *(Pop•Secret)*, 6 cups 23.0

microwave, butter flavor:

    (Chester's), 5 cups 22.0

    (Jolly Time/Jolly Time Light), 4 cups 16.0

    (Pop•Secret/Pop•Secret Jumbo Pop/*Pop•Secret* Real),
      1 cup 4.0

    (Pop•Secret), 4 cups 16.0

    (Pop•Secret Movie Theater/Pop•Secret Single Serving),
      1 cup 3.0

    (Pop•Secret Movie Theater Jumbo Pop), 1 cup 4.0

    light *(Pop•Secret/Pop•Secret Movie Theater)*, 1 cup 4.0

    light *(Pop•Secret/Pop•Secret Movie Theater)*, 6 cups . . 20.0

    light *(Pop•Secret* Single Serving), 1 cup 4.0

    94% fat free *(Pop•Secret)*, 1 cup 4.0

    94% fat free *(Pop•Secret)*, 6 cups 23.0

toffee *(Crunch 'n Munch* Fat Free), ³/₄ cup 26.0

toffee, butter:

    (Cracker Jack Fat Free), 1 cup, 1 oz. 26.0

    (Smart Snackers), .9-oz. bag 21.0

    (Wise Fat Free), 1 cup 26.0

    with peanuts *(Cracker Jack)*, 1.25-oz. box 26.0

    with pecans and almonds *(Cracker Jack)*, 1 oz. 19.0

toffee, with nuts *(Franklin)*, ²/₃ cup 24.0

toffee crunch *(Smartfood)*, ³/₄ cup 28.0

Popcorn bar, caramel or chocolate *(Pop•Secret)*, 1 bar . . . 16.0

Popcorn cake:

(Quaker Mini Lightly Salted), 7 cakes 11.0

barbecue *(Orville Redenbacher* Mini), 8 cakes, .5 oz. 12.0

butter:

    (Orville Redenbacher), 2 cakes, .6 oz. 13.0

    (Orville Redenbacher Mini), 8 cakes, .5 oz. 11.0

    (Quaker Mini), 6 cakes 11.0

caramel:
    (Orville Redenbacher), 1 cake, 4 oz. 8.0
    (Orville Redenbacher Mini), 7 cakes, .5 oz. 12.0
    (Quaker Mini), 5 cakes 12.0
cheddar:
    (Quaker Mini), 6 cakes 11.0
    white *(Lundberg* Mini), 5 cakes 12.0
    white *(Orville Redenbacher)*, 2 cakes, .6 oz. 13.0
    white *(Orville Redenbacher)*, 8 cakes, .5 oz. 12.0
cheese, nacho *(Orville Redenbacher* Mini), 8 cakes, .5 oz. . . 11.0
peanut crunch *(Orville Redenbacher* Mini), 7 cakes, .6 oz. . . 11.0
Popcorn seasoning *(Tone's)*, ¼ tsp. 0
Poppy seed:
(McCormick), ¼ tsp. 7
1 tbsp. 2.1
1 tsp. 7
Poppy seed filling, see "Pastry filling"
Porgy, see "Scup"
Pork, without added ingredients 0
Pork, barbecued, see "Pork, refrigerated"
Pork, cured (see also "Ham"):
arm (picnic), roasted, 4 oz. 0
blade roll, lean with fat, roasted, 4 oz. 4
Pork, frozen:
chops, center cut *(Schwan's)*, 5.3-oz. chop 0
patty *(Tyson)*, 3.8-oz. patty 9.0
Pork, pickled (see also "Pig's feet"), 2 oz.:
hocks *(Hormel)* 0
tidbits *(Hormel)* 0
Pork, refrigerated:
barbecued:
    shredded *(Lloyd's)*, ¼ cup 9.0
    spareribs *(Lloyd's)*, 3 ribs with sauce 15.0
    spareribs, baby back *(Lloyd's)*, 3 ribs with sauce 18.0
loin, center *(John Morrell Table Trim)*, 4 oz. 0
smoked shoulder butt *(Oscar Mayer Sweet Morsel)*, 3 oz. 0
tenderloin *(John Morrell Table Trim)*, 4 oz. 0
Pork batter, frying *(House of Tsang)*, 4 tbsp. 32.0
Pork belly, raw, 1 oz. 0
Pork dinner, frozen:
barbecue *(Swanson Hungry Man)*, 1 pkg. 78.0
patty, grilled, glazed *(Healthy Choice)*, 9.6 oz. 46.0

Pork entree, canned, chow mein *(Chun King* Bi-Pack),
1 cup 9.0
Pork entree, freeze-dried, sweet and sour, with rice
(Mountain House), 1 cup 40.0
Pork entree, frozen:
cutlet *(Banquet* Country), 10¼ oz. 37.0
ribs, BBQ *(Schwan's),* 5.7-oz. piece 20.0
ribs, barbecue sauce *(Swanson Fun Feast),* 1 pkg. 44.0
rib-shape patty, barbecue *(Swanson),* 1 pkg. 48.0
sweet and sour *(Chun King),* 13 oz. 86.0
Pork fat, roasted 0
Pork fritter *(Schwan's),* 1 piece, 4 oz. 30.0
Pork gravy, ¼ cup:
(Franco-American) 3.0
(Heinz Home Style) 3.0
mix* *(Durkee)* 3.0
mix* *(French's)* 3.0
Pork lunch meat, 2 oz.:
(Hormel Deli Pork Roast) 1.0
seasoned *(Boar's Head)* 0
Pork rind snack, ½ oz.:
(Old Dutch Bac'n Puffs) 0
all varieties *(Baken-ets/Baken-ets Cracklins)* . . . . <1.0
Pork sandwich, frozen, barbecued *(Hormel Quick Meal),*
1 piece 39.0
Pork seasoning mix:
(Durkee/French's Roasting Bag), ⅙ pkg. 5.0
(Shake'n Bake Original Recipe), ⅛ pkg. 9.0
barbecue glaze *(Shake'n Bake),* ⅛ pkg. 8.0
chops *(McCormick Bag 'n Season),* 2 tsp. mix 4.0
extra crispy *(Oven Fry),* ⅛ pkg. 11.0
hot and spicy *(Shake'n Bake),* ⅛ pkg. 8.0
sparerib *(Durkee* Roasting Bag), ⅐ pkg. 5.0
Pork and beans, see "Baked beans" and specific bean
listings
Pot roast, see "Beef dinner" and "Beef entree"
Pot roast seasoning mix, ⅙ pkg., except as noted:
(Durkee Roasting Bag) 3.0
(French's Roasting Bag) 4.0
(Lawry's), 1 tsp. 1.0
onion *(French's* Roasting Bag) 4.0
sauerbraten *(Knorr)* 5.0

Potato:
(Dole), 1 medium, 5.3 oz. 27.0
(Frieda's), ½ cup, 3 oz. 15.0
raw:
    unpeeled, 1 lb. 61.2
    peeled, 2½″-diam. potato 20.1
    peeled, diced, ½ cup 13.5
baked in skin, 1 medium, 4¾″ × 2⅓″ diam. 51.0
baked without skin, 4 oz. 24.4
baked without skin, ½ cup 13.2
boiled in skin, baby *(Frieda's),* 4 oz. 19.4
boiled in skin, peeled:
    2½″-diam. potato 27.4
    4 oz. 22.8
    ½ cup 15.7
boiled without skin, 2½″-diam. potato 27.0
boiled without skin, ½ cup 15.6
microwaved in skin:
    1 medium, 4¾″ × 2⅓″ diam. 48.7
    4 oz. 27.4
    peeled, ½ cup 18.2
    skin only, 2 oz. 16.8
mashed, with whole milk, ½ cup 18.4
mashed, with whole milk, with butter or margarine, ½ cup 17.5
Potato, canned:
(Seneca), ⅔ cup 17.0
with liquid, 4 oz. 9.8
drained, 1.2-oz. potato 4.8
whole:
    (Butterfield/Sunshine), 2½ pieces, 5.6 oz. 20.0
    (Stokely/Stokely No Salt), 5½ oz. 12.0
    new *(Del Monte),* 2 medium with liquid 13.0
    new *(S&W),* ½ cup 14.0
sliced *(Butterfield),* ½ cup 22.0
sliced *(Del Monte),* ⅔ cup 13.0
diced *(Butterfield),* ⅔ cup 22.0
mashed *(Idahoan* Complete), ⅓ cup 19.0
mashed *(Idahoan* Real), ⅓ cup 17.0
Potato, frozen (see also "Potato dishes, frozen"):
whole *(Stilwell),* 3 pieces 13.0
curls *(Schwan's),* 3 oz. 20.0

Potato, frozen *(cont.)*
fried or french-fried, 3 oz., except as noted:

    (Ore-Ida Deep Fries) 22.0
    (Ore-Ida Deep Fries Crinkle Cuts) 23.0
    (Ore-Ida Shoestrings) 22.0
    (Ore-Ida Steak Fries) 19.0
    (Ore-Ida Crispers!) 24.0
    (Ore-Ida Crispy Crowns!) 20.0
    (Ore-Ida Crispy Crunchies!) 20.0
    (Ore-Ida Fast Fries) 20.0
    (Ore-Ida Golden Crinkles) 23.0
    (Ore-Ida Golden Fries) 20.0
    (Ore-Ida Golden Pixie Crinkles) 21.0
    (Ore-Ida Golden Twirls) 23.0
    (Ore-Ida Homestyle Wedges With Skin) 19.0
    (Ore-Ida Snackin' Fries), 5-oz. pkg. 36.0
    (Ore-Ida Texas Crispers!) 20.0
    (Ore-Ida Waffle Fries) 21.0
    (Schwan's) 22.0
    cottage fries *(Ore-Ida)* 25.0
    country fries *(Ore-Ida)* 19.0
    crinkle cut *(Empire* Kosher), ½ cup 18.0
    ranch flavor *(Ore-Ida Fast Fries)* 21.0
    zesty *(Ore-Ida Snackin' Fries)*, 5-oz. pkg. 34.0
hash brown:
    (Ore-Ida Microwave), 4-oz. pkg. 26.0
    (Ore-Ida Golden Patties), 1 piece 17.0
    (Schwan's), 1 patty 14.0
    with cheddar *(Ore-Ida Cheddar Browns)*, 1 piece 14.0
    country *(Ore-Ida)*, 1 cup 14.0
    shredded *(Ore-Ida)*, 1 piece 15.0
    Southern style *(Ore-Ida)*, ¾ cup 17.0
    toaster *(Ore-Ida)*, 2 pieces 25.0
mashed *(Ore-Ida)*, ⅔ cup 16.0
O'Brien *(Ore-Ida)*, ¾ cup 15.0
puffs:
    (Hot Tots), 3 oz. 20.0
    (Schwan's Quik Taters), 13 pieces 19.0
    (Tater Tots), 3 oz. 21.0
    (Tater Tots Microwave), 4-oz. pkg. 27.0
Potato, mix:
(Betty Crocker Potato Shakers), 3 tsp. 5.0

(Betty Crocker Potato Shakers), ⅔ cup* 23.0
au gratin:
   (Betty Crocker 5.5 oz./21 oz.), ½ cup 20.0
   (Betty Crocker 5.5 oz./21 oz.), ½ cup* 22.0
   (Betty Crocker 9 oz.), ½ cup 22.0
   (Betty Crocker 9 oz.), ½ cup* 23.0
   (Hungry Jack), ½ cup 22.0
   (Hungry Jack), ⅛ pkg.* 24.0
   (Idahoan), ⅓ cup 23.0
   broccoli *(Betty Crocker),* ½ cup 19.0
   broccoli *(Betty Crocker),* ½ cup* 21.0
broccoli and cheddar *(Fantastic* Potato Cup), 1.7 oz. 35.0
cheese:
   cheddar *(Betty Crocker),* ½ cup 20.0
   cheddar *(Betty Crocker),* ½ cup* 21.0
   cheddar *(Betty Crocker Cheddar & Bac•Os),* ½ cup 20.0
   cheddar *(Betty Crocker Cheddar & Bac•Os),* ½ cup* . . . 21.0
   cheddar *(Fantastic* Potato Cup), 1.7 oz. 35.0
   cheddar *(Shake'n Bake Perfect Potatoes),* ⅙ pkg. 2.0
   cheddar, smokey *(Betty Crocker),* ½ cup 21.0
   cheddar, smokey *(Betty Crocker),* ½ cup* 22.0
   cheddar, white *(Betty Crocker),* ½ cup 21.0
   cheddar, white *(Betty Crocker),* ½ cup* 22.0
   cheddar, zesty *(Betty Crocker Potato Shakers),* 3 tsp. . . . 4.0
   cheddar, zesty *(Betty Crocker Potato Shakers),* ⅔ cup* 22.0
   cheddar and bacon *(Betty Crocker Twice Baked),* ⅓ cup 20.0
   cheddar and bacon *(Betty Crocker Twice Baked),* ⅔ cup* 22.0
   cheddar and bacon *(Hungry Jack),* ½ cup 22.0
   cheddar and bacon *(Hungry Jack),* ⅛ pkg.* 24.0
   cheddar and sour cream *(Betty Crocker),* ⅔ cup 24.0
   cheddar and sour cream *(Betty Crocker),* ½ cup* 25.0
   Parmesan and herb *(Betty Crocker Potato Shakers),*
     3 tsp. 4.0
   Parmesan and herb *(Betty Crocker Potato Shakers),*
     ⅔ cup* 23.0
   three *(Betty Crocker),* ½ cup 22.0
   three *(Betty Crocker),* ½ cup* 23.0
French country *(Good Harvest),* ⅓ cup 22.0
fries, seasoned *(Betty Crocker Potato Shakers),* 3 tsp. 4.0
fries, seasoned *(Betty Crocker Potato Shakers),* 7 fries* . . . 20.0
hash brown *(Betty Crocker),* ½ cup 30.0
hash brown *(Betty Crocker),* ½ cup* 31.0

Potato, mix *(cont.)*

garlic *(Betty Crocker Potato Shakers)*, 2 tsp. 4.0
garlic *(Betty Crocker Potato Shakers)*, ²/₃ cup* 23.0
garlic and herbs *(Fantastic Potato Cup)*, 1.7 oz. 37.0
herb garlic *(Shake'n Bake Perfect Potatoes)*, ¹/₆ pkg. 5.0
Italian, southern *(Good Harvest)*, ¹/₃ cup 23.0
julienne *(Betty Crocker)*, ¹/₂ cup 18.0
julienne *(Betty Crocker)*, ¹/₂ cup* 20.0
mashed:
   (Barbara's), ¹/₃ cup 17.0
   (Betty Crocker Potato Buds), ¹/₃ cup 18.0
   (Betty Crocker Potato Buds), ²/₃ cup* 19.0
   (Hungry Jack Flakes), ¹/₃ cup 18.0
   (Hungry Jack Flakes), ¹/₂ cup* 20.0
   (Idahoan), ¹/₃ cup 18.0
   (Martha White Spudflakes), ¹/₃ cup 17.0
   (Pillsbury Idaho Flakes), ¹/₃ cup 18.0
   (Pillsbury Idaho Flakes), ¹/₂ cup* 20.0
   (Pillsbury Idaho Granules), 2 tbsp. 20.0
   (Pillsbury Idaho Granules), ¹/₂ cup* 22.0
   all flavors except sour cream 'n chives *(Hungry Jack)*,
    ¹/₃ cup 18.0
   all flavors *(Hungry Jack)*, ¹/₂ cup* 19.0
   cheddar *(Betty Crocker Potato Buds)*, ¹/₃ cup 22.0
   cheddar *(Betty Crocker Potato Buds)*, ²/₃ cup* 23.0
   sour cream and chives *(Betty Crocker Potato Buds)*,
    ¹/₃ cup 21.0
   sour cream and chives *(Betty Crocker Potato Buds)*,
    ²/₃ cup* 23.0
   sour cream 'n chives *(Hungry Jack)*, ¹/₃ cup 17.0
ranch *(Betty Crocker)*, ¹/₂ cup 23.0
ranch *(Betty Crocker)*, ¹/₂ cup* 25.0
scalloped:
   (Betty Crocker 5 oz./20 oz.), ¹/₂ cup 21.0
   (Betty Crocker 8.25 oz.), ¹/₂ cup 22.0
   (Betty Crocker 5 oz./8.25 oz./20 oz.), ¹/₂ cup* 23.0
   (Idahoan), ¹/₃ cup 23.0
   cheesy *(Betty Crocker)*, ²/₃ cup 19.0
   cheesy *(Betty Crocker)*, ¹/₂ cup* 20.0
   cheesy *(Hungry Jack)*, ¹/₈ pkg. 22.0
   cheesy *(Hungry Jack)*, ¹/₈ pkg.* 24.0
   creamy *(Hungry Jack)*, ¹/₈ pkg. 22.0

creamy *(Hungry Jack)*, ⅛ pkg.* 24.0
and ham *(Betty Crocker)*, ½ cup 19.0
and ham *(Betty Crocker)*, ½ cup* 21.0
sour cream and chive:
   (Betty Crocker), ½ cup 21.0
   (Betty Crocker), ½ cup* 22.0
   (Fantastic Potato Cup), 1.7 oz. 36.0
   (Hungry Jack), ⅛ pkg. 22.0
   (Hungry Jack), ⅛ pkg.* 23.0
vegetable and herb *(Good Harvest)*, ⅓ cup 22.0
Western *(Idahoan)*, ¼ cup 20.0
Potato, stuffed, see "Potato dishes, frozen"
Potato, sweet, see "Sweet potato"
Potato and cheddar pocket, frozen *(Ken & Robert's Veggie*
   Pockets), 1 piece 42.0
Potato chips and crisps, 1 oz.:
(Barbara's Regular/Ripple/No Salt) 15.0
(Barrel O'Fun) 15.0
(Barrel O'Fun Ripple) 16.0
(Kettle Chips) 15.0
(Kettle Crisps) 22.0
(Lay's/Lay's Unsalted) 15.0
(Lay's Wavy Original) 15.0
(Mr. Phipps Crisps) 20.0
(Munchos) 18.0
(No Fries Original) 24.0
(Old Dutch/Old Dutch Ripl) 16.0
(Pringles Right Crisps) 19.0
(Ridgies Flat/Curlie/Super Crispy) 14.0
(Ruffles Original) 14.0
(Wise Ripple) 14.0
all varieties:
   (Lay's Baked) 23.0
   (Pringles/Pringles Ridges) 15.0
   (Ruffles Reduced Fat) 18.0
   except original *(Pringles Right Crisps)* 18.0
   except original and golden Dijon *(Ruffles)* 15.0
barbecue:
   (Barbara's) 16.0
   (Barrel O'Fun) 16.0
   (Lay's Hickory/*Lay's KC Masterpiece)* 15.0
   (Mr. Phipps Crisps) 21.0

Potato chips and crisps, barbecue *(cont.)*
    (Munchos) 15.0
    (No Fries) 24.0
    (Old Dutch) 15.0
    (Old Dutch Ripl) 16.0
barbecue, mesquite *(Krunchers!)* 16.0
barbecue, mesquite *(Old Dutch* Kettle) 19.0
Caribbean flavor *(Borden* Calypso) 15.0
cheddar *(Health Valley* Puffs) 21.0
cheddar, New York, with herbs *(Kettle* Chips) 15.0
cheddar/sour cream:
    (Barrel O'Fun Ripple) 15.0
    (Old Dutch) 16.0
    (Old Dutch Ripl) 15.0
    (Ruffles) 15.0
    (Wise) 14.0
    (Wise Super Crispy) 15.0
cheese *(Pringles Cheez Ums)* 14.0
Dijon, golden *(Ruffles)* 16.0
Dijon, honey *(Kettle* Chips) 16.0
dill pickle *(Old Dutch)* 16.0
hot *(Barrel O'Fun)* 15.0
hot *(Lay's* Flamin') 15.0
jalapeño:
    (Krunchers!) 16.0
    jack *(Kettle* Chips) 15.0
    and cheddar *(Old Dutch)* 17.0
onion, French *(Old Dutch Ripl)* 15.0
onion and garlic:
    (Barrel O'Fun) 14.0
    (Borden) 14.0
    (Lay's) 16.0
    (Old Dutch) 16.0
pesto *(Kettle* Crisps) 22.0
ranch *(Lay's Wavy Hidden Valley)* 14.0
ranch, puffs *(Health Valley)* 21.0
salsa and cheese *(Lay's)* 19.0
salsa with mesquite *(Kettle* Chips) 15.0
salt and sour *(Barrel O'Fun)* 15.0
salt and vinegar:
    (Borden) 14.0
    (Kettle Chips) 15.0

(Lay's) 15.0
(Old Dutch) 18.0
sour cream and onion:
    (Barrel O'Fun) 15.0
    (Borden) 14.0
    (Golden Ridges), 13 pieces or 1 oz. 15.0
    (Lay's) 15.0
    (Mr. Phipps Crisps) 21.0
    (Old Dutch) 17.0
    (Ruffles Reduced Fat) 18.0
yogurt and green onion (Barbara's/Barbara's No Salt) 15.0
yogurt and green onion (Kettle Chips) 15.0
Potato dishes, canned, 7.5 oz.:
au gratin, and bacon (Hormel) 23.0
scalloped, and ham (Hormel) 20.0
scalloped, and ham (Nalley) 27.0
sliced, and beef (Dinty Moore) 28.0
Potato dishes, frozen:
(Goya Rellenos de Papa), 2 pieces 36.0
(Goya Rellenos de Papa Cocktail), 6 pieces 33.0
au gratin (Schwan's), ½ cup 24.0
au gratin (Stouffer's Side Dish), 4.6 oz. 15.0
baked, 5-oz. pkg.:
    broccoli-cheese (Ore-Ida Twice Baked) 25.0
    butter flavor (Ore-Ida Twice Baked) 26.0
    cheddar (Ore-Ida Twice Baked) 26.0
    sour cream and chive (Ore-Ida Twice Baked) 27.0
cheddar (Lean Cuisine Deluxe), 1 pkg. 32.0
cheddar-broccoli (Healthy Choice), 1 pkg. 53.0
garden casserole (Healthy Choice), 1 pkg. 30.0
mozzarella, with chicken (The Budget Gourmet Italian
    Originals), 10.13 oz. 40.0
roasted, with broccoli and cheese sauce (Lean Cuisine
    Lunch Classics), 1 pkg. 31.0
scalloped (Stouffer's Side Dish), 4.6 oz. 17.0
scalloped, and ham (Swanson), 1 pkg. 29.0
stuffed (Schwan's), 1 potato 34.0
Potato entree, see "Potato dishes"
Potato flour, 1 cup 143.0
Potato pancake, frozen:
(Empire Kosher), 2-oz. cake 15.0
mini (Empire Kosher), 2 cakes, 2 oz. 16.0

Potato pancake mix:
(Hungry Jack), 2 tbsp. mix or 3 cakes*, 3″ 16.0
(Knorr), 2 tbsp. 18.0
Potato salad seasoning *(Tone's)*, 1 tsp. 3
Potato seasoning, see "Potato mix"
Potato sticks:
(Butterfield), 1.7 oz. 26.0
(Butterfield), ²⁄₃ cup 16.0
(French's), ¾ cup 16.0
(French's), 1 cup 23.0
(Pik-Nik Fabulous Fries), 1 oz. 16.0
1 oz. 15.1
hot *(Chester's Fries Flamin')*, 1 oz. 17.0
ketchup *(Pik-Nik Ket-'n Fries)*, ²⁄₃ cup 17.0
shoestring:
   (Pik-Nik), 1.75-oz. can 26.0
   (Pik-Nik), ²⁄₃ cup 15.0
   (Pik-Nik Less Salt), ¾ cup, 1.1 oz. 16.0
   BBQ *(Pik-Nik)*, ²⁄₃ cup 18.0
   sour cream and cheddar *(Pik-Nik)*, ²⁄₃ cup 17.0
Potpie, see specific entree listings
Poultry, see specific listings
Poultry seasoning, 1 tsp. 1.0
Pout, ocean, without added ingredients 0
Preserves, see "Jam and preserves"
Pretzel:
(Bachman Fat Free Thins), 11 pieces 23.0
(Bachman Twist/Butter Twist), 5 pieces 23.0
(Barbara's Honeysweet), 1 oz. 21.0
(Barrel O'Fun Minis), 1 oz. 22.0
(Borden Thins/Ultra Thins), 1 oz. 22.0
(Borden Tiny Thins/Mini), 1 oz. 23.0
(Little Debbie), 1.2 oz. 28.0
(Mister Salty Mini), 1 oz. 22.0
(Old Dutch), 1⅛-oz. bag 24.0
(Pepperidge Farm Goldfish), 45 pieces, 1.1 oz. 22.0
(Quinlan Beer), 2 pieces, 1 oz. 21.0
(Quinlan Nuggets), 1.1-oz. bag 24.0
(Quinlan Party Thins/Sticks), 1 oz. 22.0
(Quinlan Thin), 1.5-oz. bag 33.0
(Quinlan Tiny Thins/Mini), 1-oz. bag 22.0
(Quinlan Ultra Thin), 8 pieces, 1 oz. 22.0

(Thin 'n Right), 12 pieces 23.0
bagel shaped *(Manischewitz)*, 4 pieces, 1 oz. 22.0
Bavarian *(Barbara's/Barbara's* No Salt), 1 oz. 20.0
Bavarian *(Rold Gold)*, 1 oz. 21.0
cheddar *(Combos)*, 1 oz. 19.0
cheddar *(Combos)*, 1.8-oz. bag 34.0
cheese *(Handi-Snacks)*, 1.1-oz. piece 11.0
chips, 1 oz.:
    (Mr. Phipps/Mr. Phipps Lower Sodium) 21.0
    (Mr. Phipps Fat Free) 22.0
    (Mister Salty) 21.0
    (Mister Salty Fat Free) 22.0
chocolate coated or frosted, see "Candy"
Dutch *(Mister Salty)*, 2 pieces, 1.1 oz. 25.0
hard, plain, 1 oz. 22.5
hard, sourdough *(Bachman)*, 1 piece 18.0
honey mustard–onion *(Old Dutch)*, 1.1 oz. 21.0
honey mustard–onion *(Old Dutch)*, 2-oz. bag 40.0
mini *(Barbara's/Barbara's* No Salt), 1 oz. 21.0
nacho *(Combos)*, 1 oz. 19.0
nacho *(Combos)*, 1.8-oz. bag 34.0
9-grain *(Barbara's)*, 1 oz. 21.0
nuggets *(Nutzels)*, ½ cup 23.0
oat bran nuggets *(Smart Snackers)*, 1½ oz. 33.0
pizza *(Combos)*, 1 oz. 19.0
pizza *(Combos)*, 1.8-oz. bag 35.0
rods, 3 pieces, except as noted:
    (Bachman), 2 pieces 23.0
    (Old Dutch), 1.2 oz. 26.0
    (Rold Gold), 1 oz. 22.0
sourdough:
    (Quinlan/Quinlan No Salt), 1 piece 18.0
    Bavarian *(Barbara's)*, 1.1 oz. 24.0
    hard *(Rold Gold* Fat Free), 1 piece, 1 oz. 23.0
    twists *(Barbara's)*, 1.1 oz. 24.0
sticks, 1 oz.:
    (Bachman Stix) 20.0
    (Mister Salty Fat Free) 23.0
    (Old Dutch) 22.0
    (Quinlan) 22.0
    (Rold Gold Fat Free), 48 pieces 23.0
sticks, sesame *(Barbara's)*, 1.1 oz. 21.0

Pretzel *(cont.)*
thins:
    (Old Dutch Fat Free), 1.1 oz. 24.0
    (Quinlan), 1 oz. 22.0
    (Rold Gold), 10 pieces, 1 oz. 22.0
    (Rold Gold Fat Free), 12 pieces, 1 oz. 23.0
twists:
    (Old Dutch), 1 oz. 22.0
    (Mister Salty), 1 oz. 23.0
    (Planters), 1 oz. 23.0
    (Planters), 1½-oz. bag 35.0
    (Rold Gold Fat Free), 18 pieces, 1 oz. 23.0
Pretzel, soft:
    (Superpretzel/Superpretzel Added Salt), 2.3-oz. piece . . . 37.0
bites *(Superpretzel/Superpretzel* Added Salt), 4 pieces,
    1½ oz. 23.0
cheese-filled, cheddar, nacho, or pizza
    (Superpretzel Softstix), 2 pieces, 1.8 oz. 24.0
cheese-filled, frozen *(Schwan's),* 3 pieces 35.0
cinnamon raisin *(Superpretzel),* 2 pieces, 2 oz. 40.0
peanut butter and jelly filled, frozen *(Schwan's),* 3 pieces . . 42.0
Pretzel dip, 2 tbsp.:
(Nance's) 18.0
cheddar and mustard *(Heluva* Good) 2.0
Prickly pear:
(Frieda's Cactus Pear), 5 oz. 13.0
untrimmed, 1 lb. 32.6
1 medium, 4.8 oz. 9.9
Primavera entree mix, see "Entree mix, frozen"
Prosciutto *(Primissimo),* 2 oz. 0
Prune:
canned, in heavy syrup:
    (Sonoma), 3–4 pieces, 1.4 oz. 26.0
    pitted, 4 oz. 31.5
    ½ cup 32.5
    5 medium and 2 tbsp. liquid 23.9
    stewed *(S&W),* 8 pieces, 4.9 oz. 52.0
dehydrated, uncooked, ½ cup 58.8
dehydrated, cooked, ½ cup 41.6
dried, uncooked:
    (Del Monte), ¼ cup 29.0
    (Dole), 2 oz. 36.0

    with pits, ½ cup 50.5
    pitted, 10 prunes 52.7
    pitted *(Sonoma)*, ¼ cup 29.0
dried, stewed, with pits, unsweetened, ½ cup 29.8

Prune juice, 8 fl. oz.:
(Del Monte).................................. 43.0
(Goya) 40.0
(R.W. Knudsen Organic) 45.0
(Lucky Leaf/Musselman's) 40.0
(S&W) 41.0

Pudding, ready-to-serve:
banana:
    (Hunt's Snack Pack), 3.5 oz. 18.0
    (Jell-O Snack), 4 oz. 25.0
    (Thank You), ½ cup 36.0
    nondairy *(Imagine)*, 4 oz. 30.0
butterscotch:
    (Hunt's Snack Pack), 3.5 oz. 21.0
    (Rich's), 3 oz.............................. 19.0
    (Swiss Miss), 4 oz. 24.0
    (Thank You), ½ cup 27.0
    nondairy *(Imagine)*, 4 oz. 31.0
chocolate:
    (Hunt's Snack Pack), 3.5 oz. 22.0
    (Hunt's Snack Pack Fat Free), 3.5 oz. 19.0
    (Jell-O Snack), 4 oz. 28.0
    (Jell-O Free Snack), 4 oz. 23.0
    (Rich's), 3 oz............................. 19.0
    (Swiss Miss), 4 oz. 26.0
    (Swiss Miss Fat Free), 4 oz. 22.0
    (Thank You), ½ cup 33.0
    nondairy *(Imagine)*, 4 oz. 36.0
chocolate almond *(Healthy Choice)*, ½ cup 21.0
chocolate fudge:
    (Hunt's Snack Pack), 3.5 oz. 23.0
    (Swiss Miss), 4 oz. 28.0
    (Swiss Miss Fat Free), 4 oz. 23.0
    double *(Healthy Choice)*, ½ cup 20.0
chocolate marshmallow *(Hunt's Snack Pack)*, 3.5 oz. 20.5
chocolate raspberry *(Healthy Choice)*, ½ cup 19.0
chocolate swirl:
    caramel *(Hunt's Snack Pack)*, 3.5 oz. 23.0

Pudding, chocolate swirl *(cont.)*

caramel *(Jell-O Snack)*, 4 oz.	27.0
caramel *(Jell-O Free Snack)*, 4 oz.	23.0
caramel *(Swiss Miss)*, 4 oz.	26.0
milk *(Hunt's Snack Pack)*, 3.5 oz.	22.0
peanut butter *(Hunt's Snack Pack)*, 3.5 oz.	21.0
vanilla *(Jell-O Snack)*, 4 oz.	27.0
vanilla *(Jell-O Free Snack)*, 4 oz.	23.0
vanilla *(Swiss Miss)*, 4 oz.	26.0
chocolate vanilla parfait *(Swiss Miss)*, 4 oz.	25.0
chocolate vanilla parfait *(Swiss Miss Fat Free)*, 4 oz.	21.0
lemon *(Hunt's Snack Pack)*, 3.5 oz.	24.0
lemon, nondairy *(Imagine)*, 4 oz.	33.0
S'mores swirl *(Hunt's Snack Pack)*, 3.5 oz.	21.0

tapioca:

(Healthy Choice), 1/2 cup	21.0
(Hunt's Snack Pack), 3.5 oz.	21.0
(Hunt's Snack Pack Fat Free), 3.5 oz.	18.0
(Jell-O Snack), 4 oz.	26.0
(Swiss Miss), 4 oz.	24.0
(Swiss Miss Fat Free), 4 oz.	22.0
(Thank You), 1/2 cup	27.0

vanilla:

(Hunt's Snack Pack), 3.5 oz.	21.0
(Hunt's Snack Pack Fat Free), 3.5 oz.	18.0
(Jell-O Snack), 4 oz.	25.0
(Jell-O Free Snack), 4 oz.	23.0
(Rich's), 3 oz.	19.0
(Swiss Miss), 4 oz.	24.0
(Swiss Miss Fat Free), 4 oz.	21.0
(Thank You), 1/2 cup	28.0
French *(Healthy Choice)*, 1/2 cup	20.0
vanilla chocolate parfait *(Swiss Miss)*, 4 oz.	25.0
vanilla chocolate parfait *(Swiss Miss Fat Free)*, 4 oz.	21.0
vanilla-chocolate swirl *(Jell-O Snack)*, 4 oz.	26.0
vanilla-chocolate swirl *(Jell-O Free Snack)*, 4 oz.	23.0

Pudding mix, 1/2 cup*, except as noted:

banana *(Jell-O Sugar/Fat Free)*	12.0
banana cream *(Jell-O)*	26.0
banana cream *(Jell-O Instant)*	29.0
butter pecan *(Jell-O Instant)*	29.0

butterscotch:
  (Jell-O) 26.0
  (Jell-O Instant) 29.0
  (Jell-O Sugar/Fat Free) 12.0
chocolate:
  (D-Zerta) 11.0
  (Jell-O) 28.0
  (Jell-O Instant) 31.0
  (Jell-O Sugar Free) 11.0
  (Jell-O Sugar/Fat Free) 14.0
  (My*T*Fine) 22.0
  milk *(Jell-O)* 28.0
  milk *(Jell-O* Instant) 31.0
chocolate fudge:
  (Jell-O) 28.0
  (Jell-O Instant) 31.0
  (Jell-O Sugar/Fat Free) 14.0
chocolate mousse, dry, dark or white *(Alsa)*, 2 tbsp. 8.0
chocolate mousse, dry, milk *(Alsa)*, 2 tbsp. 10.0
coconut cream *(Jell-O)* 24.0
coconut cream *(Jell-O* Instant) 27.0
custard *(Jell-O Americana)* 25.0
custard, tropical *(Goya* Tembleque) 23.0
flan:
  (Alsa Creme Caramel), 1⅓ tbsp. mix, 1 tbsp. caramel . . 27.0
  (Goya) 23.0
  (Jell-O) 26.0
  with caramel *(Goya)* 21.0
lemon *(Jell-O/Jell-O* Instant) 29.0
pistachio *(Jell-O* Instant) 29.0
pistachio *(Jell-O* Sugar/Fat Free) 12.0
rice, see "Rice pudding mix"
tapioca *(Jell-O Americana)* 26.0
vanilla:
  (Jell-O) 26.0
  (Jell-O Instant) 29.0
  (Jell-O Sugar Free) 11.0
  (Jell-O Sugar/Fat Free) 12.0
  French *(Jell-O* Instant) 29.0
Pummelo:
(Frieda's), 3.5 oz. 9.6
untrimmed, 1 lb. 24.4

Pummelo *(cont.)*

1 medium, 5½″ diam., 2.4 lb. 58.6

sections, ½ cup 9.1

Pumpkin:

fresh, raw:

    untrimmed, 1 lb. 20.6

    pulp, raw, 1″ cubes, ½ cup 3.8

    pulp, boiled, drained, mashed, ½ cup 6.0

canned, ½ cup:

    (Comstock) 10.0

    (Libby's) 15.0

    (Stokely) 10.0

    with or without winter squash 9.9

pie mix, see "Pie filling"

Pumpkin flower:

raw, untrimmed, 1 lb. 5.2

raw, trimmed, ½ cup 5

boiled, drained, ½ cup 2.2

Pumpkin leaf:

raw, untrimmed, 1 lb. 4.3

raw, trimmed, ½ cup 5

boiled, drained, ½ cup 1.2

Pumpkin pie spice, 1 tsp. 1.2

Pumpkin seed:

roasted:

    in shell, 1 cup 34.4

    in shell, salted or unsalted, 1 oz. or 85 seeds 15.3

    shelled, salted or unsalted, 1 oz. 3.8

dried, shelled, 1 oz. or 142 kernels 5.1

tamari-roasted, spicy *(Eden),* 1 oz. 5.0

Punch, see "Fruit drink blends," and "Fruit juice blends"

Purslane:

raw, untrimmed, 1 lb. 11.8

raw, ½ cup 7

boiled, drained, ½ cup 2.1

FOOD AND MEASURE	CARBOHYDRATE GRAMS

Quail, without added ingredients 0
Quince:
(Frieda's), 4.9 oz. 21.0
1 medium, 5.3 oz. 14.1
peeled, seeded, 1 oz. 4.3
Quincy's Family Steakhouse, 1 serving:
breakfast items:
    apples, escalloped, 3.5 oz. 26.0
    bacon, ¼ oz. 0
    corned beef hash, 4.5 oz. 11.0
    eggs, scrambled, 2 oz. 1.0
    ham, 1.5 oz. 1.0
    oatmeal, 1 oz. 18.0
    pancakes, 1.5 oz. 12.0
    sausage gravy, 4 oz. 20.0
    sausage links, 2 oz. 3.0
    sausage patties, 2 oz. 0
    steak fingers, 3.5 oz. 0
    syrup, 1 oz. 18.0
beef entrees:
    fillet with bacon, 8 oz.[1] 2.0
    sirloin tips with mushroom gravy, 6 oz. 5.0
    sirloin tips with pepper and onions, 5 oz. 4.0
    steak, chopped, 8 oz.[1] 0
    steak, country, with gravy, 9 oz. 44.0
    steak, cowboy, 14 oz.[1] 9.0
    steak, New York strip, 10 oz. 1.0
    steak, porterhouse, 17 oz.[1] 0
    steak, ribeye, 10 oz.[1] 0
    steak, sirloin, regular, 8 oz.[1] 0
    steak, sirloin, large, 10 oz.[1] 2.0
    steak, strip, smothered, 10 oz.[1] 12.0
    steak, T-bone, 13 oz.[1] 0

[1] *Weight before cooking.*

Quincy's Family Steakhouse *(cont.)*

other entree items:

chicken, grilled, 5 oz.	1.0
chicken, roasted, with herbs, 14 oz.	4.0
chicken, roasted BBQ, 14 oz.	21.0
chicken fillet, homestyle, 3 oz.	21.0
salmon, grilled, 7 oz.	1.0
shrimp, breaded, 7 oz.	47.0
steak and shrimp, 9 oz.	33.0

sandwiches, 1 piece:

burger, ⅓ lb.	32.0
burger, bacon cheese	33.0
chicken, grilled	39.0
chicken, spicy BBQ	45.0
steak, Philly cheese	38.0
steak, smothered	36.0

side dishes, 4 oz., except as noted:

apples, with cinnamon	34.0
beans, barbecue	21.0
beans, green	6.0
broccoli spears	5.0
broccoli spears, with cheese sauce, 5 oz.	6.0
corn	24.0
potatoes:	
baked, plain, 6 oz.	30.0
fries, steak	45.0
mashed	11.0
rice pilaf	23.0

bread, 2 oz.:

banana nut bread	22.0
biscuit	29.0
corn bread	19.0
roll, yeast	29.0

soups, 6 oz.:

broccoli, cream of	18.0
chili	21.0
clam chowder	21.0
vegetable beef	14.0

salad dressings, 1 oz.:

blue cheese	2.0
French	4.0
French, light	13.0

honey mustard 10.0
Italian 3.0
Italian, light 2.0
Italian, light, creamy 8.0
Parmesan peppercorn 4.0
ranch 1.0
Thousand Island, light 8.0
desserts:
  brownie pudding cake, 4 oz. 66.0
  cobbler, 6 oz.:
      apple 49.0
      cherry 55.0
      peach 50.0
  cookie, chocolate chip or sugar, ½ oz. 8.0
  pudding, banana, 5 oz. 30.0
  yogurt, frozen, 4 oz. 25.0
  yogurt topping, caramel, 1 oz. 24.0
  yogurt topping, fudge, 1 oz. 15.0
Quinoa:
(Eden), ¼ cup 31.0
(Frieda's), ⅓ cup 31.0
1 oz. 19.5
¼ cup 29.3
Quinoa seeds *(Arrowhead Mills),* ¼ cup 25.0

R

FOOD AND MEASURE   **CARBOHYDRATE GRAMS**

Rabbit, without added ingredients 0
Radiatore entree, vegetarian, frozen *(Hain* Bolognese),
    10 oz. 52.0
Radicchio, fresh:
(Frieda's), 2 cups 4.0
trimmed, 1 oz. 1.3
1 medium leaf, .3 oz. 4
shredded, ½ cup 9
Radish:
(Dole), 7 pieces 3.0
untrimmed, 1 lb. 14.6
10 medium, ¾″–1″ diam., 1.8 oz. 1.6
sliced, ½ cup 2.1
Radish, black:
1 lb. 16.3
1 oz. 1.0
Radish, Oriental:
raw:
     untrimmed, 1 lb. 14.7
     1 medium, 7″ × 2¼″ diam. 13.9
     sliced, ½ cup 1.8
     Chinese *(Frieda's* Lo Bok), ⅔ cup, 3 oz. 5.0
     Japanese *(Frieda's* Daikon), ⅔ cup, 3 oz. 3.0
boiled, drained, sliced, ½ cup 2.5
dried, 1 oz. 18.0
Radish, white-icicle:
untrimmed, 1 lb. 7.7
1 medium, .6 oz. 5
sliced, ½ cup 1.3
Radish leaves, 1 oz. 2.8
Radish seeds, sprouted:
(Jonathan's), 1 cup 3.0
1 lb. 13.9
½ cup 6
Rainbow baking morsels *(Nestlé),* 1 tbsp. 10.0

Raisin, ¼ cup, except as noted:
golden seedless:
    (Del Monte) 33.0
    (Dole), ½ cup 66.0
    (S&W) 31.0
    (Sun•Maid) 31.0
    not packed 28.9
monukka/Thompson *(Sonoma)* 31.0
muscat *(Sun•Maid)* 31.0
seeded, not packed 28.5
seedless:
    (Del Monte) 33.0
    (Del Monte), 1.5-oz. box 36.0
    (Dole), ½ cup 66.0
    (S&W) 31.0
    (Sun•Maid) 31.0
    not packed 28.7
chocolate or yogurt coated, see "Candy"
Raisin sauce *(Reese),* ¼ cup 36.0
Ranch dip, 2 tbsp.:
(Heluva Good Classic) 2.0
(Heluva Good Fat Free) 3.0
(Kraft) 3.0
(Marie's Creamy/Homestyle) 3.0
(Nalley) 2.0
(Old Dutch) 3.0
(Ruffles) 4.0
(Ruffles Low Fat) 6.0
bacon *(Marie's)* 3.0
peppercorn *(Marie's* Fat Free) 7.0
vegetable *(Bernstein's)* 2.0
Ranch dip mix, cracked pepper *(Knorr),* ½ tsp. 1.0
Rapini, see "Broccoli rabe"
Raspberry:
fresh:
    (Dole), 3 oz. 10.0
    untrimmed, 1 lb. 50.4
    ½ cup 7.1
canned, in heavy syrup *(Comstock),* ½ cup 23.0
canned, in heavy syrup *(Oregon),* ½ cup 30.0
frozen, red:
    (Big Valley), ⅔ cup 12.0

Raspberry, frozen, red *(cont.)*
   (Birds Eye), ½ cup 22.0
   (Schwan's), 1¼ cups 13.0
   sweetened, ½ cup 32.7
Raspberry baking chips *(Hershey's)*, 1 tbsp. 10.0
Raspberry drink, 8 fl. oz.:
   (Farmer's Market) 30.0
   hibiscus *(R.W. Knudsen)* 23.0
   lemon *(Santa Cruz)* 29.0
   black, frozen* *(Schwan's Vita Sun)* 26.0
Raspberry juice, 8 fl. oz.:
   (Heinke's) 30.0
   blend *(Dole* Country) 34.0
   cranberry *(Apple & Eve)* 30.0
   peach *(R.W. Knudsen)* 31.0
Raspberry nectar, 8 fl. oz.:
   (Santa Cruz) 26.0
   frozen* *(R.W. Knudsen)* 30.0
Raspberry syrup:
   (Fox's No Cal), 2 tbsp. 0
   (R.W. Knudsen), ¼ cup 38.0
Rattlesnake beans, dried *(Frieda's)*, ½ cup 22.0
Ravioli, frozen or refrigerated:
   (Monterey Pasta Company Mediterranean), 3 oz. 35.0
   beef and garlic *(Contadina)*, 1¼ cups 44.0
   cheddar roasted garlic *(Monterey Pasta Company)*, 3 oz. . . . 33.0
   cheese:
      (Amy's), 9.5 oz. 44.0
      (Celentano), ½ of 13-oz. pkg. 61.0
      (Celentano Great Choice), ½ of 13-oz. pkg. 69.0
      (Contadina Family Pack), 1 cup 35.0
      (Schwan's), 5 pieces 35.0
      four *(Contadina)*, 1 cup 35.0
      four *(Contadina* Light), 1 cup 38.0
      four *(Wolfgang Puck's)*, 13 oz. 16.0
      and garlic *(Di Giorno* Light), 1 cup 45.0
      herb *(Di Giorno)*, 1 cup 44.0
      mini or round mini *(Celentano)*, 4 oz. 42.0
   chicken and rosemary *(Contadina)*, 1¼ cups 47.0
   chicken and rosemary *(Real Torino)*, 1 cup 49.0
   crab, snow *(Monterey Pasta Company)*, 3 oz. 41.0
   garden vegetable *(Contadina* Light), 1 cup 39.0

garlic basil cheese *(Monterey Pasta Company)*, 3 oz. 34.0
Gorgonzola *(Contadina)*, 1¼ cups 45.0
Gorgonzola roasted walnut *(Monterey Pasta Company)*,
    3 oz. 33.0
Monterey Jack, smoked *(Monterey Pasta Company)*, 3 oz. . . 33.0
mushroom and spinach *(Wolfgang Puck's)*, 13 oz. 15.0
parsley *(Putney)*, 1 cup 39.0
with sausage, Italian *(Di Giorno)*, ¾ cup 41.0
spinach and ricotta *(Real Torino)*, 1 cup 44.0
tofu *(Tofutti)*, 1 cup 54.0
tomato and cheese *(Di Giorno Light)*, 1 cup 49.0
Ravioli entree, canned, 1 cup, except as noted:
beef, tomato sauce:
    (Franco-American) 40.0
    (Libby's), 7¾ oz. 29.0
    (Nalley) 40.0
    (Nalley), 7½ oz. 33.0
    (Nalley Microwave), 7½ oz. 26.0
    (Progresso) 45.0
    (Top Shelf), 10 oz. 35.0
    with meat *(Chef Boyardee)* 37.0
    with meat *(Franco-American)* 42.0
    with meat sauce *(Hunt's Homestyle)* 31.5
    mini, with meat *(Franco-American)* 36.0
    mini with meat *(Chef Boyardee Bowl)*, 7½ oz. 34.0
cheese, tomato sauce:
    (Chef Boyardee) 44.0
    (Progresso) 43.0
    with cheese *(Chef Boyardee Bowl)*, 7½ oz. 35.0
    with meat *(Chef Boyardee Bowl)*, 7½ oz. 33.0
mini *(Kid's Kitchen)*, 7½ oz. 35.0
tomato sauce *(Hormel Micro Cup)*, 7½ oz. 34.0
Ravioli entree, frozen:
cheese:
    (Kid Cuisine Raptor), 9.8 oz. 63.0
    (Lean Cuisine), 8.5 oz. 34.0
    (Stouffer's), 10⅝ oz. 51.0
    (Swanson Fun Feast Roaring), 1 pkg. 73.0
    Florentine *(Smart Ones)*, 8.5 oz. 43.0
    in marinara sauce *(Marie Callender's)*, 1 cup, 8 oz. 47.0
    parmigiana *(Healthy Choice)*, 9 oz. 44.0
mushroom and spinach *(Wolfgang Puck's)*, 13 oz. 15.0

Red beans (see also "Kidney beans" and "Mexican beans"):
dried *(Goya* Dominican), ¼ cup 32.0
canned, ½ cup:
    (Allens) 19.0
    (Green Giant/Joan of Arc) 19.0
    (Stokely) 20.0
    (Van Camp's) 20.0
    small *(Hunt's)* 19.0
Red beans, mix:
Barcelona, with radiatore *(Bean Cuisine)*, ½ cup* 27.0
New Orleans *(Fantastic* One Pot Meals), ⅜ cup 31.0
rice and, see "Rice dishes, mix"
Red snapper, without added ingredients 0
Redfish, without added ingredients 0
Refried beans, canned, ½ cup:
(Allens) 24.0
(Chi-Chi's) 16.0
(Chi-Chi's Fat Free) 14.0
(Gebhardt) 20.0
(Gebhardt No Fat) 19.5
(Goya) 20.0
(Las Palmas) 17.0
(Las Palmas No Fat) 19.0
(Old El Paso) 17.0
(Old El Paso Fat Free) 20.0
(Rosarita) 19.0
(Rosarita No Fat) 28.0
bacon *(Rosarita)* 19.0
black beans:
    (Las Palmas) 18.0
    (Old El Paso) 18.0
    (Rosarita Low Fat) 22.5
cheese *(Old El Paso)* 18.0
cheese, nacho *(Rosarita)* 19.0
green chili:
    (Old El Paso) 17.0
    (Rosarita) 20.0
    and lime *(Rosarita* No Fat) 22.0
jalapeño *(Gebhardt)* 19.0
onion *(Rosarita)* 21.0
salsa, zesty *(Rosarita* No Fat) 24.0
sausage *(Old El Paso)* 14.0

spicy *(Old El Paso)* 22.0
spicy *(Rosarita)* 22.0
vegetarian:
   (Chi-Chi's) 14.0
   (Gebhardt) 20.0
   (Old El Paso) 17.0
   (Rosarita) 42.0
Refried beans, mix *(Fantastic)*, ½ cup* 29.0
Relish, see "Pickle relish" and specific listings
Remoulade sauce *(Zararain's)*, ¼ cup 9.0
Rennet *(Junket)*, 1 tablet 0
Rhubarb:
fresh:
   (Frieda's), ⅔ cup, 3 oz. 4.0
   untrimmed, 1 lb. 15.4
   diced, ½ cup 2.8
frozen:
   (Big Valley), ⅔ cup 4.0
   (Stilwell), 1 cup 5.0
   cooked, sweetened, ½ cup 37.4
Rice, dry, ¼ cup, except as noted:
Arborio *(Fantastic)* 45.0
Arborio *(Frieda's)* 45.0
basmati, brown:
   (Arrowhead Mills) 33.0
   (Fantastic) 36.0
   (Lundberg Organic) 34.0
   (Lundberg Nutra-Farmed/Lundberg Royal) 38.0
basmati, white:
   (Casbah) 36.0
   (Fantastic) 38.0
   (Lundberg Organic) 38.0
   (Lundberg Nutra-Farmed) 41.0
blend:
   (Lundberg Black Japonica) 38.0
   (Lundberg Countrywild/Wild Blend) 35.0
   (Lundberg Jubilee) 39.0
brown:
   (Carolina/Mahatma/River) 32.0
   (Lundberg Wehani) 38.0
   (Success), ½ cup 33.0

Rice *(cont.)*
brown, long grain:
  (Arrowhead Mills) 33.0
  (Lundberg Organic) 38.0
  (Lundberg Nutra-Farmed) 37.0
  (S&W) 32.0
  (Uncle Ben's Whole Grain) 35.0
  (Uncle Ben's Instant), ½ cup 42.0
brown, medium grain:
  (Arrowhead Mills) 35.0
  (Arrowhead Mills Quick) 32.0
  (Lundberg) 34.0
brown, quick *(Lundberg)* 32.0
brown, short grain *(Arrowhead Mills)* 36.0
brown, short grain *(Lundberg* Organic/*Lundberg Nutra-
  Farmed)* 40.0
brown, precooked *(S&W* Quick), ½ cup 33.0
brown, sweet *(Lundberg* Organic/Premium) 35.0
glutinous or sweet *(Goya* Fancy Blue Rose/Valencia) 37.0
glutinous or sweet, ½ cup cooked 37.8
jasmine *(Fantastic)* 38.0
white, long grain:
  (Canilla) 35.0
  (Carolina) 35.0
  (Mahatma) 35.0
  (Martha White) 38.0
  (River/Water Maid) 37.0
  (Success), ½ cup 44.0
  ½ cup cooked 22.3
  extra *(Goya)* 35.0
  instant *(Carolina)* 36.0
  instant *(Mahatma)* 36.0
  instant *(Minute)*, ½ cup 37.0
  instant *(Minute* Boil-in Bag), ½ cup 42.0
  instant *(Minute* Premium), ½ cup 36.0
  instant *(Uncle Ben's)*, ½ cup 43.0
  parboiled *(Uncle Ben's Converted)* 38.0
white, medium grain, ½ cup cooked 26.6
Rice, wild, see "Wild rice"
Rice beverage, see " 'Milk,' nondairy"
Rice bran, crude, 1 cup 41.2

Rice cake (see also "Popcorn cake"), 1 cake, except as noted:

(Mother's/Mother's Sodium Free)	7.0
(Quaker Salted/Salt Free)	7.0

all varieties:

(Crispy Cakes)	7.0
(Lundberg/Lundberg Unsalted)	14.0
(Pritikin/Pritikin Unsalted)	7.0
bars *(Health Valley* Crisp Fat Free)	26.0
except white cheddar *(Quaker* Mini), 5 cakes	12.0
apple, crisp *(Pritikin* Mini), 5 cakes	12.0
apple cinnamon *(Quaker)*	11.0
banana nut *(Mother's)*	11.0
banana nut *(Quaker)*	11.0
blueberry crunch *(Quaker)*	12.0
brown *(Lundberg* Mini), 5 cakes	14.0
butter *(Mother's* Sodium Free)	7.0
butter popped corn *(Mother's)*	7.0
butter popped corn *(Quaker)*	7.0
caramel nut *(Pritikin* Mini), 5 cakes	12.0
caramel popped corn *(Mother's)*	12.0

cheese:

cheddar, white *(Quaker)*	12.0
cheddar, white *(Quaker* Mini), 6 cakes	11.0
cheddar, white, popped corn *(Mother's)*	8.0
Monterey Jack *(Quaker)*	8.0
nacho *(Lundberg* Mini), 5 cakes	13.0
chocolate crunch *(Quaker)*	11.0
cinnamon crunch *(Quaker)*	11.0
dill, creamy *(Lundberg* Mini), 5 cakes	13.0
sesame *(Mother's/Mother's* Sodium Free)	7.0

Rice chips, brown *(Eden)*, 50 chips, 1.1 oz.	19.0

Rice dishes, canned:

Chinese fried *(La Choy)*, 1 cup	53.0
Spanish *(Old El Paso)*, 1 cup	28.0
Spanish *(Van Camp's)*, ½ cup	18.5

Rice dishes, freeze-dried, wild, pilaf, with almonds

(AlpineAire), 1⅓ cups	89.0

Rice dishes, frozen (see also "Rice entree, frozen" and specific listings):

and broccoli *(Green Giant)*, 10-oz. pkg.	44.0

Rice dishes, frozen *(cont.)*
and broccoli, au gratin *(Freezer Queen* Family Side Dish),
  1 cup 32.0
and vegetables, 10-oz. pkg.:
  (Green Giant Medley) 46.0
  pilaf *(Green Giant)* 44.0
  white and wild *(Green Giant)* 45.0
Rice dishes, mix, 2 oz. dry[1], except as noted:
(Lipton Rice & Sauce Original Recipe), ½ cup or 1 cup* . . 48.0
and beans:
  black *(Carolina/Mahatma)* 39.0
  black or red *(Goya)* 34.0
  black, Mediterranean, pilaf *(Near East)* 52.0
  black, savory *(Good Harvest)*, ⅓ cup 31.0
  black, spicy *(Spice Islands* Quick), 1 pkg. 35.0
  Cajun *(Lipton* Rice & Sauce), ½ cup or 1 cup* 52.0
  pinto *(Mahatma)* 40.0
  red *(Carolina/Mahatma)* 40.0
  red *(Rice-A-Roni)*, 1 cup* 51.0
  red, pilaf *(Near East)* 41.0
  red, spicy *(Good Harvest)*, ⅓ cup 32.0
  red, spicy *(Spice Islands* Quick Meal), 1 pkg. 35.0
  tomato herb, pilaf *(Near East)* 52.0
  vegetables, garden, pilaf *(Near East)* 52.0
beef/beef flavor:
  (Country Inn) 43.0
  (Lipton Rice & Sauce), ½ cup or 1 cup* 47.0
  (Rice-A-Roni), 1 cup* 51.0
  (Rice-A-Roni Less Salt), 1 cup* 53.0
  (Success) 51.0
  and mushroom *(Rice-A-Roni)*, 1 cup* 51.0
  pilaf *(Near East)* 42.0
broccoli:
  Alfredo *(Lipton* Rice & Sauce), ½ cup 43.0
  Alfredo *(Lipton* Rice & Sauce), 1 cup* 46.0
  cheese *(Mahatma)* 41.0
  cheese *(Success)* 40.0
broccoli au gratin:
  (Country Inn) 41.0
  (Rice-A-Roni), 1 cup* 47.0

[1]*Yields approximately 1 cup prepared.*

(Rice-A-Roni Less Salt), 1 cup* 49.0
(Savory Classics), 1 cup* 47.0
brown and wild *(Success)* 40.0
brown and wild, herb *(Arrowhead* Quick), ¼ pkg. 28.0
Cajun *(Lipton* Rice & Sauce), ½ cup or 1 cup* 46.0
cheddar, white, with herbs *(Rice-A-Roni)*, 1 cup* 49.0
cheddar broccoli *(Lipton* Rice & Sauce), ½ cup or 1 cup* 46.0
cheese *(Country Inn)* 41.0
chicken/chicken flavor:
   (Country Inn) 42.0
   (Lipton Rice & Sauce), ½ cup or 1 cup* 45.0
   (Rice-A-Roni), 1 cup* 52.0
   (Rice-A-Roni Less Salt), 1 cup* 53.0
   (Savory Classics), 1 cup* 52.0
   (Success Classic) 32.0
   creamy *(Lipton* Rice & Sauce), ½ cup or 1 cup* 45.0
   pilaf *(Eastern Traditions)* 45.0
   pilaf *(Knorr)*, ⅓ cup 47.0
   pilaf *(Lundberg* Quick Country) 47.0
   pilaf *(Near East)* 42.0
   pilaf *(Spice Islands* Quick), 1 pkg. 38.0
   pilaf, with wild rice, Mediterranean *(Near East)* 43.0
   roasted *(Lipton* Seasoned Rice), ⅓ cup or 1 cup* 46.0
   Southwestern *(Lipton* Seasoned Rice), ⅓ cup or 1 cup* 47.0
chicken and broccoli:
   (Country Inn) 43.0
   (Lipton Rice & Sauce), ½ cup or 1 cup* 46.0
   (Rice-A-Roni), 1 cup* 51.0
chicken and mushrooms *(Rice-A-Roni)*, 1 cup* 52.0
chicken with vegetables *(Country Inn)* 42.0
chicken with vegetables *(Rice-A-Roni)*, 1 cup* 52.0
chicken and wild rice *(Country Inn)* 41.0
chicken and wild rice, almond *(Savory Classics)*, 1 cup* ... 53.0
chili *(Lundberg One Step)* 42.0
curry:
   (Lundberg One Step) 38.0
   basmati, with lentils *(Fantastic* One Pot Meals), ⅜ cup .. 35.0
   pilaf *(Near East)* 42.0
fried:
   (Chun King), ½ cup 29.0
   (Rice-A-Roni), 1 cup* 51.0
   (Rice-A-Roni Less Salt), 1 cup* 52.0

Rice dishes, mix *(cont.)*

garlic basil *(Lundberg One Step)* 37.0
gumbo *(Mahatma)* 31.0
herb and butter *(Lipton Rice & Sauce)*, ½ cup or 1 cup* . . 43.0
herb and butter *(Rice-A-Roni)*, 1 cup* 53.0
jambalaya *(Mahatma)* 43.0
long grain and wild:
   (Mahatma) 41.0
   (Rice-A-Roni), 1 cup* 43.0
   (Uncle Ben's Fast/Original) 41.0
   butter and herb *(Uncle Ben's)* 51.0
   chicken with almonds *(Rice-A-Roni)*, 1 cup* 51.0
   chicken and herb *(Uncle Ben's)* 40.0
   pilaf *(Near East)* 42.0
   pilaf *(Rice-A-Roni)*, 1 cup* 51.0
   vegetable herb *(Uncle Ben's)* 40.0
medley *(Lipton* Rice & Sauce), ½ cup or 1 cup* 44.0
Mexican:
   (Goya) 37.0
   (Pritikin) 43.0
   (Savory Classics Fiesta), 1 cup* 55.0
   cheesy *(Old El Paso)*, ½ pkg. 89.0
mushroom:
   (Lipton Rice & Sauce), ½ cup or 1 cup* 45.0
   brown *(Uncle Ben's)* 40.0
   and herb *(Lipton* Rice & Sauce), ½ cup or 1 cup* 49.0
Oriental:
   (Pritikin) 43.0
   (Rice-A-Roni), 1 cup* 54.0
   (Savory Classics), 1 cup* 43.0
   stir fry *(Lipton* Seasoned Rice), ⅓ cup or 1 cup* 16.0
   and vegetables *(Spice Islands* Quick), 1 pkg. 39.0
pilaf (see also specific listings):
   (Casbah), 1 oz. 22.0
   (Country Inn) 44.0
   (Eastern Traditions) 43.0
   (Eastern Traditions Harvest) 40.0
   (Knorr Original), ⅓ cup 47.0
   (Lipton Rice & Sauce), ½ cup or 1 cup* 47.0
   (Mahatma) 43.0
   (Near East) 42.0
   (Rice-A-Roni), 1 cup* 53.0

(Success) 44.0
almond, toasted *(Near East)* 41.0
brown rice *(Near East)* 41.0
brown rice, with miso *(Fantastic)*, ½ cup 55.0
four grain with wild rice *(Fantastic* Healthy
   Complements)*, ½ cup 35.0
garden *(Savory Classics)*, 1 cup* 41.0
garlic herb *(Lundberg* Quick) 47.0
lemon herb, with jasmine rice *(Knorr)*, ⅓ cup 56.0
Mediterranean *(Good Harvest)*, ⅓ cup 32.0
mushroom, savory *(Lundberg* Quick) 41.0
nutted *(Casbah)*, 1 oz. 20.0
primavera *(Goya)* 35.0
three grain with herbs *(Fantastic)*, ⅓ cup 49.0
risotto:
   broccoli au gratin *(Knorr)*, ⅓ cup 54.0
   chicken and Parmesan *(Lipton* Rice & Sauce)*, ½ cup or
     1 cup* 43.0
   classico *(Fantastic* Healthy Complements)*, ¼ cup 31.0
   herb, Italian *(Lundberg)*, ¼ pkg. 28.0
   Milanese *(Knorr)*, ⅓ cup 61.0
   mushroom *(Fantastic* Healthy Complements)*, ¼ cup . . . 33.0
   mushroom *(Knorr)*, ⅓ cup 66.0
   onion herb *(Knorr)*, ⅓ cup 66.0
   Parmesan, creamy *(Lundberg)*, ¼ pkg. 27.0
   primavera *(Knorr)*, ⅓ cup 61.0
   primavera, garlic *(Lundberg)*, ¼ pkg. 29.0
   tomato basil *(Lundberg)*, ¼ pkg. 30.0
   tomato–wild mushroom *(Good Harvest)*, ⅓ cup 31.0
salsa style *(Lipton* Seasoned Rice)*, ⅓ cup or 1 cup* 37.0
scampi style *(Lipton* Rice & Sauce)*, ½ cup or 1 cup* 44.0
Spanish:
   (Country Inn) 43.0
   (Fantastic Healthy Complements)*, ⅜ cup 36.0
   (Good Harvest), ⅓ cup 49.0
   (Lipton Rice & Sauce)*, ½ cup or 1 cup* 47.0
   (Mahatma) 42.0
   (Old El Paso), ½ pkg. 90.0
   (Rice-A-Roni), 1 cup* 46.0
   (Success) 43.0
brown *(Arrowhead Mills* Quick)*, ¼ pkg. 30.0
brown rice pilaf *(Fantastic)*, ½ cup 55.0

Rice dishes, mix, Spanish *(cont.)*
pilaf *(Casbah)*, 1 oz. 22.0
pilaf *(Knorr)*, 1/3 cup 50.0
pilaf *(Near East)* 42.0
pilaf, brown *(Lundberg* Quick Fiesta) 47.0
sticky, with coconut milk *(Thai Kitchen)*, 1/2 cup* 51.0
Stroganoff *(Rice-A-Roni)*, 1 cup* 50.0
teriyaki *(Lipton* Rice & Sauce), 1/2 cup or 1 cup* 45.0
vegetable, country *(Spice Islands* Quick), 1 pkg. 38.0
vegetable, herb *(Arrowhead Mills* Quick), 1/4 pkg. 30.0
wild, and bean *(Good Harvest)*, 1/3 cup 31.0
wild, and vegetables *(Spice Islands* Quick), 1 pkg. 35.0
yellow *(Goya)* 37.0
yellow, saffron *(Carolina/Mahatma)* 43.0
Rice entree, frozen (see also "Rice dishes, frozen"):
and beans, Santa Fe *(Weight Watchers* International
    Selections), 10 oz. 41.0
cheese, four, with pasta and chicken *(The Budget Gourmet*
    Italian Originals), 10.5 oz. 36.0
fried, with chicken *(Chun King)*, 8 oz. 44.0
fried, with pork *(Chun King)*, 8 oz. 48.0
Italian style, and chicken and mozzarella *(The Budget
    Gourmet* Italian Originals), 10 oz. 39.0
pilaf Florentine *(Weight Watchers* International Selections),
    10.13 oz. 47.0
risotto, with cheese and mushrooms *(Weight Watchers)*,
    10 oz. 44.0
and vegetables:
    Hunan *(Weight Watchers* International Selections),
        10.34 oz. 39.0
    paella *(Weight Watchers* International Selections),
        10.33 oz. 48.0
    Peking *(Weight Watchers* International Selections),
        10.5 oz. 48.0
    stir-fry *(The Budget Gourmet* Value Classics), 8.5 oz. . . . 54.0
    Szechuan, and chicken *(Smart Ones)*, 9 oz. 39.0
    wild, pilaf *(The Budget Gourmet* Value Classics), 8.5 oz. . 56.0
Rice flour:
(Goya), 3 tbsp. 26.0
brown *(Arrowhead Mills)*, 1/4 cup 27.0
brown, 1/2 cup 60.4
white *(Arrowhead Mills)*, 1/4 cup 33.0

white, ½ cup 63.3
Rice pudding, canned *(Thank You),* ½ cup 32.0
Rice pudding mix, dry, except as noted:
(Goya), ½ cup* 20.0
(Jell-O Americana), ½ cup* 20.0
cinnamon raisin *(Lundberg* Elegant), ½ cup 16.0
cinnamon and raisin *(Uncle Ben's),* 1.5 oz. 37.0
coconut *(Lundberg* Elegant), ½ cup 13.0
honey almond *(Lundberg* Elegant), ½ cup 15.0
Rice puffs, five flavor *(Eden),* 30 puffs, 1.1 oz. 24.0
Rice seasoning mix:
fried *(Durkee),* ¼ pkg. 2.0
Mexican *(Lawry's),* 1½ tbsp. 9.0
Rice syrup *(Lundberg Nutra-Farmed/Lundberg* Organic),
¼ cup 42.0
Rigatoni, refrigerated *(Tutta Pasta),* 1 cup 58.0
Rigatoni dishes, mix, approx. 1 cup*:
cheddar and broccoli *(Pasta Roni).* 48.0
tomato basil *(Pasta Roni)* 35.0
Rigatoni entree, frozen:
(Freezer Queen Family), 1 cup, 8.3 oz. 36.0
cream sauce, with broccoli and chicken *(The Budget*
  Gourmet Special Selections), 9 oz. 35.0
creamy, with broccoli and chicken *(Smart Ones),* 9 oz. 40.0
parmigiana *(Marie Callender's/Marie Callender's* Multi-
  Serve), 1 cup 32.0
Risotto, see "Rice dishes, mix"
Rockfish, without added ingredients 0
Roe (see also "Caviar"):
raw, 1 oz. 4
raw, 1 tbsp. 2
baked, broiled, or microwaved, 4 oz. 2.2
Roll (see also "Biscuit" and "Bun, sweet"), 1 roll, except as
  noted:
(Arnold Bran'nola Buns) 27.0
(Arnold Francisco 3″) 18.0
assorted *(Brownberry* Hearth) 22.0
brown and serve:
  (Pepperidge Farm Hearth), 3 rolls 28.0
  (Roman Meal), 2 rolls 26.0
  club *(Pepperidge Farm)* 22.0
  French *(Pepperidge Farm* 3) 45.0

Roll, brown and serve *(cont.)*
    French *(Pepperidge Farm* 2), ½ roll 34.0
    sourdough *(Arnold Francisco)* 17.0
crescent, butter *(Pepperidge Farm* Heat & Serve) 13.0
croissant, see "Croissant"
dill and onion *(Awrey's* Deli Rounds) 30.0
dinner:
    (Arnold 12 Pack) 19.0
    (Arnold 24 Pack) 20.0
    (Arnold August Bros.) 18.0
    (Arnold Bran'nola) 13.0
    (Brownberry Francisco Intl.) 26.0
    (Pepperidge Farm Country Style), 3 rolls 22.0
    (Roman Meal), 2 rolls 27.0
    all varieties *(Awrey's)*, 2 rolls, 1.6 oz. 19.0
    finger *(Pepperidge Farm)*, 3 rolls 20.0
    parker house *(Pepperidge Farm)*, 3 rolls 20.0
    potato *(Arnold)*, 2 rolls 21.0
    potato *(Pepperidge Farm* Deli Classic) 12.0
    sesame seed *(Arnold)*, 2 rolls 19.0
    wheat or white *(Arnold August Bros.)* 19.0
egg, twist *(Arnold Levy* Old Country) 30.0
French:
    (Arnold 6″) 35.0
    (Brownberry Francisco Intl. 6″) 35.0
    mini *(Arnold Francisco)* 22.0
    7 grain *(Pepperidge Farm* 9) 19.0
    sourdough *(Pepperidge Farm)* 18.0
garlic and pepper *(Awrey's* Deli Rounds) 30.0
hamburger:
    (Arnold 8 Pack) 26.0
    (Arnold 12 Pack) 24.0
    (Arnold August Bros.) 26.0
    (Pepperidge Farm) 22.0
    (Roman Meal) 22.0
    (Wonder) 21.0
    (Wonder 4″) 24.0
    wheat *(Arnold August Bros.)* 25.0
hoagie (see also "sub," below):
    (Awrey's) 46.0
    (Merita) 43.0
    (Pepperidge Farm Deli Classic/Multi-Grain) 32.0

(Wonder Deli) 34.0
hot dog/frankfurter:
    (Arnold 11 oz.) 19.0
    (Arnold 12 oz./12 Pack) 21.0
    (Arnold Bran'nola/Arnold New England) 21.0
    (Brownberry) 22.0
    (Pepperidge Farm) 24.0
    (Roman Meal) 20.0
    (Wonder) 21.0
    (Wonder Foot Long Coney) 34.0
    Dijon *(Pepperidge Farm)* 23.0
    potato *(Arnold)* 23.0
    wheat *(Brownberry)* 21.0
Italian *(Arnold Savoni* 8″) 56.0
kaiser:
    (Arnold August Bros.) 32.0
    (Arnold Francisco 6″/*Arnold Levy* Old Country) 35.0
    (Awrey's) 37.0
    (Brownberry Hearth) 30.0
    (Brownberry Francisco) 35.0
    sesame *(Arnold* Sandwich) 25.0
onion:
    (Arnold Deli) 35.0
    (Arnold August Bros.) 33.0
    (Arnold Levy Old Country) 31.0
party *(Pepperidge Farm* 20), 5 rolls 26.0
potato *(Arnold)* 28.0
potato, sesame *(Arnold)* 27.0
sandwich roll/bun:
    (Pepperidge Farm Hearty) 39.0
    (Roman Meal) 35.0
    multigrain *(Pepperidge Farm)* 24.0
    onion *(Pepperidge Farm)* 26.0
    potato *(Brownberry)* 28.0
    potato *(Pepperidge Farm)* 28.0
    sesame, soft *(Arnold)* 23.0
    sesame seed *(Pepperidge Farm)* 23.0
    soft *(Arnold* 8/12 Pack) 24.0
    sourdough *(Pepperidge Farm)* 28.0
    wheat *(Brownberry)* 24.0
    white *(Brownberry)* 25.0
sesame *(Arnold August Bros.)* 33.0

Roll *(cont.)*
sourdough *(Arnold Francisco)* 17.0
steak *(Arnold* Premium*/Arnold August Bros.)* 33.0
steak *(Arnold Francisco)* 33.0
sub:
   (Arnold August Bros.) 33.0
   (Arnold Levy Old Country) 30.0
   super loaf *(Arnold Francisco)*, 1 oz. 14.0
tea *(Wonder)* 25.0
Roll, frozen or refrigerated, 1 roll, except as noted:
(Rich's Homestyle), 2 rolls 27.0
crescent, regular or cheese *(Pillsbury)* 11.0
crescent, reduced fat *(Pillsbury)* 12.0
dinner, wheat or white *(Pillsbury)* 18.0
Roll, mix, hot:
(Dromedary), 1/16 pkg. 20.0
(Pillsbury), 1/4 cup or 1/15 pkg.* 21.0
Roll, sweet, see "Bun, sweet"
Roman beans, 1/4 cup:
dry *(Goya)* 24.0
canned *(Goya)* 20.0
Roseapple:
untrimmed, 1 lb. 17.3
trimmed, 1 oz. 1.6
Roselle:
untrimmed, 1 lb. 31.3
trimmed, 1 oz. or 1/2 cup 3.2
Rosemary, dried:
(McCormick), 1/4 tsp. 3
1 tbsp. 2.1
1 tsp. 8
Rotini dishes, mix:
cheese, three *(Lipton* Pasta & Sauce), 3/4 cup 41.0
cheese, three *(Lipton* Pasta & Sauce), 1 cup* 44.0
mushroom sauce *(Knorr)*, 2/3 cup 50.0
primavera *(Lipton* Pasta & Sauce), 3/4 cup 42.0
primavera *(Lipton* Pasta & Sauce), 1 cup* 45.0
Roughy, orange:
fresh, without added ingredients 0
frozen *(Schwan's)*, 4 oz. 0

Roy Rogers, 1 serving:

breakfast items:

bagel, plain	60.0
bagel, cinnamon raisin	63.0
Big Country Breakfast Platter, with bacon	61.0
Big Country Breakfast Platter, with ham	67.0
Big Country Breakfast Platter, with sausage	61.0
biscuit, plain	44.0
biscuit, bacon or bacon and egg	44.0
biscuit, *Cinnamon 'N' Raisin*	48.0
biscuit, ham, with cheese, egg, or cheese and egg	48.0
biscuit, sausage or sausage and egg	44.0
hash rounds	24.0
pancakes, 3 pieces, plain	56.0
pancakes, 3 pieces, with bacon or sausage	56.0
sourdough sandwich, ham, egg, and cheese	45.0

sandwiches:

bacon cheeseburger	29.0
bacon cheeseburger, sourdough	43.0
cheeseburger	34.0
cheeseburger, ¼ lb.	42.0
chicken, grilled	32.0
chicken, grilled, sourdough	46.0
chicken fillet	49.0
Fisherman's Fillet, seasonal	56.0
hamburger	33.0
hamburger, ¼ lb.	41.0
roast beef	30.0

chicken, fried:

breast	29.0
leg	15.0
thigh	30.0
wing	23.0

¼ *Roy's Roaster:*

dark meat	2.0
dark meat, with skin off	1.0
white meat	3.0
white meat, with skin off	2.0
chicken nuggets, 6 pieces	20.0
chicken nuggets, 9 pieces	32.0

salads:

chicken, grilled	2.0

Roy Rogers, salads *(cont.)*
garden 3.0
side salad 3.0
potatoes:
baked, plain or with margarine 27.0
baked, with margarine and sour cream 28.0
fries, regular 49.0
fries, large 59.0
mashed, 5 oz. 20.0
gravy for mashed potatoes 3.0
sides:
baked beans, 5 oz. 30.0
coleslaw, 5 oz. 16.0
corn bread 35.0
vanilla frozen yogurt cone 29.0
Rum runner mixer, raspberry, frozen* *(Bacardi)*, 8 fl. oz. . . 33.0
Rutabaga:
fresh:
untrimmed, 1 lb. 31.4
raw, cubed, 1/2 cup 5.7
boiled, drained, 1/2 cup 7.4
boiled, drained, mashed, 1/2 cup 10.5
canned *(Sunshine)*, 1/2 cup 7.0
Rye, whole-grain:
(Arrowhead Mills), 1/4 cup 34.0
1 cup 117.9
Rye flakes, rolled *(Arrowhead Mills)*, 1/3 cup 24.0
Rye flour:
(Arrowhead Mills), 1/4 cup 20.0
dark, 1 cup 88.0
light, 1 cup 81.8
medium, 1 cup 79.0
medium *(Pillsbury)*, 1/4 cup 22.0
Rye-Wheat flour *(Pillsbury* Bohemian Style), 1/4 cup 22.0

S

FOOD AND MEASURE	CARBOHYDRATE GRAMS

Sablefish, without added ingredients 0
Safflower seed kernel, dried, 1 oz. 9.7
Safflower seed meal, partially defatted, 1 oz. 13.8
Saffron:
1 tbsp. 1.4
1 tsp. 5
Sage, ground:
(McCormick), ¼ tsp. 1
1 tbsp. 1.2
1 tsp. 4
Salad, complete, with dressing, fresh:
Caesar:
    (Dole Complete Salads), 3½ oz. 8.0
    (Dole Lunch for One), 5.75 oz. 18.0
    low-fat *(Dole* Complete Salads), 3½ oz. 10.0
    low-fat *(Dole* Lunch for One), 6 oz. 18.0
herb ranch, low-fat *(Dole* Complete Salads), 3½ oz. 10.0
Italian, low-fat *(Dole* Lunch for One), 7 oz. 23.0
Italian, zesty, low-fat *(Dole* Complete Salads), 3½ oz. 11.0
Oriental *(Dole* Complete Salads), 3½ oz. 13.0
ranch *(Dole* Lunch for One), 7 oz. 18.0
ranch, sunflower *(Dole* Complete Salads), 3½ oz. 6.0
raspberry romaine *(Dole* Complete Salads), 3½ oz. 13.0
Romano *(Dole* Complete Salads), 3½ oz. 8.0
spinach bacon *(Dole* Complete Salads), 3½ oz. 18.0
Salad blend mix, fresh, 3 oz.:
American or European *(Dole Special Blends)* 3.0
French *(Dole Special Blends)* 4.0
Italian or romaine *(Dole Special Blends)* 2.0
Salad dressing, 2 tbsp.:
bacon and tomato *(Kraft)*. 2.0
bacon and tomato *(Kraft Deliciously Right)* 3.0
balsamic vinegar *(S&W Vintage)* 8.0
berry vinaigrette *(Knott's Berry Farm)* 7.0

Salad dressing *(cont.)*

blue cheese:

(Bernstein's Dressing/Dip)	0
(Bernstein's Dressing/Dip Lite)	1.0
(Hellmann's)	1.0
(Kraft Free)	12.0
(Kraft Roka)	5.0
(Marie's Salad Bar Reduced Calorie)	7.0
creamy *(Bernstein's)*	2.0
creamy *(Marie's* Low Fat)	6.0
vinaigrette *(Herb Magic)*	0

blue cheese, chunky:

(Marie's)	3.0
(Marie's Reduced Calorie)	7.0
(Seven Seas)	5.0
(Wish-Bone 8 oz./12 oz.)	3.0
(Wish-Bone 16 oz./24 oz.)	2.0
(Wish-Bone Free)	7.0
(Wish-Bone Lite)	3.0

Caesar:

(Bernstein's)	1.0
(Bernstein's Extra Rich)	2.0
(Cardini's Original)	1.0
(Hidden Valley Ranch Fat Free)	6.0
(Kraft/Kraft Deliciously Right)	2.0
(Kraft Classic)	1.0
(Salad Celebrations)	1.0
(Wish-Bone)	2.0
(Wish-Bone Free)	5.0
cheese, three *(Salad Celebrations)*	5.0
creamy *(Hellmann's)*	2.0
creamy *(Seven Seas)*	1.0
creamy *(Seven Seas Viva)*	2.0
creamy *(Wish-Bone)*	1.0
creamy, with cracked pepper *(Lawry's)*	1.0
garlic, roasted *(Knott's Berry Farm)*	2.0
ranch *(Kraft)*	1.0
cheese *(Bernstein's* Fantastico!)	2.0
cheese *(Bernstein's Light Fantastic* Fantastico!)	5.0
chicken salad, Oriental *(Knott's Berry Farm)*	4.0
citrus vinaigrette *(Knott's Berry Farm)*	8.0
coleslaw *(Kraft)*	8.0

coleslaw *(Marie's)* 6.0
cucumber, creamy *(Herb Magic)* 4.0
Dijon, creamy *(Bernstein's Light Fantastic)* 9.0
Dijon vinaigrette, balsamic *(Pritikin)* 3.0
dill, creamy *(Bernstein's Light Fantastic)* 6.0
dill, creamy *(Nasoya Vegi-Dressing)* 3.0
French:
   (Hellmann's Fat Free) 12.0
   (Kraft) 4.0
   (Kraft Catalina) 8.0
   (Kraft Deliciously Right) 6.0
   (Kraft Deliciously Right Catalina) 9.0
   (Kraft Free) 12.0
   (Kraft Free Catalina) 11.0
   (Nalley) 6.0
   (Salad Celebrations) 9.0
   (Wish-Bone Deluxe) 5.0
   (Wish-Bone Lite) 8.0
   herbal, creamy *(Bernstein's)* 8.0
   with honey *(Kraft Catalina)* 8.0
   honey *(Pritikin)* 11.0
   honey and bacon *(Hidden Valley Ranch)* 10.0
   style *(Pritikin)* 8.0
   style *(Wish-Bone* Free Deluxe) 7.0
   sweet 'n spicy *(Wish-Bone)* 6.0
   sweet 'n spicy style *(Wish-Bone* Fat Free) 7.0
   tangy *(Marie's)* 8.0
   vinaigrette, true *(Herb Magic)* .... <1.0
fruit salad *(Knott's Berry Farm)* 8.0
fruit vinaigrette *(Knott's Berry Farm)* 9.0
garden, zesty *(Kraft Salsa)* 1.0
garlic:
   creamy *(Kraft)* 2.0
   creamy *(Wish-Bone* Free) 9.0
   roasted, creamy *(Wish-Bone)* 3.0
   zesty *(Cardini's)* 2.0
green goddess *(Seven Seas)* 1.0
herb, garden *(Nasoya Vegi-Dressing)* 3.0
herb, vinaigrette, zesty *(Marie's* Free) 7.0
herbs and spices *(Seven Seas)* 1.0
honey Dijon:
   (Hellmann's Fat Free) 12.0

Salad dressing, honey Dijon *(cont.)*
   (Hidden Valley Ranch Fat Free) 7.0
   (Kraft) 4.0
   (Kraft Free) 11.0
   (Pritikin) 11.0
   (Salad Celebrations) 11.0
   (Wish-Bone Free) 10.0
   vinaigrette, zesty *(Marie's* Free) 11.0
honey mustard:
   (Bernstein's Dressing/Dip) 7.0
   (Knott's Berry Farm) 4.0
   (Marie's) 8.0
   (Nalley) 7.0
Italian:
   (Bernstein's) 1.0
   (Bernstein's Reduced Calorie) 3.0
   (Bernstein's Restaurant Recipe) 12.0
   (Bernstein's Wine Country) 2.0
   (Bernstein's Light Fantastic) 6.0
   (Hellmann's) 3.0
   (Herb Magic) 2.0
   (Kraft House) 3.0
   (Kraft Oil/Fat Free) 2.0
   (Kraft Presto) 2.0
   (Kraft Deliciously Right) 3.0
   (Kraft Free) 2.0
   (Ott's Zesty) 1.0
   (Pritikin) 5.0
   (Salad Celebrations) 2.0
   (Seven Seas Free) 2.0
   (Seven Seas Viva) 2.0
   (Seven Seas Viva Reduced Calorie) 2.0
   (Wish-Bone) 3.0
   (Wish-Bone Classic House) 2.0
   (Wish-Bone Free) 2.0
   (Wish-Bone Lite) 2.0
   (Wish-Bone Rubusto) 4.0
   with cheese *(Bernstein's* Reduced Calorie) 1.0
   cheese, 2 *(Seven Seas)* 3.0
   cheese and garlic *(Bernstein's)* 2.0
   creamy *(Hellmann's)* 2.0
   creamy *(Kraft)* 3.0

creamy *(Kraft Deliciously Right)* 3.0
creamy *(Nasoya Vegi-Dressing)* 3.0
creamy *(Salad Celebrations)* 7.0
creamy *(Seven Seas)* 2.0
creamy *(Seven Seas* Reduced Calorie) 2.0
creamy *(Wish-Bone)* 4.0
creamy *(Wish-Bone* Free) 9.0
garlic, creamy *(Marie's)* 3.0
garlic, creamy *(Marie's* Reduced Calorie) 6.0
herb, creamy *(Marie's* Low Fat) 7.0
herb and cheese *(Hidden Valley Ranch* Fat Free) 6.0
herb and garlic, creamy *(Bernstein's)* 3.0
olive oil *(Seven Seas* Reduced Calorie) 2.0
olive oil *(Wish-Bone* Classic) 4.0
Parmesan *(Hidden Valley Ranch* Fat Free) 4.0
vinaigrette, zesty *(Marie's* Free) 8.0
zesty *(Kraft)* 2.0
mango–key lime vinegar *(S&W* Vintage Lite) 7.0
mayonnaise type, see "Mayonnaise"
olive oil vinaigrette *(Wish-Bone)* 4.0
Oriental *(Bernstein's Light Fantastic)* 11.0
Oriental rice wine vinegar *(S&W* Vintage Lite) . . 8.0
(Ott's Famous Original) 9.0
(Ott's Famous Free) 9.0
(Ott's Famous Reduced Calorie) 8.0
Parmesan:
creamy *(Marie's* Low Fat) 7.0
and onion *(Wish-Bone)* 5.0
and onion *(Wish-Bone* Free) 9.0
peppercorn, ground *(Knott's Berry Farm)* 1.0
poppy seed:
(Herb Magic) 8.0
(Knott's Berry Farm) 10.0
(Marie's) 8.0
(Ott's Free) 12.0
(Ott's Reduced Calorie) 9.0
herb *(Cardini's* Low Fat Low Calorie) 2.0
potato salad *(Best Foods/Hellmann's One Step)* 2.0
potato salad *(Best Foods/Hellmann's One Step* ⅓ Less Fat) . 4.0
ranch:
(Bernstein's Dressing/Dip) 1.0
(Bernstein's Dressing/Dip Lite) 2.0

Salad dressing, ranch *(cont.)*
   (Bernstein's Light Fantastic) 7.0
   (Hellmann's Fat Free) 11.0
   (Herb Magic) 4.0
   (Hidden Valley Ranch Original) 1.0
   (Kraft/Kraft Deliciously Right) 2.0
   (Kraft Free) 11.0
   (Kraft Salsa) 1.0
   (Marie's Salad Bar Reduced Calorie) 7.0
   (Nalley) 6.0
   (Nalley Fat Free) 8.0
   (Ott's Buttermilk) 1.0
   (Salad Celebrations) 7.0
   (Seven Seas) 2.0
   (Seven Seas Reduced Calorie) 5.0
   (Seven Seas Free) 12.0
   (Wish-Bone) 1.0
   (Wish-Bone Free) 9.0
   (Wish-Bone Lite) 5.0
   with bacon *(Hidden Valley Ranch)* 1.0
   buttermilk *(Kraft)* 2.0
   buttermilk *(Marie's)* 4.0
   creamy *(Hellmann's)* 1.0
   creamy *(Marie's* Reduced Calorie) 7.0
   cucumber *(Kraft/Kraft Deliciously Right)* 2.0
   Italian *(Bernstein's)* 3.0
   Parmesan *(Marie's)* 2.0
   Parmesan garlic *(Bernstein's)* 3.0
   Parmesan garlic *(Bernstein's Light Fantastic)* 7.0
   peppercorn *(Kraft)* 1.0
   peppercorn *(Kraft Free)* 11.0
   sour cream and onion *(Kraft)* 1.0
   zesty *(Marie's* Low Fat) 7.0
raspberry:
   blush vinegar *(S&W* Vintage Lite) 10.0
   vinaigrette *(Knott's Berry Farm* Low Fat) 8.0
   vinaigrette *(Pritikin)* 11.0
   vinaigrette, zesty *(Marie's* Free) 8.0
red wine vinaigrette:
   (Wish-Bone) 9.0
   (Wish-Bone Free) 7.0
   zesty *(Marie's* Free) 10.0

red wine vinegar:
- (Kraft Free) 3.0
- (Seven Seas Free) 3.0
- with herbs (S&W Vintage Lite) 8.0
- and oil (Seven Seas/Seven Seas Reduced Calorie) 2.0

Roquefort (Bernstein's Dressing/Dip) 1.0

Russian:
- (Kraft) 10.0
- (Salad Celebrations) 8.0
- (Seven Seas Viva) 3.0
- (Wish-Bone) 15.0

salsa and sour cream (Bernstein's Dressing/Dip) 2.0
sesame garlic (Nasoya Vegi-Dressing) 3.0
sour cream and dill (Marie's) 3.0
sweet and sour (Herb Magic) 9.0
sweet and sour (Old Dutch) 13.0

Thousand Island:
- (Bernstein's Dressing/Dip) 4.0
- (Herb Magic) 4.0
- (Kraft) 5.0
- (Kraft Deliciously Right) 8.0
- (Kraft Free) 11.0
- (Marie's) 7.0
- (Marie's Salad Bar) 6.0
- (Nalley) 4.0
- (Nalley Fat Free) 8.0
- (Nasoya Vegi-Dressing) 6.0
- (Salad Celebrations) 8.0
- (Wish-Bone) 7.0
- (Wish-Bone Free) 9.0
- (Wish-Bone Lite) 8.0
- with bacon (Kraft) 5.0

tomato, sun-dried, vinaigrette (Knott's Berry Farm) 3.0
tuna salad (Best Foods/Hellmann's One Step) 4.0
vinaigrette (see also specific listings), (Herb Magic) 3.0
white wine vinaigrette, zesty (Marie's Free) 10.0
white wine vinegar with herbs (S&W Vintage Lite) 10.0

Salad dressing mix, 2 tbsp.*, except as noted:
buttermilk (Tone's), ½ tsp. 1.0
buttermilk, farm (Good Seasons) 2.0
Caesar, gourmet (Good Seasons) 3.0
cheese garlic (Good Seasons) 1.0

Salad dressing mix *(cont.)*
garlic and herbs *(Good Seasons)* 1.0
herb, zesty *(Good Seasons Free)* 2.0
honey mustard *(Good Seasons)* 3.0
honey mustard *(Good Seasons Free)* 5.0
Italian:
    (Good Seasons) 1.0
    (Good Seasons Free) 3.0
    (Good Seasons Reduced Calorie) 2.0
    creamy *(Good Seasons Free)* 3.0
    mild *(Good Seasons)* 2.0
    zesty *(Good Seasons)* 1.0
    zesty *(Good Seasons Reduced Calorie)* 2.0
Mexican spice *(Good Seasons)* 2.0
Oriental sesame *(Good Seasons)* 3.0
ranch *(Good Seasons)* 2.0
ranch *(Good Seasons Reduced Calorie)* 3.0
Salad seasoning *(McCormick)*, ½ tsp. 0
Salad toppers (see also "Croutons"), all varieties:
(McCormick Salad Toppin's), 1⅓ tbsp. 2.0
all varieties *(Pepperidge Farm)*, 1 tbsp. 4.0
Salami, 2 oz., except as noted:
beef:
    (Boar's Head Chub) 0
    (Hebrew National) 0
    (Hebrew National Lean) 1.0
    (Hebrew National Reduced Fat) 0
    (Oscar Mayer Machiach), 2 slices, 1.6 oz. 1.0
beer *(Oscar Mayer)*, 2 slices, 1.6 oz. 1.0
cooked *(Boar's Head)* 0
cotto *(Oscar Mayer)*, 2 slices, 1.6 oz. 0
cotto, beef *(Oscar Mayer)*, 2 slices, 1.6 oz. 1.0
dry or hard *(Boar's Head)*, 1 oz. . . . . <1.0
dry or hard *(Hormel Homeland/Sandwich Maker)*, 1 oz. 0
Genoa:
    (Boar's Head) 1.0
    (Di Lusso), 1 oz. 0
    (Hormel Pillow Pack/Hormel Sandwich Maker), 1 oz. 1.0
    (Oscar Mayer), 1 oz. 0
    (San Remo Brand), 1 oz. 0
hard *(Oscar Mayer)*, 3 slices, 1 oz. 0
"Salami," vegetarian, frozen *(Worthington)*, 3 slices 2.0

Salisbury steak, see "Beef dinner" and "Beef entree"
Salmon, fresh, canned, or **frozen,** without added
    ingredients 0
Salmon, refrigerated, boneless, skinless:
burger *(Salmon Chef),* 3-oz. burger 0
cuts *(Salmon Chef),* 5-oz. piece 0
cuts, in dill-sorrel-chive marinade *(Salmon Chef),* 5-oz.
    piece 1.0
kabob *(Salmon Chef),* 3.3 oz. 4.0
kabob, in teriyaki sesame marinade *(Salmon Chef),* 3.3 oz. . . 0
loin *(Salmon Chef),* 2 pieces, 4 oz. 0
loin, in chili-cilantro marinade *(Salmon Chef),* 2 pieces,
    4 oz. 0
tenderloin *(Salmon Chef),* 6-oz. piece 0
tenderloin, in sweet pepper-sage marinade *(Salmon Chef),*
    6-oz. piece 1.0
Salmon, smoked:
chinook, regular or lox, 4 oz. 0
lox, natural Nova or Nova with color *(Vita),* 2 oz. . . . . <1.0
lox, natural Nova or Nova with color *(Vita),* 3-oz. pkg. 1.0
Salmon, smoked, spread:
(Vita), ¼ cup, 2 oz. 2.9
cream cheese *(Vita),* ¼ cup, 2 oz. 2.0
Salsa, 2 tbsp., except as noted:
(Gracias Original/Hot) 2.0
(Kaukauna Extra Chunky) 3.0
(La Victoria Ranchera) 2.0
(La Victoria Victoria) 1.0
(Marie's Tomato) 2.0
all varieties:
    (Clemente Jacques) 2.0
    (Del Monte Traditional/Thick & Chunky/Fire Roasted/
        Garlic) 2.0
    (Heluva Good Thick & Chunky) 2.0
    (Hunt's Alfresco Homestyle) 2.0
    (Hunt's Homestyle/Squeeze) 6.0
    (La Victoria Thick N Chunky) 1.0
    (Nalley Superba) 2.0
    (Old El Paso Homestyle) 2.0
    (Old El Paso Thick n' Chunky) 2.0
    (Pace Thick & Chunky) 2.0
    (Progresso) 2.0

Salsa, all varieties *(cont.)*
   (S&W Ready-Cut), ¼ cup 4.0
   (Tostitos) 3.0
and cheese, see "Cheese dip"
garlic, roasted *(Marie's)* 2.0
green *(Goya)* 2.0
green *(La Victoria* Jalapeña) 1.0
green chili *(La Victoria)* 1.0
green chili *(Old El Paso)* 2.0
hot *(Chi-Chi's)* 1.0
hot *(Guiltless Gourmet)* 2.0
medium:
   (La Victoria Suprema) 1.0
   (Las Palmas Mexicana) 2.0
   (Porino's) 2.0
   (Rosarita) 2.0
   (Rosarita Extra Chunky) 1.0
mild:
   (Chi-Chi's) 1.0
   (La Victoria Suprema) 2.0
   (Las Palmas Mexicana) 1.0
picante (see also "Picante sauce"):
   (Old Dutch) 2.0
   (Old El Paso) 2.0
   medium or mild *(La Victoria* Suprema) 1.0
pico de gallo *(Chi-Chi's)* 2.0
red *(La Victoria* Jalapeña) 2.0
roasted *(Rosarita)* 2.0
taco, see "Taco sauce"
tomatillo, green *(Rosarita)* 2.0
verde *(Old El Paso)* 2.0
verde, medium or mild *(Chi-Chi's)* 3.0
Salsa seasoning *(Lawry's)*, ½ tsp. 1.0
Salsify, fresh:
raw:
   (Frieda's), ¾ cup, 3 oz. 16.0
   untrimmed, 1 lb. 73.4
   sliced, ½ cup 12.5
boiled, drained, sliced, ½ cup 10.5
Salt (see also specific listings):
(McCormick Season-All), ¼ tsp. 0
1 tbsp. 0

seasoned, ¼ tsp.:
    (House of Tsang Hong Kong) 0
    (Morton/Morton Nature's Seasons) 0
    regular or red pepper *(Lawry's)* 0
Salt, substitute:
(Morton), ¼ tsp. 0
seasoned *(Lawry's* Salt Free), ¼ tsp. 0
seasoned *(Morton),* 1 tsp. 5
Salt pork, raw 0
Sandwich, see specific listings
Sandwich dressing, 2 tbsp.:
bell pepper salsa *(Vlasic Sandwich Zesters)* 4.0
garden onion *(Vlasic Sandwich Zesters)* 4.0
Italian tomato *(Vlasic Sandwich Zesters)* 3.0
jalapeño salsa *(Vlasic Sandwich Zesters)* 4.0
mushroom and onion *(Vlasic Sandwich Zesters)* 4.0
Sandwich sauce, ¼ cup, except as noted:
(Durkee Famous), 1 tbsp. 2.0
(Hunt's Manwich Original) 6.0
(Hunt's Manwich Bold) 13.0
(Hunt's Manwich Thick & Chunky) 8.5
Mexican *(Hunt's Manwich)* 5.0
Sloppy joe:
    (Del Monte Original) 16.0
    (Del Monte Hickory Flavor) 18.0
    (Green Giant) 11.0
    (Heinz), ½ cup 14.0
    (Hormel Not-So-Sloppy Joe Sauce) 15.0
    (Libby's), ⅓ cup 10.0
    barbecue *(Hunt's Manwich* Sloppy Joe) 14.0
taco, see "Taco sauce"
Sandwich sauce seasoning mix:
(Hunt's Manwich), ¼ oz. 5.0
Sloppy joe *(Lawry's),* 1 tsp. 3.0
Sandwich spread (see also "Sandwich sauce" and specific
    listings):
(Blue Plate), 1 tbsp. 3.0
(Hellmann's), 1 tbsp. 3.0
(Kraft Spread & Burger Sauce), 1 tbsp. 3.0
(Loma Linda), ¼ cup 7.0
Sapodilla:
untrimmed, 1 lb. 72.5

Sapodilla *(cont.)*
1 medium, 3″ × 2½″, approx. 7.5 oz. 33.0
trimmed, ½ cup 24.1
Sapote:
(Frieda's), 5 oz. 47.0
untrimmed, 1 lb. 108.7
1 medium, 11.2 oz. 76.0
trimmed, 1 oz. 9.6
Sardine, fresh, see "Herring"
Sardine, canned:
in lemon *(Goya)*, ¼ cup 0
in mustard sauce *(Underwood)*, 3¾-oz. can . . . . . . : . . . 2.0
in oil, 4 oz. . . . . : 0
in olive oil, drained, 4 oz. 0
in soy oil, drained *(Underwood)*, 3 oz. 1.0
in soy oil, drained, skinless, boneless *(King Oscar)*, 3 pieces . . 0
spiced *(Goya)*, ¼ cup 0
in tomato sauce:
   (Del Monte), 2 oz., ½ fish, with sauce 1.0
   (Goya/Goya Oval), ¼ cup 1.0
   (Goya Tinapa), 2 pieces 2.0
   (Underwood), 3¾ oz. 4.0
Sauce, see specific listings
Sauerkraut, 2 tbsp., except as noted:
(Boar's Head) 1.0
(Claussen), ¼ cup 1.0
(Del Monte) . . . . <1.0
(Eden Organic), ½ cup 4.0
(Frank's/Snowfloss) 1.0
(Hebrew National) 1.0
(Hebrew National), ½ cup 4.0
(Hebrew National/Shorr's New), ½ cup 11.0
(Pickle Eater's Kozmic Kraut) 1.0
(Pickle Eater's Reduced Sodium) 6
(Rosoff Home Style), ½ cup 11.0
(S&W) 2.0
(Seneca) 1.0
(Silverfloss) 1.0
(Stokely) 1.0
(Stokely), ½ cup 5.0
Bavarian style:
   (Del Monte) 4.0

(Frank's/Snowfloss) 3.0
(Seneca) 3.0
(Silverfloss) 2.0
(Stokely) 2.0
(Stokely), ½ cup 7.0
sweet and sour *(Stokely)* 5.0
sweet and sour *(Stokely)*, ½ cup 18.0
with liquid, ½ cup 5.1
Sauerkraut juice:
(S&W), 10-oz. can 7.0
(Stokely), 8 fl. oz. 4.0
Sausage (see also specific listings), cooked:
(Hormel Special Recipe), 1 link 0
(Hormel Special Recipe), 1 patty 0
beef:
   (Jones Dairy Farm Golden Brown), 2 links 1.0
   roll *(Jones Dairy Farm* All Natural), 2 oz. 0
   smoked *(Oscar Mayer* Smokies), 1 link 1.0
brown and serve:
   (Little Sizzlers), 3 links 1.0
   (Little Sizzlers), 2 patties 1.0
   beef, smoked *(Jones Dairy Farm)*, 2 links 1.0
   light *(Jones Dairy Farm)*, 2 links 1.0
   pork or pork and bacon *(Jones Dairy Farm)*, 2 links 1.0
cheese, smoked *(Oscar Mayer* Smokies), 1 link 1.0
cheese, smoked *(Oscar Mayer* Little Smokies), 6 links 1.0
dinner, 1 link or patty:
   (Jones Dairy Farm/Jones Dairy Farm All Natural) 1.0
   Italian *(Jones Dairy Farm)* 1.0
   sandwich patty *(Jones Dairy Farm)* 1.0
pickled, smoked or hot *(Hormel)*, 6 links 1.0
pork, crumbles, Italian or Mexican style *(Johnsville)*, 2 oz. . 2.0
pork, Italian, 1 oz. 4
pork, link:
   (Garden State Breakfast), 3 links 2.0
   (Jones Dairy Farm All Natural Light), 2 links 1.0
   (Jones Dairy Farm All Natural Little Links), 3 links 1.0
   (Little Sizzlers), 3 links 0
   (Oscar Mayer), 2 links 1.0
   (Schwan's), 3 links 0
   fresh, .5 oz. (1 oz. raw link) 1
   apple 'n cinnamon *(Johnsville)*, 3 links 1.0

Sausage, pork, link *(cont.)*

hot and spicy *(Little Sizzlers)*, 3 links 0
Italian style, hot or sweet *(Garden State)*, 1 link 1.0
light *(Jones Dairy Farm* Golden Brown), 2 links 1.0
maple *(Jones Dairy Farm* Golden Brown), 2 links 1.0
maple, Vermont *(Johnsville)*, 3 links 1.0
mild, milk or spicy *(Jones Dairy Farm* Golden Brown),
   2 links 2.0

pork, patty:

(Jones Dairy Farm All Natural), 1 patty 0
(Jones Dairy Farm Golden Brown), 1 patty 1.0
(Little Sizzlers), 2 patties 0
(Schwan's), 2-oz. patty 0
fresh, 1 oz. (2 oz. raw patty) 3

pork roll, regular or hot *(Jones Dairy Farm* All Natural),
   2 oz. 1.0

smoked:

(Boar's Head), 4.5 oz. 2.0
(John Morrell Bun Size), 1 link 4.0
(John Morrell Bun Size Less Fat), 1 link 9.0
(Light & Lean 97 Dinner Link), 1 link 2.0
(Oscar Mayer Little Smokies), 6 links 1.0
(Oscar Mayer Smokie Links), 1 link 1.0
hot *(Boar's Head)*, 3.2 oz. 1.0

Sausage, canned:

(Diana Salchichas), 3 links 1.0
Vienna, see "Vienna sausage"

"Sausage," vegetarian:

.9-oz. link 2.5
1.3-oz. patty 3.7
canned *(Loma Linda* Little Links), 2 links 2.0
canned *(Worthington Saucettes)*, 1 link 1.0

frozen:

(Green Giant Harvest Burger Breakfast), 3 links 6.0
(Green Giant Harvest Burger Breakfast), 2 patties 5.0
(Morningstar Farms Breakfast), 2 links 2.0
(Morningstar Farms Breakfast), 1 patty 2.0
(Morningstar Farms Recipe Crumbles), 2/3 cup 5.0
(Natural Touch Crumbles), 1/2 cup 4.0
(Worthington Vegetarian), 1/2 cup 3.0
(Worthington Prosage Links), 2 links 2.0
(Worthington Prosage Patties), 1 patty 3.0

roll *(Worthington Prosage)*, ⅝″ slice 2.0
mix* *(Fantastic Nature's Sausage)*, 2 tbsp., 1 patty or
  2 links 7.0
Sausage biscuit, frozen, 1 piece:
(Hormel Quick Meal) 30.0
(Schwan's), 1 pkg. 22.0
(Weight Watchers) 20.0
with cheese *(Hormel Quick Meal)* 30.0
with egg *(Hormel Quick Meal)* 31.0
with gravy *(Schwan's)*, 4.4-oz. piece 28.0
Sausage gravy mix *(Durkee/French's)*, ¼ cup* 5.0
Sausage hash, canned *(Mary Kitchen)*, 1 cup 29.0
Sausage seasoning, pork *(Tone's)*, 1 tsp. 2.7
Sausage stick, 1 piece, except as noted:
(Tombstone Snappy Sticks) . . . . <1.0
beef:
    (Boar's Head), .6 oz. 2.0
    (Old Dutch), 1 oz. 1.0
    (Rustlers Roundup Jerky) 1.0
    (Tombstone Jerky) . . . . <1.0
    (Tombstone Stick) 0
hot *(Rustlers Roundup)* 1.0
smoked *(Rustlers Roundup Steak Stick)* 1.0
smoked, mild or spicy *(Slim Jim)*, 1.4-oz. box 2.0
spicy *(Rustlers Roundup)* . . . . <1.0
summer sausage *(Old Dutch)*, 1 oz. 0
Savory, ground:
(McCormick), ¼ tsp. 4
1 tbsp. 3.0
1 tsp. 1.0
summer *(Tone's)*, 1 tsp. 1.0
Scallion, see "Onion, green"
Scallop, meat only:
raw, 4 oz. 2.7
raw, 2 large or 5 small, 1.1 oz. 7
frozen *(Tyson Delight)*, ½ cup 11.0
Scallop, fried, frozen *(Mrs. Paul's)*, 12 pieces 20.0
"Scallop," imitation, from surimi, 4 oz. 12.1
"Scallop," vegetarian, canned:
(Loma Linda Tender Bits), 6 pieces 7.0
(Worthington Vegetable Skallops), ½ cup 3.0

Scallop squash:
raw, untrimmed, 1 lb. 17.1
raw, sliced, ½ cup 2.5
boiled, drained, sliced, ½ cup 3.0
boiled, drained, mashed, ½ cup 4.0
Scrapple *(Jones Dairy Farm)*, 2 oz. 7.0
Scrod, fresh, without added ingredients 0
Scup, without added ingredients 0
Sea bass, without added ingredients 0
Sea trout, without added ingredients 0
Seafood, see specific listings
Seafood sauce (see also specific listings), cocktail, ¼ cup,
    except as noted:
(Bookbinder's Restaurant Style) 15.0
(Crosse & Blackwell) 25.0
(Del Monte) 24.0
(Heinz) 14.0
(Heluva Good) 10.0
(Maull's), 2 tbsp. 10.0
(Nalley) 15.0
(S&W), 1 tsp. 5.0
(Sauceworks) 13.0
hot and spicy *(Bookbinder's)* 15.0
Seafood seasoning, see "Fish seasoning and coating mix"
Seasoning (see also specific listings), ¼ tsp., except as
    noted:
(Ac'cent), ⅛ tsp. 0
(Sa-son con Ajo Cebolla/con Azafran/con Culantro) 0
(Sa-son Ac'cent) 0
Seasoning and coating mix (see also specific listings),
    ⅛ pkt.:
country *(Shake'n Bake)* 5.0
glaze, honey mustard *(Shake'n Bake)* 9.0
glaze, tangy honey *(Shake'n Bake)* 10.0
Italian herb *(Shake'n Bake)* 7.0
Seaweed:
agar:
    raw, 1 oz. 1.9
    dried, 1 oz. 22.9
    flakes or bar *(Eden)*, 1 tbsp. 2.0
arame *(Eden)*, ½ cup 7.0
hiziki *(Eden)*, ½ cup 6.0

Irish moss, raw, 1 oz. 3.5
kelp, raw, 1 oz. 2.7
kombu *(Eden),* ½ of 7″ piece 2.0
laver, raw, 1 oz. 1.4
nori *(Eden),* 1 sheet 1.0
spirulina, raw, 1 oz. 7
spirulina, dried, 1 oz. 6.8
wakame, raw, 1 oz. 2.6
wakame, flakes or regular *(Eden),* ½ cup 4.0
Seitan mix *(Arrowhead Mills),* ⅓ cup 14.0
Semolina, whole-grain, 1 cup 121.6
Semolina flour, mix *(Arrowhead Mills),* ½ cup 50.0
Serrano chili, see "Pepper, chili"
Sesame butter *(Roaster Fresh),* 1 oz. 6.0
Sesame flour, 1 oz.:
high-fat 7.6
partially defatted 10.0
low-fat 10.1
Sesame meal, partially defatted, 1 oz. 7.4
Sesame paste (see also "Tahini"), from whole sesame
   seeds, 1 tbsp. 4.1
Sesame seasoning, all varieties *(Eden),* ½ tsp. 0
Sesame seeds:
raw *(McCormick),* ¼ tsp. 4
whole, brown *(Arrowhead Mills),* ¼ cup 8.0
whole, roasted and toasted, 1 oz. 7.3
kernels, decorticated:
   (Arrowhead Mills), ¼ cup 5.0
   dried, 1 tsp. 3
   toasted, 1 oz. 7.4
Shad, without added ingredients 0
Shaddock, see "Pummelo"
Shallot:
(Frieda's), 1 tbsp. 5.0
fresh or stored, peeled, 1 oz. 4.8
fresh or stored, chopped, 1 tbsp. 1.7
freeze-dried, 1 tbsp. 7
freeze-dried *(McCormick),* ¼ tsp. 1
Shark, without added ingredients 0
Sheepshead, without added ingredients 0
Shellie beans, canned, ½ cup:
(Stokely) 8.0

Shellie beans *(cont.)*
with liquid 7.6
Shells, pasta:
dry, see "Pasta"
refrigerated *(Tutta Pasta)*, 7/8 cup 60.0
stuffed, frozen, without sauce:
    (Celentano), 4 shells 32.0
    (Celentano Value Pack), 3 shells 23.0
    (Schwan's), 3 shells 30.0
Shells, pasta, dinner, marinara, frozen
(Healthy Choice), 12 oz. 55.0
Shells, pasta, entree, frozen:
and cheese *(Stouffer's)*, 1/2 of 12-oz. pkg., approx. 1 cup . . 31.0
stuffed:
    (Celentano), 10 oz. 34.0
    (Celentano), 1/2 of 14-oz. pkg. 30.0
    (Celentano Great Choice), 10 oz. 41.0
    (Celentano Value Pack), 3 shells, 8 oz. 35.0
    broccoli *(Celentano* Great Choice), 10 oz. 31.0
    cheese *(Lean Cuisine* 80 oz.), 8.9 oz. 30.0
    Florentine *(Celentano)*, 10 oz. 32.0
Shells, pasta, mix, white cheddar *(Pasta Roni)*, approx.
1 cup* 48.0
Sherbet (see also "Ice" and "Sorbet"), 1/2 cup, except as
noted:
(Edy's/Dreyer's Raz Chip) 30.0
orange:
    (Breyers) 26.0
    (Carnation Cup), 3 fl. oz. 19.0
    (Carnation Plastic), 5 fl. oz. 32.0
    (Schwan's) 27.0
    Swiss *(Edy's/Dreyer's)* 30.0
pink lemonade *(Dreyer's)* 27.0
rainbow *(Breyers)* 26.0
rainbow *(Schwan's)* 27.0
raspberry *(Breyers)* 27.0
strawberry kiwi *(Edy's/Dreyer's)* 27.0
tangerine *(Edy's)* 28.0
tropical *(Breyers)* 26.0
tropical *(Edy's/Dreyer's)* 28.0
Sherbet cup, orange *(Sealtest)*, 4-oz. cup 28.0

Sherbet pop, 1 piece:
(Popsicle Big Stick) 24.0
(Popsicle Cyclone) 11.0
(Schwan's Push-Ems) 20.0
orange *(Popsicle Pop Ups)* 19.0
rainbow *(Popsicle Pop Ups)* 19.0
smoothie, strawberry fields *(Dreyer's)* 22.0
smoothie, tropical oasis *(Dreyer's)* 21.0
Shortening, 1 tbsp.:
(Jewel/Snowdrift/Swiftening) 0
all varieties *(Crisco)* 0
hydrogenated soybean and cottonseed or palm 0
lard and vegetable oil 0
Shrimp, meat only, raw:
1 lb. 4.1
4 oz. 1.0
4 large, 1 oz. 3
Shrimp, canned:
drained, 1 cup 1.3
all sizes *(Goya)*, 2 oz. 0
deveined, small or medium *(S&W)*, ¼ cup 0
Shrimp, frozen:
cooked, regular or tail on *(Contessa)*, approx. 1 cup, 3 oz. . . 0
jumbo *(Schwan's)*, 6 pieces 1.0
medium *(Schwan's)*, 4 oz. . . . . <1.0
"Shrimp," imitation:
from surimi, 4 oz. 10.4
frozen, jumbo *(Captain Jac Shrimp Tasties)*, 3 pieces, 3 oz. 12.0
Shrimp cocktail:
(Sau-Sea), 4-oz. jar 17.0
(Sau-Sea), 6-oz. jar 26.0
(Vita), 4-oz. jar 20.0
Shrimp dinner, frozen, 1 pkg.:
marinara *(Healthy Choice)*, 10.5 oz. 44.0
mariner *(The Budget Gourmet)*, 11 oz. 40.0
and vegetables Maria *(Healthy Choice)*, 12.5 oz. 46.0
Shrimp entree, canned, chow mein *(La Choy* Bi-Pack),
1 cup 9.0
Shrimp entree, freeze-dried, 1½ cups:
Alfredo *(AlpineAire)* 44.0
Newburg *(AlpineAire)* 49.0

Shrimp entree, frozen:
batter, beer *(Gorton's)*, 6 pieces 19.0
breaded:
  (Gorton's), 6 pieces 18.0
  (Schwan's), approx. 11 pieces, 4 oz. 37.0
  (Van de Kamp's), 7 pieces, 4 oz. 28.0
  butterfly *(Van de Kamp's)*, 7 pieces 28.0
  fantail *(Schwan's)*, 4 pieces, 4 oz. 37.0
  oven-ready *(Schwan's)*, 7 pieces, 3 oz. 19.0
  with pasta *(Marie Callender's)*, 1 cup, 7.5 oz. 27.0
  scampi *(Gorton's)*, 6 pieces 18.0
marinara *(Smart Ones)*, 9 oz. 35.0
popcorn, breaded:
  (Gorton's), 1 cup, 3.2 oz. 21.0
  (Van de Kamp's), 20 pieces, 4 oz. 28.0
  garlic and herb *(Gorton's)*, 1¼ cups, 3.5 oz. 26.0
Shrimp entree mix, Creole *(Luzianne)*, ⅕ pkg. 34.0
Shrimp sauce *(Crosse & Blackwell)*, ¼ cup 25.0
Shrimp spice *(Tone's Craboil)*, 1 tsp. 1.2
Sizzler, 1 serving:
hot entrees:
  hamburger on bun, with lettuce, tomato 36.0
  chicken breast, hibachi, with pineapple, 5 oz. 13.0
  chicken breast, lemon-herb, 5 oz. 0
  chicken breast, Santa Fe, 5 oz. 0
  chicken patty, Malibu 11.0
  salmon, 8 oz. 0
  shrimp, broiled, 5 oz. 0
  shrimp, fried, 4 pieces 35.0
  shrimp, mini, 4 oz. 24.0
  shrimp scampi, 5 oz. 0
  steak, Dakota Ranch, all sizes 0
  swordfish, 8 oz. 0
side dishes:
  cheese toast 16.0
  french fries, 4 oz. 45.0
  potato, baked, pulp 24.0
  rice pilaf, 6 oz. 47.0
sauces, 1½ oz.:
  buttery dipping 0
  cocktail sauce 8.0
  hibachi sauce 11.0

Malibu sauce 0
sour dressing 0
tartar sauce 6.0

hot bar:
chicken wings, 1 oz. 4.0
focaccia bread, 2 pieces 9.0
marinara sauce, 1 oz. 3.0
meatballs, 4 pieces 5.0
nacho sauce, 2 oz. 3.0
pasta, fettuccine, 2 oz. 15.0
pasta, spaghetti, 2 oz. 16.0
potato skins, 2 oz. 22.0
refried beans, ¼ cup 11.0
saltines, 2 pieces 4.0
taco filling, 2 oz. 3.0
taco shells, 1 piece 7.0

hot bar, soup, 4 oz.:
broccoli cheese 10.0
chicken noodle 4.0
clam chowder 11.0
minestrone 7.0
vegetable sirloin 6.0

salads, prepared, 2 oz.:
carrot and raisin 10.0
chicken, Chinese 6.0
jicama, spicy 4.0
Mediterranean Minted Fruit 7.0
Mexican Fiesta 10.0
pasta, seafood Louis 9.0
potato, old-fashioned 10.0
potato, red herb 9.0
seafood Louis 4.0
teriyaki beef 5.0
tuna pasta 6.0

dressings, 1 oz.:
blue cheese 1.0
guacamole 2.0
honey mustard 4.0
Italian, lite 2.0
Parmesan, Italian 2.0
ranch 2.0
ranch, lite 4.0

Sizzler, **dressings** *(cont.)*

    rice vinegar, Japanese 2.0

    salsa 2.0

    sour dressing 0

    Thousand Island 3.0

Sloppy joe entree, frozen *(Swanson Fun Feast),* 1 pkg. . . . 41.0

Sloppy joe sauce, see "Sandwich sauce"

Smelt, rainbow, without added ingredients 0

Snack bar (see also "Cookie" and "Granola and cereal

    bar"), 1 bar, except as noted:

(Figurines S'Mores Diet Bars), 2 bars 25.0

(Little Debbie Star Crunch) 44.0

blueberry *(Little Debbie Fruit Boosters)* 41.0

blueberry *(Sweet Rewards)* 29.0

brownie *(Sweet Rewards)* 22.0

brownie *(Sweet Success* Chewy) 23.0

chocolate *(Figurines* Diet Bars), 2 bars 24.0

chocolate caramel *(Figurines* Diet Bars), 2 bars 24.0

chocolate chip *(Sweet Success* Chewy) 23.0

chocolate peanut butter *(Figurines* Diet Bars), 2 bars 23.0

chocolate raspberry *(Sweet Success* Chewy) 23.0

fig *(Little Debbie Figaroos)* 45.0

peanut butter *(Sweet Success* Chewy) 23.0

strawberry *(Little Debbie Fruit Boosters)* 42.0

strawberry *(Sweet Rewards)* 29.0

vanilla *(Figurines* Diet Bars), 2 bars 25.0

Snack chips and crisps (see also specific listings), 1 oz.,

    except as noted:

(Zings Chips), 1.8-oz. bag 34.0

apple cinnamon *(Crunchwells Crumpet Chips)* 21.0

cheddar *(Old Dutch Multicrisps)* 20.0

hot and spicy *(Eden* Wasabi), 1.1 oz. 24.0

mixed *(Terra* Chips) 18.0

onion *(Funyons)* 18.0

onion, French *(Old Dutch Multicrisps)* 21.0

Parmesan garlic *(Crunchwells Crumpet Chips)* 20.0

raspberry *(Crunchwells Crumpet Chips)* 21.0

spicy barbecue *(Crunchwells Crumpet Chips)* 20.0

Snack mix:

(Cheez-It), ½ cup 19.0

(Chex Mix), ⅔ cup 22.0

(Chex Mix Bold n' Zesty), ½ cup 17.0

(Old Dutch Party Mix), ⅔ cup 19.0
(Pepperidge Farm Light Season), ½ cup 22.0
(Pepperidge Farm Goldfish), ½ cup 21.0
cheddar *(Chex Mix),* ⅔ cup 24.0
cheddar, zesty *(Pepperidge Farm Goldfish),* ½ cup 19.0
honey mustard and onion *(Pepperidge Farm),* ½ cup 19.0
nutty, extra *(Pepperidge Farm),* ½ cup 20.0
Snail, sea, see "Whelk"
Snapper, without added ingredients 0
Snow peas, see "Peas, edible-podded"
Snow pea sprouts *(Jonathan's),* 1 cup 8.0
Soft drinks, carbonated, 12 fl. oz., except as noted:
all varieties:
   (R.W. Knudsen Fruit TeaZer) 26.0
   except pineapple-cherry *(Shasta Plus)* 42.0
   sparkling *(Santa Cruz)* 38.0
amaretto almond *(After the Fall* Spritzer) 36.0
apple:
   (R.W. Knudsen Spritzer) 42.0
   (Welch's Sparkling) 56.0
   spiced *(Natural Brew)* 42.0
berry *(After the Fall* Berrymeister Spritzer) 40.0
berry *(Jeff's Berry Dream),* 9.5 fl. oz. 38.0
birch beer *(Canada Dry),* 8 fl. oz. 27.0
blackberry *(Clearly Canadian),* 8 fl. oz. 24.0
boysenberry *(R.W. Knudsen* Spritzer) 42.0
cafe mocha *(Natural Brew)* 34.0
(Canada Dry Cactus Cooler), 8 fl. oz. 27.0
(Canada Dry Hi-Spot), 8 fl. oz. 28.0
cherry:
   (After the Fall American Pie Spritzer) 35.0
   (Crush) 52.0
   (Sundrop) 46.0
   (Sunkist), 8 fl. oz. 35.0
   amaretto *(Natural Brew)* 40.0
   black *(After the Fall* Spritzer) 42.0
   black *(Canada Dry),* 8 fl. oz. 32.0
   black *(R.W. Knudsen* Spritzer) 42.0
   black *(Shasta)* 41.0
   French *(Snapple),* 8 fl. oz. 29.0
   spice *(Slice)* 40.0
   wild *(Canada Dry),* 8 fl. oz. 28.0

Soft drinks, cherry *(cont.)*
    wild *(Clearly Canadian)*, 8 fl. oz. 23.0
cherry-lime:
    (Slice) 43.0
    (Spree) 45.0
    rickey *(Snapple)*, 8 fl. oz. 27.0
chocolate *(Jeff's Chocolate Dream)*, 9.5 fl. oz. 45.0
citrus *(Canada Dry* Half & Half), 8 fl. oz. 27.0
citrus *(Sunkist)*, 8 fl. oz. 25.0
club soda:
    (Canada Dry) 0
    (Schweppes) 0
    (Shasta) 0
cola:
    (Canada Dry Jamaica), 8 fl. oz. 27.0
    (Coca-Cola Classic), 8 fl. oz. 27.0
    (Juice Fizz Cooler), 8 fl. oz. 28.0
    (Pepsi/Pepsi Caffeine Free) 41.0
    (Shasta) 42.0
    (Slice) 43.0
    (Spree) 42.0
cola, cherry:
    (R.W. Knudsen Spritzer) 42.0
    (Shasta) 43.0
    wild *(Pepsi)* 43.0
cola, ginseng *(Natural Brew)* 42.0
collins mixer *(Canada Dry)*, 8 fl. oz. 21.0
collins mixer *(Schweppes)*, 8 fl. oz. 25.0
cranberry:
    (After the Fall Tart 'n Sweet Spritzer) 40.0
    (R.W. Knudsen Spritzer) 45.0
    (Shasta) 44.0
cran-orange *(After the Fall* Tart 'n Sweet Spritzer) 40.0
cran-raspberry *(After the Fall* Tart 'n Sweet Spritzer) 40.0
cream/creme:
    (A&W), 8 fl. oz. 28.0
    (Hires) 48.0
    (IBC) 42.0
    (Mug) 48.0
    (Shasta) 47.0
    vanilla *(Canada Dry)*, 8 fl. oz. 30.0
    vanilla *(Crush)* 44.0

vanilla *(R.W. Knudsen* Spritzer) 35.0
vanilla *(Natural Brew)* 42.0
vanilla *(Snapple)*, 8 fl. oz. 33.0
(Doc Shasta) 39.0
(Dr Pepper) 40.0
(Dr. Slice) 39.0
fruit punch/blend:
  (Canada Dry Tahitian), 8 fl. oz. 36.0
  (Juice Fizz), 8 fl. oz. 32.0
  (Juice Fizz Wild Red), 8 fl. oz. 30.0
  (Shasta) 50.0
  (Slice) 50.0
  (Sunkist), 8 fl. oz. 33.0
  (Welch's Sparkling) 53.0
  tropical *(Juice Fizz)*, 8 fl. oz. 30.0
  tropical *(Spree)* 42.0
ginger ale:
  (After the Fall Nantucket) 35.0
  (Canada Dry), 8 fl. oz. 25.0
  (Canada Dry Golden), 8 fl. oz. 24.0
  (R.W. Knudsen Spritzer) 40.0
  (Natural Brew Outrageous) 42.0
  (Schweppes), 8 fl. oz. 22.0
  (Shasta) 32.0
ginger ale–cherry *(Canada Dry)*, 8 fl. oz. 27.0
ginger ale–cranberry *(After the Fall)* 35.0
ginger ale–cranberry *(Canada Dry)*, 8 fl. oz. 25.0
ginger ale–grape, dry *(Schweppes)*, 8 fl. oz. 25.0
ginger ale–lemon *(Canada Dry)*, 8 fl. oz. 25.0
ginger ale–raspberry *(After the Fall)* 36.0
ginger ale–raspberry *(Schweppes)*, 8 fl. oz. 26.0
ginger beer *(Goya)* 27.0
ginger beer *(Schweppes)*, 8 fl. oz. 25.0
grape:
  (After the Fall Concord Spritzer) 45.0
  (Canada Dry Concord), 8 fl. oz. 29.0
  (Crush) 52.0
  (Juice Fizz Purple Thunder), 8 fl. oz. 34.0
  (R.W. Knudsen Spritzer) 41.0
  (Schweppes), 8 fl. oz. 33.0
  (Shasta) 48.0
  (Slice) 51.0

Soft drinks, grape *(cont.)*
  (Welch's Sparkling) 51.0
grapefruit:
  (Schweppes), 8 fl. oz. 27.0
  (Shasta Ruby Red) 47.0
  (Spree) 41.0
  (Wink), 8 fl. oz. 31.0
  (Wink Diet), 8 fl. oz. 1.0
guava–passion fruit *(Shasta)* 45.0
kiwi-lime *(R.W. Knudsen* Spritzer) 40.0
kiwi-strawberry:
  (After the Fall Spritzer) 40.0
  (Shasta) 43.0
  (Snapple), 8 fl. oz. 33.0
lemon:
  bitter *(Schweppes)*, 8 fl. oz. 26.0
  sour *(Canada Dry)*, 8 fl. oz. 21.0
  sour *(Schweppes)*, 8 fl. oz. 26.0
  spicy *(After the Fall* Spritzer) 37.0
lemon-lime:
  (R.W. Knudsen Spritzer) 41.0
  (Schweppes), 8 fl. oz. 25.0
  (Slice) 40.0
  (Slice Diet) 1.0
  (Spree) 42.0
lemon-tangerine *(Spree)* 45.0
lemonade:
  (Country Time), 8 fl. oz. 26.0
  (Sunkist), 8 fl. oz. 30.0
  Jamaican *(R.W. Knudsen* Spritzer) 41.0
  kiwi berry *(Country Time)*, 8 fl. oz. 27.0
  raspberry *(Country Time)*, 8 fl. oz. 27.0
  tangerine *(Country Time)*, 8 fl. oz. 27.0
lime *(After the Fall* Caribbean Spritzer) 42.0
lime *(Canada Dry* Island), 8 fl. oz. 33.0
lime-lemon *(Shasta* Twist) 38.0
mandarin-lime *(R.W. Knudsen* Spritzer) 42.0
mandarin-lime *(Spree)* 42.0
mandarin-pineapple *(After the Fall* Spritzer) ... 37.0
mango *(After the Fall* Hawaiian Spritzer) 45.0
mango *(R.W. Knudsen* Fandango Spritzer) 45.0
mango-ginger *(After the Fall* Spritzer) 38.0

(Mountain Dew/Mountain Dew Caffeine Free) 46.0
orange:
    (After the Fall Icicle Spritzer) 42.0
    (After the Fall Zudachi Spritzer) 40.0
    (Canada Dry Sunripe), 8 fl. oz. 35.0
    (Crush) 52.0
    (Jeff's Orange Dream), 9.5 fl. oz. 38.0
    (Orangina), 10 fl. oz. 28.0
    (Shasta) 49.0
    (Sunkist), 8 fl. oz. 51.0
    (Welch's Sparkling) 51.0
    mandarin *(Slice)* 51.0
    mandarin *(Slice* Diet) 1.0
orange–passion fruit *(R.W. Knudsen* Spritzer) 40.0
passion fruit *(Snapple),* 8 fl. oz. 29.0
peach:
    (Canada Dry), 8 fl. oz. 30.0
    (R.W. Knudsen Spritzer) 37.0
    (Shasta) 43.0
    (Snapple Melba), 8 fl. oz. 31.0
    (Sunkist), 8 fl. oz. 30.0
    (Welch's Sparkling) 52.0
peach-vanilla *(After the Fall* Spritzer) 42.0
pear *(Kristian Regale* Swedish Sparkler), 8 fl. oz. 26.0
pineapple:
    (Canada Dry), 8 fl. oz. 26.0
    (Crush) 52.0
    (Shasta) 51.0
    (Slice) 51.0
    (Sunkist), 8 fl. oz. 35.0
    (Welch's Sparkling) 53.0
pineapple-cherry *(Shasta Plus)* 41.0
pineapple-orange *(Shasta)* 46.0
raspberry:
    (After the Fall Spritzer) 42.0
    (Snapple Royal), 8 fl. oz. 31.0
    creme *(Shasta)* 44.0
    red *(R.W. Knudsen* Spritzer) 42.0
red *(Shasta)* 43.0
red *(Slice)* 51.0
root beer:
    (A&W), 8 fl. oz. 20.0

Soft drinks, root beer *(cont.)*

(Hires)	46.0
(IBC)	42.0
(Mug)	43.0
(Shasta)	42.0
(Snapple Tru), 8 fl. oz.	42.0
(Spree)	42.0
seltzer, plain or flavored *(Canada Dry)*	0
seltzer, plain or flavored *(Schweppes)*	0
(7Up)	39.0
(7Up Cherry)	39.0
sour mixer *(Canada Dry)*, 8 fl. oz.	22.0
spritzer, see specific soda listings	

strawberry:

(After the Fall Twist O' Spritzer)	37.0
(Canada Dry California), 8 fl. oz.	27.0
(Clearly Canadian), 8 fl. oz.	19.0
(Crush)	46.0
(R.W. Knudsen Spritzer)	42.0
(Shasta)	46.0
(Slice)	47.0
(Sunkist), 8 fl. oz.	34.0
(Welch's Sparkling)	51.0
strawberry-peach *(Shasta)*	42.0
strawberry-vanilla *(After the Fall* Spritzer)	42.0
(Sundrop)	46.0

tangerine:

(Clearly Canadian), 8 fl. oz.	23.0
spritzer *(After the Fall)*	40.0
spritzer *(R.W. Knudsen)*	39.0

tonic:

(Canada Dry), 8 fl. oz.	24.0
(Schweppes), 8 fl. oz.	22.0
(Shasta)	42.0
with fruit flavors *(Schweppes)*, 8 fl. oz.	20.0
with lime *(Canada Dry)*, 8 fl. oz.	24.0
vanilla, see "cream," above	
vanilla bean *(After the Fall* Spritzer)	42.0
Vichy water *(Canada Dry)*	0

Sole:

fresh, without added ingredients	0
frozen *(Van de Kamp's* Natural), 4-oz. fillet	0

Sole entree, breaded, frozen, 1 fillet:
(Mrs. Paul's Premium) 16.0
(Van de Kamp's Light) 17.0
Sopressata *(Boar's Head Cinghiale Mini)*, 1 oz. . . . . <1.0
Sorbet (see also "Ice" and "Sherbet"), ½ cup:
banana-strawberry *(Häagen-Dazs)* 34.0
(Ben & Jerry's Doonesbury) 33.0
cherry cordial *(Edy's/Dreyer's Whole Fruit)* 38.0
chocolate *(Häagen-Dazs)* 30.0
chocolate *(Tofutti)* 16.0
coconut *(Sharon's)* 15.0
coffee *(Tofutti)* 19.0
cranberry-orange *(Ben & Jerry's)* 32.0
and cream, orange *(Häagen-Dazs)* 24.0
and cream, raspberry *(Häagen-Dazs)* 23.0
devil's food *(Ben & Jerry's)* 36.0
lemon:
    (Edy's/Dreyer's Whole Fruit) 36.0
    (Häagen-Dazs Zesty Lemon) 31.0
    (Tofutti) 22.0
mango *(Häagen-Dazs)* 30.0
mango-lime *(Ben & Jerry's)* 32.0
mango-orange *(Edy's/Dreyer's Whole Fruit)* 30.0
orange-peach-mango *(Tofutti)* 21.0
peach *(Edy's/Dreyer's Whole Fruit)* 33.0
peach, orchard *(Häagen-Dazs)* 35.0
piña colada *(Ben & Jerry's)* 33.0
purple passion *(Ben & Jerry's)* 33.0
raspberry:
    (Edy's/Dreyer's Whole Fruit) 33.0
    (Häagen-Dazs) 29.0
    (Tofutti) 21.0
strawberry:
    (Edy's/Dreyer's Whole Fruit) 31.0
    (Edy's/Dreyer's Whole Fruit No Sugar) 29.0
    (Häagen-Dazs) 33.0
    (Tofutti) 19.0
strawberry-kiwi *(Ben & Jerry's)* 36.0
Sorbet bar, 1 bar:
berry, wild *(Häagen-Dazs)* 22.0
chocolate *(Häagen-Dazs)* 20.0

Sorbet and yogurt bar, 1 bar:
banana and strawberry *(Häagen-Dazs)* 20.0
chocolate and cherry *(Häagen-Dazs)* 21.0
raspberry and vanilla *(Häagen-Dazs)* 20.0
Sorghum, whole-grain, 1 cup 143.3
Sorghum syrup:
½ cup 123.7
1 tbsp. 15.7
Sorrel, see "Dock"
Soup, canned, ready-to-serve, 1 cup, except as noted:
bean:
   (Grandma Brown's) 31.0
   black *(Goya)* 34.0
   black *(Progresso)* 30.0
   black, and vegetable *(Health Valley)* 24.0
   salsa *(Campbell's Home Cookin')* 31.0
bean with bacon *(Campbell's Microwave),* 10½ oz. 40.0
bean and ham:
   (Campbell's Chunky) 29.0
   (Campbell's Chunky), 11 oz. 42.0
   (Campbell's Home Cookin') 33.0
   (Healthy Choice) 31.0
   (Progresso) 25.0
beef:
   barley *(Progresso)* 13.0
   barley *(Progresso 99% Fat Free)* 20.0
   broth *(College Inn/College Inn Low Sodium)* 0
   broth *(Health Valley)* 0
   broth *(Swanson)* 2.0
   chowder, chunky *(Nalley),* 7½-oz. can 17.0
   minestrone *(Progresso)* 14.0
   noodle *(Progresso)* 15.0
   pasta *(Campbell's Chunky)* 18.0
   pasta *(Campbell's Chunky),* 10¾ oz. 23.0
   and potato *(Healthy Choice)* 16.0
   Stroganoff *(Campbell's Chunky),* 10¾ oz. 28.0
beef vegetable:
   (Progresso 99% Fat Free) 24.0
   country *(Campbell's Chunky)* 18.0
   country *(Campbell's Chunky),* 10¾ oz. 22.0
   and rotini *(Progresso)* 14.0
borscht *(Gold's)* 16.0

broccoli:
  carotene *(Health Valley)* 16.0
  cheddar *(Healthy Choice)* 22.0
  and shells *(Progresso* Pasta Soup) 13.0
cheddar potato, white *(Progresso* 99% Fat Free) 26.0
chicken:
  (Progresso Chickarina) 11.0
  barley *(Progresso)* 13.0
  broccoli cheese *(Campbell's* Chunky) 14.0
  broccoli cheese *(Campbell's* Chunky), 10¾ oz. 17.0
  hearty *(Healthy Choice)* 20.0
  minestrone *(Progresso)* 14.0
  rotisserie, seasoned *(Progresso)* 13.0
  with vegetables, hearty *(Campbell's* Chunky) 12.0
  with vegetables, hearty *(Campbell's* Chunky), 10¾ oz. . . 15.0
  with vegetables, homestyle *(Progresso)* 9.0
chicken, cream of *(Campbell's* Home Cookin') 8.0
chicken, cream of, with vegetables *(Healthy Choice)* 21.0
chicken broth:
  (Campbell's Low Sodium), 10¾ oz. 2.0
  (Campbell's Healthy Request) 1.0
  (College Inn/College Inn Less Sodium) 1.0
  (Health Valley) 0
  (Pritikin) 1.0
  (Progresso) 1.0
  (Swanson/Swanson Natural Goodness) 1.0
chicken chowder:
  (Nalley), 7½ oz. 15.0
  corn *(Campbell's* Chunky) 18.0
  corn *(Campbell's* Chunky), 10¾ oz. 22.0
  corn *(Healthy Choice)* 30.0
  mushroom *(Campbell's* Chunky) 15.0
chicken noodle:
  (Campbell's Chunky Classic) 16.0
  (Campbell's Chunky Classic), 10¾ oz. 20.0
  (Campbell's Home Cookin') 11.0
  (Campbell's Home Cookin'), 10¾ oz. 14.0
  (Campbell's Low Sodium), 7¼ oz. 10.0
  (Healthy Choice Old Fashioned) 19.0
  (Progresso) 7.0
  (Progresso 99% Fat Free) 12.0
  (Weight Watchers), 10½ oz. 25.0

Soup, canned, ready-to-serve, chicken noodle *(cont.)*
 chunky *(Campbell's* Microwave), 1 cont. 18.0
 hearty *(Campbell's Healthy Request)* 25.0
chicken pasta:
 (Campbell's Glass Jar) 14.0
 (Healthy Choice) 17.5
 (Pritikin) 18.0
 Alfredo *(Healthy Choice)* 17.5
 with mushroom *(Campbell's* Chunky) 10.0
 with mushroom *(Campbell's* Chunky), 10¾ oz. 13.0
chicken and penne, spicy *(Progresso* Pasta Soup) 14.0
chicken rice:
 (Campbell's Chunky) 18.0
 (Campbell's Home Cookin') 17.0
 (Campbell's Home Cookin'), 10¾ oz. 21.0
 (Campbell's Microwave), 10¾ oz. 20.0
 (Campbell's Healthy Request) 15.0
 (Healthy Choice) 19.0
 (Pritikin) 18.0
 (Weight Watchers), 10½ oz. 17.0
 with vegetables *(Progresso)* 11.0
 with vegetables *(Progresso* 99% Fat Free) 13.0
 wild rice *(Progresso)* 13.0
chicken and rotini *(Progresso* Pasta Soup) 8.0
chicken vegetable:
 (Campbell's Chunky) 12.0
 (Campbell's Home Cookin') 20.0
 (Campbell's Home Cookin'), 10¾ oz. 24.0
 (Progresso) 13.0
 hearty *(Campbell's Healthy Request)* 18.0
 spicy *(Campbell's* Chunky) 13.0
chili beef *(Healthy Choice)* 32.0
chili beef, with beans *(Campbell's* Chunky), 11 oz. 38.0
clam chowder, Manhattan:
 (Campbell's Chunky) 20.0
 (Progresso) 11.0
clam chowder, New England:
 (Campbell's Chunky) 21.0
 (Campbell's Chunky), 10¾ oz. 26.0
 (Campbell's Home Cookin') 16.0
 (Campbell's Healthy Request) 17.0
 (Healthy Choice) 23.0

(Nalley), 7½ oz. 14.0
(Progresso) 21.0
(Progresso 99% Fat Free) 22.0
clam and rotini chowder *(Progresso)* 21.0
corn, country, and vegetable *(Health Valley)* 17.0
egg flower *(Rice Road)* 15.0
escarole, in chicken broth *(Progresso)* 2.0
hot and sour *(Rice Road)* 15.0
Italian, carotene *(Health Valley* Fat Free) 19.0
lentil:
    (Healthy Choice) 27.5
    (Pritikin) 24.0
    (Progresso) 22.0
    (Progresso 99% Fat Free) 20.0
    and carrots *(Health Valley* Fat Free) 25.0
    savory *(Campbell's* Home Cookin') 24.0
    and shells *(Progresso* Pasta Soup) 23.0
macaroni and bean *(Progresso)* 23.0
meatballs and pasta pearls *(Progresso)* 13.0
minestrone:
    (Campbell's Chunky) 22.0
    (Campbell's Glass Jar) 23.0
    (Campbell's Home Cookin') 19.0
    (Healthy Choice) 24.0
    (Pritikin) 19.0
    (Progresso) 21.0
    (Progresso 99% Fat Free) 23.0
    (Weight Watchers), 10½ oz. 23.0
    hearty *(Campbell's Healthy Request)* 24.0
    Italian *(Health Valley)* 21.0
    Parmesan *(Progresso)* 16.0
    and shells *(Progresso* Pasta Soup) 20.0
    Tuscany *(Campbell's* Home Cookin') 21.0
mushroom, cream of:
    (Campbell's Glass Jar) 10.0
    (Campbell's Home Cookin') 9.0
    (Campbell's Low Sodium), 10¾ oz. 18.0
    (Healthy Choice) 14.0
    (Progresso) 12.0
mushroom chicken, creamy *(Progresso* 99% Fat Free) 12.0
mushroom rice, country *(Campbell's* Home Cookin') 16.0

Soup, canned, ready-to-serve *(cont.)*
pasta:
    Bolognese *(Health Valley Healthy Pasta)* 17.0
    cacciatore *(Health Valley Healthy Pasta)* 19.0
    Chinese *(Rice Road)* 12.0
    fagioli *(Health Valley Healthy Pasta)* 17.0
    primavera *(Health Valley Healthy Pasta)* 21.0
    Romano *(Health Valley Healthy Pasta)* 32.0
pea, split:
    (Campbell's Low Sodium), 10¾ oz. 38.0
    (Grandma Brown's) 31.0
    (Pritikin) 29.0
    (Progresso 99% Fat Free) 29.0
    and carrots *(Health Valley)* 17.0
    green *(Progresso)* 25.0
pea, split, with ham:
    (Campbell's Chunky) 27.0
    (Campbell's Chunky), 10¾ oz. 33.0
    (Campbell's Home Cookin') 30.0
    (Campbell's Healthy Request) 28.0
    (Healthy Choice) 26.0
    (Progresso) 20.0
penne, hearty, in chicken broth *(Progresso Pasta Soup)* . . . 14.0
penne, zesty *(Campbell's Healthy Request)* 17.0
pepper steak *(Campbell's Chunky)* 18.0
potato, with roasted garlic *(Campbell's Home Cookin')* 21.0
potato ham chowder *(Campbell's)* 16.0
potato ham chowder *(Campbell's Chunky)*, 10¾ oz. 20.0
sirloin burger, with vegetable *(Campbell's Chunky)* 20.0
sirloin burger, with vegetable *(Campbell's Chunky)*, 10¾ oz. 25.0
steak and potato *(Campbell's Chunky)* 20.0
steak and potato *(Campbell's Chunky)*, 10¾ oz. 24.0
tomato:
    (Campbell's Low Sodium), 10½ oz. 28.0
    garden *(Campbell's Home Cookin')*, 10¾ oz. 27.0
    garden *(Healthy Choice)* 19.0
    hearty, and rotini *(Progresso Pasta Soup)* 23.0
    tortellini *(Progresso Pasta Soup)* 13.0
    vegetable *(Campbell's Glass Jar)* 14.0
    vegetable *(Health Valley)* 17.0
    vegetable *(Progresso)* 15.0
    vegetable, garden *(Progresso 99% Fat Free)* 19.0

vegetable, with pasta *(Campbell's Healthy Request)* 22.0
tortellini, in chicken broth *(Progresso)* 10.0
tortellini, with chicken and vegetables *(Campbell's)*. 18.0
turkey with wild rice *(Healthy Choice)* 8.5
turkey with wild rice, vegetable *(Campbell's Healthy
    Request)* 17.0
vegetable:
    (Campbell's Chunky) 22.0
    (Campbell's Chunky), 10¾ oz. 28.0
    (Progresso) 15.0
    (Progresso 99% Fat Free) 13.0
    (Weight Watchers), 10½ oz. 27.0
    barley *(Health Valley* Fat Free) 19.0
    carotene *(Health Valley* Fat Free) 17.0
    country *(Campbell's* Home Cookin') 19.0
    country *(Campbell's* Home Cookin'), 10¾ oz. 26.0
    country *(Healthy Choice)*. 23.5
    5 bean *(Health Valley)* 32.0
    14 garden *(Health Valley* Fat Free) 17.0
    garden *(Healthy Choice)* 22.5
    harborside *(Campbell's* Home Cookin') 13.0
    hearty *(Campbell's Healthy Request)* 20.0
    hearty *(Pritikin)* 20.0
    hearty, with pasta *(Campbell's* Chunky) 21.0
    hearty, with rotini *(Progresso* Pasta Soup) 20.0
    Italian *(Campbell's* Home Cookin') 14.0
    and pasta *(Campbell's* Glass Jar) 21.0
    Southwestern *(Campbell's* Home Cookin') 24.0
    Southwestern, with black bean *(Campbell's Healthy
        Request)* 28.0
    vegetarian *(Pritikin)* 23.0
vegetable beef:
    (Campbell's Chunky) 17.0
    (Campbell's Chunky), 10¾ oz. 20.0
    (Campbell's Home Cookin') 18.0
    (Campbell's Home Cookin'), 10¾ oz. 22.0
    (Campbell's Low Sodium), 10¾ oz. 19.0
    (Campbell's Microwave), 1 cont. 26.0
    (Healthy Choice) 14.0
    hearty *(Campbell's Healthy Request)* 20.0
vegetable broth *(Pritikin)* 2.0
vegetable broth *(Swanson)*. 3.0

Soup, canned, condensed (see also "Soup, canned, semi-condensed"), undiluted, ½ cup:

asparagus, cream of *(Campbell's)* 11.0
bean:
   with bacon *(Campbell's)* 25.0
   with bacon *(Campbell's Healthy Request)* 26.0
   black *(Campbell's)* 19.0
beef:
   broth, double rich *(Campbell's)* 1.0
   consommé *(Campbell's)* 2.0
   noodle *(Campbell's)* 8.0
   with vegetables, barley *(Campbell's)* 11.0
broccoli:
   cream of *(Campbell's/Campbell's Healthy Request)* 9.0
   cream of *(Campbell's 98% Fat Free)* 12.0
   creamy *(Campbell's Healthy Request Creative Chef)* 11.0
   cheddar and onion *(Healthy Choice)* 15.0
   cheese *(Campbell's)* 9.0
   cheese *(Campbell's 98% Fat Free)* 11.0
celery, cream of:
   (Campbell's/Campbell's 98% Fat Free) 9.0
   (Campbell's Healthy Request) 11.0
   (Healthy Choice) 14.0
cheese, cheddar *(Campbell's)* 10.0
cheese, nacho *(Campbell's)* 11.0
chicken:
   alphabet, with vegetables *(Campbell's)* 11.0
   broth *(Campbell's)* 2.0
   cream of *(Campbell's)* 11.0
   cream of *(Campbell's 98% Fat Free)* 10.0
   cream of *(Campbell's Healthy Request)* 12.0
   cream of *(Campbell's Healthy Request Creative Chef)* ... 12.0
   cream of, and broccoli *(Campbell's)* 9.0
   cream of, and broccoli *(Campbell's Healthy Request)* ... 10.0
   cream of, roasted *(Healthy Choice)* 12.5
   dumplings *(Campbell's)* 10.0
   gumbo *(Campbell's)* 9.0
   mushroom, creamy *(Campbell's)* 9.0
   noodle *(Campbell's/Campbell's Healthy Request)* 9.0
   noodle *(Campbell's Homestyle)* 9.0
   noodle *(Campbell's Noodle O's)* 10.0
   noodle, creamy *(Campbell's)* 12.0

noodle, curly *(Campbell's)* 12.0
with rice *(Campbell's)* 9.0
with rice *(Campbell's Healthy Request)* 10.0
and stars *(Campbell's)* 9.0
vegetable *(Campbell's/Campbell's Healthy Request)* 10.0
vegetable, Southwestern *(Campbell's)* 18.0
white and wild rice *(Campbell's)* 9.0
chili beef with beans *(Campbell's)* 24.0
clam chowder:
  Manhattan *(Bookbinder's)* 12.0
  Manhattan *(Campbell's)* 12.0
  New England *(Bookbinder's)* 16.0
  New England *(Campbell's)* 15.0
  New England *(Doxsee)* 18.0
corn, golden *(Campbell's)* 20.0
crab bisque *(Bookbinder's)* 10.0
garlic, roasted, cream of *(Healthy Choice)* 13.0
lobster bisque *(Bookbinder's)* 10.0
minestrone *(Campbell's)* 16.0
minestrone *(Campbell's Healthy Request)* 17.0
mushroom:
  beefy *(Campbell's)* 6.0
  cream of *(Campbell's/Campbell's 98% Fat Free)* 9.0
  cream of *(Campbell's Healthy Request)* 10.0
  cream of *(Campbell's Healthy Request Creative Chef)* . . . 10.0
  cream of *(Healthy Choice)* 13.0
  golden *(Campbell's)* 10.0
noodle, double, chicken broth *(Campbell's)* 15.0
noodle and ground beef *(Campbell's)* 11.0
onion, cream of *(Campbell's)* 13.0
onion, French, with beef stock *(Campbell's)* 10.0
oyster stew *(Bookbinder's)* 8.0
oyster stew *(Campbell's)* 6.0
pea, green *(Campbell's)* 29.0
pea, split, with ham and bacon *(Campbell's)* 28.0
pepper, Mexican, cream of *(Campbell's)* 10.0
pepperpot *(Campbell's)* 9.0
potato, cream of *(Campbell's)* 14.0
potato, cream of *(Campbell's Healthy Request Creative Chef)* 14.0
Scotch broth *(Campbell's)* 9.0
seafood bisque *(Bookbinder's)* 9.0
shrimp, cream of *(Campbell's)* 8.0

Soup, canned, condensed *(cont.)*

shrimp bisque *(Bookbinder's)* 9.0
snapper *(Bookbinder's)* 11.0
tomato:
    (Campbell's/Campbell's Healthy Request) 18.0
    bisque *(Campbell's)* 24.0
    fiesta *(Campbell's)* 16.0
    garden, with herbs *(Healthy Choice)* 18.0
    with herbs *(Campbell's Healthy Request Creative Chef)* . . 20.0
    Italian, with basil, oregano *(Campbell's)* 23.0
    rice *(Campbell's Old Fashioned)* 23.0
turkey, noodle *(Campbell's)* 10.0
turkey vegetable *(Campbell's)* 11.0
vegetable:
    (Campbell's 10¾ oz.) 14.0
    (Campbell's 26¼ oz.) 15.0
    (Campbell's Old Fashioned) 10.0
    (Campbell's Healthy Request) 16.0
    beef *(Campbell's)* 10.0
    beef *(Campbell's Healthy Request)* 11.0
    California style *(Campbell's)* 10.0
    hearty, with pasta *(Campbell's)* 18.0
    hearty, with pasta *(Campbell's Healthy Request)* 16.0
    vegetarian *(Campbell's)* 14.0
won ton *(Campbell's)* 5.0

Soup, canned, semi-condensed, undiluted, ⅔ cup:

bacon, lettuce, tomato with chicken broth *(Pepperidge
    Farm)* 14.0
black bean with sherry *(Pepperidge Farm)* 19.0
broccoli, cream of *(Pepperidge Farm)* 11.0
chicken curry *(Pepperidge Farm)* 16.0
chicken with rice *(Pepperidge Farm)* 8.0
clam chowder, Manhattan *(Pepperidge Farm)* 12.0
clam chowder, New England *(Pepperidge Farm)* 13.0
consommé Madrilene *(Pepperidge Farm)* 6.0
corn chowder *(Pepperidge Farm)* 14.0
crab *(Pepperidge Farm)* 9.0
gazpacho *(Pepperidge Farm)* 12.0
hunter's, with turkey and beef *(Pepperidge Farm)* 9.0
lobster bisque *(Pepperidge Farm)* 12.0
minestrone *(Pepperidge Farm)* 12.0
mushroom, shiitake *(Pepperidge Farm)* 10.0

onion, French *(Pepperidge Farm)* 7.0
oyster stew *(Pepperidge Farm)* 12.0
pea, green, with ham *(Pepperidge Farm)* 28.0
vichyssoise *(Pepperidge Farm)* 11.0
watercress *(Pepperidge Farm)* 11.0
Soup, frozen, 7.5 oz., except as noted:
barley mushroom *(Tabatchnick/Tabatchnik No Salt)* 13.0
bean, Yankee *(Tabatchnick)* 27.0
broccoli, cream of *(Schwan's)* 16.0
broccoli, cream of *(Tabatchnick)* 12.0
cabbage *(Tabatchnick)* 14.0
cheddar vegetable, Wisconsin *(Tabatchnick)* 12.0
cheese, Wisconsin *(Schwan's)*, 1 cup 20.0
chicken with noodles and dumplings *(Tabatchnick)* 13.0
chicken with noodles and vegetables *(Tabatchnick)* 6.0
clam chowder, Boston *(Schwan's)*, 1 cup 19.0
corn chowder *(Tabatchnick)* 22.0
lentil, Tuscany *(Tabatchnick)* 25.0
minestrone *(Tabatchnick)* 27.0
pea *(Tabatchnick/Tabatchnick No Salt)* 31.0
potato, New England *(Tabatchnick)* 21.0
potato, old-fashioned *(Tabatchnick)* 16.0
spinach, cream of *(Tabatchnick)* 11.0
vegetable *(Tabatchnick/Tabatchnick No Salt)* 20.0
Soup base, bottled, 1 tsp.:
(Goya Recaito) 0
(Goya Sofrito) 1.0
Soup base mix, 1/8 pkg., except as noted:
beef, ground, vegetable *(Soup Starter)* 17.0
beef, ground, vegetable *(Soup Starter Quick Cook)*, 1/4 pkg. 17.0
beef barley vegetable *(Soup Starter)* 20.0
beef stew, hearty *(Soup Starter)*, 1/7 pkg. 17.0
beef vegetable *(Soup Starter)* 19.0
chicken noodle *(Soup Starter)* 17.0
chicken noodle *(Soup Starter Quick Cook)*, 1/4 pkg. 16.0
chicken and rice *(Soup Starter)* 14.0
chicken and rice *(Soup Starter Quick Cook)*, 1/4 pkg. 12.0
chicken vegetable *(Soup Starter)*, 1/7 pkg. 16.0
chicken with white and wild rice *(Soup Starter)* 15.0
Soup mix, dry, 1 pkg., except as noted:
barley, beef *(Buckeye Beans)*, 2 tbsp. 15.0
barley, better *(Aunt Patsy's Pantry)*, 2 tbsp. 17.0

Soup mix *(cont.)*
bean:
    (Bean Cuisine Bouillabaisse), 1 serving 18.0
    (Buckeye Beans), 3 tbsp. 19.0
    black *(Aunt Patsy's Pantry)*, ⅙ pkg. 36.0
    black *(Bean Cuisine* Island), 1 serving 24.0
    black *(Knorr* Cup) 36.0
    black *(Smart Soup)* 32.0
    black, hearty *(Fantastic)*, 2.2 oz. 39.0
    black, spicy, with couscous *(Health Valley)*, ⅓ cup 29.0
    black, zesty, with rice *(Health Valley)*, ⅓ cup 22.0
    5, hearty *(Fantastic)*, 2.3 oz. 43.0
    navy *(Aunt Patsy's Pantry)*, 3 tbsp. 21.0
    navy *(Knorr* Cup) 30.0
    pasta, see "pasta and beans," below
    rice, see "rice and beans," below
    vegetable *(Buckeye Beans)*, 3 tbsp. 18.0
    white *(Bean Cuisine* Provençal), 1 serving 19.0
bean and ham *(Hormel* Micro Cup) 28.0
beef vegetable *(Hormel* Micro Cup) 14.0
broccoli, cream of *(Knorr* Chef's), 2 tbsp. 9.0
broccoli-cheese:
    cheddar, creamy *(Fantastic)*, 1.5 oz. 23.0
    creamy *(Cup-a-Soup)* 9.0
    with ham *(Hormel* Micro Cup) 10.0
    and rice *(Uncle Ben's* Hearty) 26.0
chicken:
    broth *(Cup-a-Soup)* 3.0
    broth, with pasta *(Cup-a-Soup)* 8.0
    country, with pasta and herbs *(Lipton Soup Secrets*
      Kettle Style), ¼ cup or 1 cup* 18.0
    cream of *(Cup-a-Soup)* 12.0
    noodle *(Campbell's* Real Chicken Broth), 3 tbsp. 17.0
    noodle *(Campbell's* Soup and Recipe), 3 tbsp. 15.0
    noodle *(Cup-a-Soup)* 8.0
    noodle *(Hormel* Micro Cup) 12.0
    noodle, hearty *(Cup-a-Soup)* 10.0
    'n onion *(Lipton Soup Secrets* Kettle Style), ¼ cup
      or 1 cup* 24.0
    pasta and beans *(Lipton Soup Secrets* Kettle Style),
      ¼ cup or 1 cup* 19.0
    rice *(Hormel* Micro Cup) 17.0

rice *(Mrs. Grass)*, ¼ pkg. 15.0
thyme *(Aunt Patsy's Pantry)*, 2 tbsp. 20.0
thyme *(Buckeye Beans)*, 2 tbsp. 21.0
vegetable *(Smart Soup)* 24.0

chili:
    (Aunt Patsy's Pantry Cowgirl), 4 tbsp. 29.0
    black bean *(Aunt Patsy's Pantry)*, 3 tbsp. 20.0
    black bean *(Buckeye Beans)*, 3 tbsp. 26.0
    chicken *(Aunt Patsy's Pantry)*, 4 tbsp. 33.0
    chicken, white *(Buckeye Beans)*, ¼ cup 36.0
    hearty *(Fantastic Cha-Cha Cup)*, 2.4 oz. 37.0

clam chowder, New England *(Hormel Micro Cup)* 16.0
clam chowder, New England *(Knorr Chef's)*, 3 tbsp. 12.0

corn chowder:
    (Knorr Cup) 26.0
    (Smart Soup) 23.0
    and potato, creamy *(Fantastic)*, 1.7 oz. 34.0
    with tomatoes *(Health Valley)*, ½ cup 20.0

couscous:
    (Casbah Moroccan Stew Cup) 38.0
    black bean salsa *(Fantastic)*, 2.4 oz. 46.0
    cheddar, nacho *(Fantastic)*, 1.9 oz. 36.0
    corn, sweet *(Fantastic)*, 1.8 oz. 36.0
    with lentil *(Fantastic Only a Pinch)*, 2.3 oz. 47.0
    with lentil, hearty *(Fantastic)*, 2.3 oz. 44.0
    vegetable, Creole *(Fantastic)*, 2.1 oz. 41.0

herb:
    fiesta, with red pepper *(Lipton Recipe Secrets)*, 1⅓ tbsp.
       or 1 cup* 6.0
    fine *(Knorr Box)*, 2 tbsp. 13.0
    with garlic, savory *(Lipton Recipe Secrets)*, 1 tbsp. or
       1 cup* 6.0
    golden, with lemon *(Lipton Recipe Secrets)*, ½ tbsp. or
       1 cup* 7.0
    Italian, with tomato *(Lipton Recipe Secrets)*, 2 tbsp. or
       1 cup* 9.0

hot and sour *(Knorr Box)*, 2 tbsp. 8.0
leek *(Knorr Box)*, 2 tbsp. 9.0

lentil:
    (Smart Soup) 35.0
    with couscous *(Health Valley)*, ⅓ cup 28.0

Soup mix, lentil *(cont.)*
  hearty *(Fantastic)*, 2.3 oz. 41.0
  hearty *(Knorr* Cup) 42.0
  homestyle *(Lipton Soup Secrets* Kettle Style), ¼ cup or
    1 cup* 22.0
  red *(Aunt Patsy's Pantry)*, 2 tbsp. 15.0
minestrone:
  (Lipton Soup Secrets Kettle Style), ¼ cup or 1 cup* . . . 21.0
  (Smart Soup) 24.0
  hearty *(Fantastic)*, 1.5 oz. 29.0
  hearty *(Knorr* Cup) 28.0
mushroom:
  beefy *(Lipton Recipe Secrets)*, 1½ tbsp. 7.0
  creamy *(Cup-a-Soup)* 10.0
  creamy *(Fantastic)*, 1.2 oz. 24.0
noodle:
  (Nissin Top Ramen Damae/Oriental) 27.0
  (Nissin Top Ramen Low Fat Oriental) 31.0
  with chicken broth *(Mrs. Grass)*, ¼ pkg. 10.0
  chicken free *(Fantastic)*, 1.5 oz. 26.0
  extra *(Lipton Soup Secrets)*, 3 tbsp. or 1 cup* 15.0
  homestyle *(Borden)*, ¼ pkg. 11.0
  ring noodle *(Cup-a-Soup)* 9.0
noodle, beef:
  (Campbell's Baked Ramen), 1 pkg. 44.0
  (Campbell's Baked Ramen), ½ block 30.0
  (Campbell's/Sanwa Ramen), ½ block 26.0
  (Nissin Cup Noodles) 39.0
  (Nissin Cup Noodles Twin), 1.2 oz. 20.0
  (Nissin Top Ramen) 27.0
  (Nissin Top Ramen Low Fat) 31.0
  onion *(Nissin Cup Noodles)* 40.0
  spicy *(Nissin Top Ramen)* 27.0
noodle, chicken:
  (Campbell's Ramen) 43.0
  (Knorr Box), 2 tbsp. 17.0
  (Knorr Cup) 19.0
  (Lipton Soup Secrets Giggle Noodle), 2 tbsp. or 1 cup* 11.0
  (Lipton Soup Secrets Ring-O-Noodle), 2 tbsp. or 1 cup* 10.0
  (Nissin Cup Noodles) 39.0
  (Nissin Cup Noodles Twin), 1.2 oz. 20.0
  (Nissin Top Ramen) 27.0

(Nissin Top Ramen Low Fat) 31.0
(Sanwa Ramen Pride), ½ block 26.0
broth *(Lipton Soup Secrets)*, 2 tbsp. 9.0
broth *(Mrs. Grass)*, ¼ pkg. 10.0
with chicken meat *(Lipton Soup Secrets)*, 3 tbsp. or
    1 cup* 12.0
mushroom *(Nissin Cup Noodles)* 39.0
mushroom *(Nissin Top Ramen)* 27.0
regular or spicy *(Campbell's* Baked Ramen), ½ block . . . 30.0
sesame *(Nissin Top Ramen)* 27.0
spicy *(Campbell's/Sanwa* Ramen), ½ block 26.0
spicy *(Nissin Cup Noodles)* 38.0
spicy *(Nissin Cup Noodles* Twin), 1.2 oz. 20.0
with vegetables *(Health Valley)*, ⅓ cup 18.0
noodle, crab *(Nissin Cup Noodles)* 39.0
noodle, lobster *(Nissin Cup Noodles)* 40.0
noodle, Oriental:
    (Campbell's Ramen) 45.0
    (Campbell's Ramen), ½ block 30.0
    Sanwa Ramen), ½ block 26.0
noodle, pork:
    (Campbell's Ramen), ½ block 26.0
    (Nissin Cup Noodles) 39.0
    (Nissin Top Ramen) 27.0
noodle, shrimp:
    (Campbell's/Sanwa Ramen), ½ block 26.0
    (Nissin Cup Noodles) 39.0
    (Nissin Cup Noodles Twin), 1.2 oz. 20.0
    (Nissin Top Ramen) 27.0
    picante *(Nissin Cup Noodles)* 40.0
noodle, vegetable:
    beef *(Mrs. Grass)*, ¼ pkg. 11.0
    curry *(Fantastic)*, 1.5 oz. 28.0
    garden *(Nissin Cup Noodles)* 40.0
    miso *(Fantastic)*, 1.3 oz. 25.0
    tomato *(Fantastic)*, 1.5 oz. 40.0
onion:
    (Campbell's Soup and Recipe), 1 tbsp. 5.0
    (Knorr Box), 2 tbsp. 8.0
    (Lipton Recipe Secrets), 1 tbsp. or 1 cup* 4.0
    (Mrs. Grass Soup/Recipe), ¼ pkg. 6.0
    beefy *(Lipton Recipe Secrets)*, 1 tbsp. or 1 cup* 5.0

Soup mix, onion *(cont.)*

golden *(Lipton Recipe Secrets)*, 1⅔ tbsp. 10.0
onion-mushroom *(Lipton Recipe Secrets)*, 2 tbsp. or 1 cup* . 6.0
onion-mushroom *(Mrs. Grass Soup/Recipe)*, ¼ pkg. 10.0
oxtail *(Knorr Box)*, 2 tbsp. 9.0
pasta:

Italiano *(Health Valley Fat Free)*, ½ cup 31.0
marinara *(Health Valley Pasta Cup Fat Free)*, ½ cup . . . 20.0
Mediterranean *(Health Valley Pasta Cup Fat Free)*, ½ cup 20.0
Parmesan *(Health Valley Pasta Cup Fat Free)*, ½ cup . . . 20.0
spiral *(Lipton Soup Secrets)*, 3 tbsp. 12.0
pasta and beans:

(Bean Cuisine Ultima)*, 1 serving 22.0
(Casbah Pasta Fasul) 12.0
white bean *(Uncle Ben's* Hearty)*, ⅕ oz. 27.0
pea, green *(Cup-a-Soup)* 12.0
pea, snow, cream of *(Knorr* Chef's)*, 3 tbsp. 10.0
pea, split:

(Aunt Patsy's Pantry), 3 tbsp. 28.0
(Bean Cuisine Thick as Fog)*, 1 serving 21.0
(Buckeye Beans), 4 tbsp. 35.0
(Knorr Cup) 29.0
(Smart Soup) 28.0
with carrots *(Health Valley)*, ½ cup 25.0
hearty *(Fantastic)*, 2 oz. 35.0
potato:

with broccoli *(Health Valley)*, ⅓ cup 15.0
cheese, with ham *(Hormel* Micro Cup)* 16.0
leek *(Knorr Cup)* 24.0
leek *(Smart Soup)* 23.0
rice *(Casbah Thai Yum)* 30.0
rice and beans:

(Casbah La Fiesta)* 34.0
black *(Uncle Ben's* Hearty)* 28.0
Cajun *(Casbah* Jambalaya)* 27.0
Cajun *(Fantastic)*, 2.3 oz. 47.0
Caribbean *(Fantastic)*, 2.1 oz. 44.0
curry *(Fantastic)*, 2.3 oz. 46.0
Italian, northern *(Fantastic)*, 2.2 oz. 49.0
red *(Smart Soup)* 35.0
Spanish *(Fantastic* Only a Pinch)*, 2.2 oz. 49.0
Szechuan *(Fantastic)*, 1.9 oz. 41.0

Tex-Mex *(Fantastic)*, 2.4 oz. 53.0
spinach, cream of *(Knorr* Box), 2 tbsp. 9.0
tomato:
   (Cup-a-Soup) 20.0
   basil *(Knorr* Box), 2 tbsp. 14.0
   basil *(Uncle Ben's* Hearty) 18.0
   rice Parmesano *(Fantastic)*, 1.9 oz. 41.0
vegetable:
   (Knorr Box), 2 tbsp. 6.0
   (Lipton Recipe Secrets), 1⅔ tbsp. or 1 cup* 7.0
   (Mrs. Grass Soup/Recipe), ¼ pkg. 7.0
   barley, hearty *(Fantastic)*, 1.5 oz. 29.0
   beef *(Mrs. Grass)*, ¼ pkg. 11.0
   chicken flavor *(Cup-a-Soup)* 10.0
   chicken flavor *(Knorr* Cup) 19.0
   chicken flavor, creamy *(Cup-a-Soup)* 10.0
   spring *(Cup-a-Soup)* 8.0
   spring *(Knorr)*, 2 tbsp. 5.0
Sour cream, see "Cream, sour"
Sour cream dip mix *(Durkee)*, 2 tsp. 4.0
Soursop:
untrimmed, 1 lb. 51.2
1 medium, approx. 2.1 lb. 105.3
trimmed, ½ cup 18.9
Soy beverage, 8 fl. oz.:
(EdenSoy/EdenSoy Extra) 13.0
(Soy Moo Fat Free) 22.0
carob *(EdenSoy)* 23.0
vanilla *(EdenSoy/EdenSoy* Extra) 23.0
Soy beverage mix, ¼ cup:
(Loma Linda Soyagen All Purpose/No Sucrose) 12.0
carob *(Loma Linda Soyagen)* 13.0
Soy butter, mix *(Morningstar Farms/Natural Touch*
   SoyButter), 2 tbsp. 10.0
Soy flour:
(Arrowhead Mills), ½ cup 16.0
stirred, 1 cup:
   full-fat, raw 29.9
   full-fat, roasted 28.6
   defatted 38.4
   low-fat 33.4
Soy meal, defatted, raw, 1 cup 49.0

Soy milk, see "Soy beverage"
Soy protein, concentrate, 1 oz. 8.8
Soy sauce, 1 tbsp., except as noted:
(Chun King) 1.0
(Chun King Lite) 2.0
(House of Tsang), .5-oz. pkt. . . . . <1.0
(House of Tsang Light/Low Sodium) 0
(Just Rite) 1.0
(Kikkoman) 0
(Kikkoman Light) 1.0
(La Choy) 1.0
(La Choy Lite) 2.0
dark *(House of Tsang)* 1.0
ginger flavor *(House of Tsang)* 4.0
ginger flavor *(House of Tsang* Low Sodium) 2.0
hot *(Try Me Dragon Sauce),* 1 tsp. . . . . <1.0
mushroom flavor *(House of Tsang* Low Sodium) 2.0
tamari 1.0
tamari *(Eden* Domestic/Imported) 2.0
shoyu 1.5
shoyu *(Eden Natural/Organic)* 2.0
Soybean cake or curd, see "Tofu"
Soybean kernels, roasted, toasted:
1 oz. or 95 kernels 8.7
whole, 1 cup 33.0
Soybean sprouts *(Jonathan's),* 1 cup, 3 oz. 8.0
Soybeans, ½ cup, except as noted:
green:
   raw, in pods, 1 lb. 26.6
   raw, shelled 14.1
   boiled, drained 10.0
canned, black *(Eden* Organic) 9.0
dried:
   raw 28.1
   raw *(Arrowhead Mills),* ¼ cup 14.0
   boiled 8.5
   dry-roasted 28.1
   roasted 28.9
Soybeans, fermented, see "Miso" and "Natto"
Spaghetti, see "Pasta"
Spaghetti dinner, and meatballs, frozen *(Swanson),* 1 pkg. 36.0

Spaghetti dishes, mix:
with meat sauce *(Kraft* Dinner), 5.5 oz. 46.0
mild *(Kraft* American Dinner), 2 oz. 40.0
tangy *(Kraft* Italian Dinner), 2 oz. 38.0
Spaghetti entree, canned:
(Franco-American Garfield Pizzos), 1 cup 36.0
with beef *(Franco-American Garfield* Pizzos), 1 cup 31.0
with franks:
   (Franco-American SpaghettiO's), 1 cup 32.0
   (Van Camp's Weenee), 1 can 34.0
   rings *(Kid's Kitchen),* 7½ oz. 36.0
with meatballs:
   (Campbell's Superiore/Franco-American), 1 cup 35.0
   (Franco-American SpaghettiO's), 1 cup 31.0
   (Hormel Micro Cup), 7½ oz. 28.0
   (Libby's Diner), 7¾ oz. 27.0
   (Top Shelf), 10 oz. 35.0
   mini meatballs *(Kid's Kitchen),* 7½ oz. 28.0
   rings *(Kid's Kitchen),* 7½ oz. 35.0
rings *(Kid's Kitchen),* 7½ oz. 34.0
tomato-cheese sauce *(Franco-American),* 1 cup 41.0
tomato-cheese sauce *(Franco-American* SpaghettiO's), 1 cup 36.0
Spaghetti entree, freeze-dried, with meat, sauce *(Mountain*
   House), 1 cup 27.0
Spaghetti entree, frozen:
Bolognese *(Banquet),* 10.5 oz. 40.0
marinara:
   (The Budget Gourmet Value Classics), 9 oz. 59.0
   (Marie Callender's), 1 cup, 8 oz. 35.0
   (Weight Watchers), 9 oz. 46.0
with meat sauce:
   (The Budget Gourmet Special Selections), 10 oz. 50.0
   (Lean Cuisine), 11.5 oz. 51.0
   (Marie Callender's), 1 cup, 6.8 oz. 32.0
   (Morton), 8.5 oz. 30.0
   (Stouffer's), 10 oz. 46.0
   (Weight Watchers), 10 oz. 41.0
with meatballs *(Lean Cuisine),* 9.5 oz. 43.0
with meatballs *(Stouffer's),* 12⅝ oz. 56.0
and sauce, with seasoned beef *(Healthy Choice),* 10 oz. . . . 43.0
Spaghetti sauce, see "Pasta sauce"

Spaghetti squash:

raw, untrimmed, 1 lb. 22.3

raw, cubed, ½ cup 3.5

baked or boiled, drained, ½ cup 5.0

Spareribs, see "Pork" and "Pork, refrigerated"

Spearmint, dried *(McCormick)*, ¼ tsp. 1

Spelt flakes *(Arrowhead Mills)*, 1 cup 22.0

Spelt flour *(Arrowhead Mills)*, ¼ cup 24.0

Spinach:

fresh:

   raw, untrimmed, 1 lb. 11.4

   raw, chopped *(Dole)*, 1 cup, 2 oz. 2.0

   raw, chopped, ½ cup 1.0

   boiled, drained, ½ cup 3.4

canned, ½ cup:

   (Allens/Popeye) 7.0

   (Allens/Popeye Low Sodium) 4.0

   (Del Monte/Del Monte No Salt) 4.0

   (S&W) 4.0

   chopped *(Allens/Popeye/Sunshine)* 6.0

   with liquid 3.4

frozen (see also "Spinach dishes"):

   (Green Giant), ¾ cup 3.0

   (Green Giant Harvest Fresh), ½ cup 3.0

   leaf *(Seabrook)*, 1 cup 2.0

   leaf or chopped *(Birds Eye)*, ⅓ cup 3.0

   chopped *(Seabrook)*, ⅓ cup 2.0

   in butter sauce, cut *(Green Giant)*, ½ cup 5.0

Spinach, mustard:

raw, untrimmed, 1 lb. 16.5

raw, chopped, ½ cup 2.9

boiled, drained, chopped, ½ cup 2.5

Spinach, New Zealand:

raw, untrimmed, 1 lb. 8.2

raw, trimmed, 1 oz. or ½ cup chopped 7

boiled, drained, chopped, ½ cup 2.0

Spinach, vine, see "Vine spinach"

Spinach, water *(Frieda's* Ong Choy), 2 cups, 3 oz. 3.0

Spinach dip *(Marie's)*, 2 tbsp. 3.0

Spinach dishes, frozen:

creamed, ½ cup, except as noted:

   (Birds Eye) 7.0

(Green Giant) 10.0
(Schwan's) 6.0
(Seabrook) 10.0
(Stouffer's Side Dish), ½ of 9-oz. pkg. 8.0
(Tabatchnick), 7.5 oz. 8.0
Indian *(Deep* Palak Paneer), 5 oz. 7.0
soufflé *(Stouffer's* Side Dish), 4 oz. 9.0
Spinach salad, see "Salad, complete"
Spinach-feta pocket *(Amy's Pocketfuls)*, 4.5-oz. piece 27.0
Spiny lobster, meat only:
raw, 4 oz. 2.8
boiled or steamed, 2-lb. lobster with shell 5.1
boiled or steamed, 4 oz. 3.5
Split peas:
uncooked, ¼ cup:
   green *(Arrowhead Mills)* 31.0
   green *(Goya)* 27.0
   yellow *(Goya)* 28.0
boiled, ½ cup 20.7
Sports drinks, all flavors:
(All Sport), 8 fl. oz. 20.0
(Body Works), 12 fl. oz. 23.0
(Recharge), 8 fl. oz. 18.0
Spot, without added ingredients 0
Spring onion, see "Onion, green"
Sprouts (see also "Bean sprouts" and specific listings):
hot and spicy *(Jonathan's)*, 1 cup, 4 oz. 4.0
mixed:
   (Jonathan's Gourmet), 1 cup, 3 oz. 3.0
   (Shaw's), 2 oz. 0
   lentil, adzuki, and pea *(Jonathan's)*, 3 oz. 21.0
Squab, without added ingredients 0
Squash (see also specific squash listings), ½ cup:
canned *(Stokely)* 10.0
frozen *(Birds Eye)* 12.0
frozen *(Stilwell)* 2.0
Squid:
meat only, raw, 4 oz. 3.5
canned *(Goya)*, ⅓ can 1.0
canned, in juice *(Goya)*, ¼ cup 2.0
Star fruit, see "Carambola"
Steak, see "Beef"

Steak sandwich, see "Beef sandwich"
Steak sauce, 1 tbsp.:
(A.1.) 3.0
(A.1. Bold) 5.0
(A.1. Thick and Hearty) 6.0
(Alanna Irish) 4.0
(Heinz Traditional) 2.0
(Heinz 57) 4.0
(HP) 3.0
(Hunt's) 2.0
(Maull's) 5.0
(Texas Best) 4.0
(Trappey's Great American) 4.0
and burger *(Try Me Bullfighter)* 4.0
Caribbean style *(Tabasco)* 4.0
garlic peppercorn *(Lea & Perrins)* 6.0
New Orleans style *(Tabasco)* 2.0
New Orleans style *(Trappey's Chef-Magic)* 2.0
sweet, mild *(Maull's)* 4.0
sweet, spicy *(Lea & Perrins)* 6.0
Stir-fry entree, see "Entree mix, frozen" and specific entree
 listings
Stir-fry sauce (see also "Marinade," and specific listings),
 1 tbsp., except as noted:
(House of Tsang Classic) 4.0
(House of Tsang Saigon Sizzle) 8.0
(House of Tsang Szechuan Spicy) 4.0
(Ka•Me) 1.0
(Ken's Steak House) 5.0
(Kikkoman) 3.0
(Lawry's) 4.0
(S&W Oriental) 5.0
garlic and ginger *(Rice Road)* 3.0
honey *(Ken's Steak House)* 5.0
lemon *(Rice Road)* 4.0
mandarin soy *(La Choy)*, ½ cup 16.0
and marinade *(Mary Rose* Halu) 6.0
and rib, garlic *(Mi-Kee)* 10.0
sesame and ginger *(Rice Road)* 4.0
spicy *(La Choy* Szechwan), ½ cup 18.0
sweet and sour *(House of Tsang)* 8.0
sweet and sour, spicy *(La Choy)*, ½ cup 36.0

teriyaki *(La Choy),* ½ cup 22.0
teriyaki *(Rice Road)* 4.0
Stir-fry seasoning, teriyaki flavor *(Adolph's Meal Makers),*
　1 tbsp. 7.0
Stomach, pork, without added ingredients 0
Strawberry:
fresh:
　(Dole), 8 berries, 5.3 oz. 17.0
　untrimmed, 1 lb. 30.0
　trimmed, ½ cup 5.2
canned, ½ cup:
　in light syrup *(Oregon)* 23.0
　in heavy syrup 29.9
　whole, in syrup *(Comstock)* 33.0
dried *(Frieda's),* ½ cup, 1.4 oz. 34.0
frozen:
　unsweetened, ½ cup 6.8
　(Big Valley), ⅔ cup 12.0
　(Birds Eye), ½ cup 17.0
　(Schwan's), 1¼ cups 13.0
　(Stilwell), ⅔ cup 13.0
Strawberry drink:
(Capri Sun Cooler), 6.75 fl. oz. 26.0
(Farmer's Market), 8 fl. oz. 30.0
nectar *(Libby's/Kern's),* 11.5 fl. oz. 52.0
Strawberry drink blends, 8 fl. oz.:
banana:
　(R.W. Knudsen) 30.0
　cactus *(R.W. Knudsen)* 29.0
　nectar *(Kern's)* 36.0
guava *(R.W. Knudsen)* 27.0
guava *(Santa Cruz)* 24.0
kiwi *(R.W. Knudsen)* 30.0
melon *(Veryfine* Shivering Chillers) 29.0
orange banana *(Tree Top)* 29.0
Strawberry drink mix*, 8 fl. oz.:
(Kool-Aid) 25.0
(Kool-Aid with Sugar) 16.0
Strawberry juice, 8 fl. oz.:
(Veryfine Juice-Ups) 36.0
nectar *(R.W. Knudsen)* 30.0

Strawberry milk:
(Nestlé Quik), 1 cup 31.0
low-fat:
   (Nestlé Quik), 1 cup 32.0
   (Nestlé Quik Aseptic), 8-fl.-oz. cont. 35.0
   banana *(Nestlé Quik)*, 8 fl. oz. 31.0
shake *(Nestlé Killer)*, 14 oz. 62.0
shake *(Nestlé Quik)*, 9 oz. 40.0
Strawberry milk drink, canned, 10 fl. oz.:
(Sego) 37.0
(Sego Lite) 18.0
creme *(Carnation Instant Breakfast)* 35.0
Strawberry milk drink mix, dry:
(Nestlé Quik), 2 tbsp. 22.0
1 oz. 28.1
creme *(Carnation Instant Breakfast)*, 1 pkt. 28.0
creme *(Carnation Instant Breakfast* No Sugar), 1 pkt. 12.0
Strawberry syrup:
(Fox's No Cal), 2 tbsp. 0
(Hershey's), 2 tbsp. 26.0
(Knott's Berry Farm), 2 tbsp. 30.0
(R.W. Knudsen), ¼ cup 38.0
(S&W Reduced Calorie), ¼ cup 15.0
Strawberry topping, 2 tbsp.:
(Kraft) 29.0
(Mrs. Richardson's Fat Free) 18.0
(Smucker's) 26.0
Melba *(Dickinson's)* 23.0
String beans, see "Green beans"
Stroganoff gravy *(Pepperidge Farm)*, ¼ cup 4.0
Stroganoff mix (see also "Tofu dishes, mix"), vegetarian
   (Natural Touch), 4 tbsp. 10.0
Stroganoff sauce, beef *(Lawry's)*, 1 tbsp. 5.0
Stroganoff seasoning mix *(Durkee)*, ⅛ pkg. 3.0
Strudel, apple *(Entenmann's)*, ¼ strudel 44.0
Stuffing (see also "Stuffing mix"):
(Arnold Unspiced), 2 cups 50.0
apple and raisin *(Pepperidge Farm)*, ½ cup 27.0
Cajun rice *(Good Harvest)*, ½ cup 24.0
chicken, classic *(Pepperidge Farm)*, ½ cup 24.0
corn bread:
   (Arnold), 2 cups 49.0

  (Brownberry), 2 cups 51.0
  (Pepperidge Farm), ¾ cup 33.0
  honey pecan *(Pepperidge Farm)*, ½ cup 23.0
country style *(Pepperidge Farm)*, ¾ cup 27.0
cube *(Pepperidge Farm)*, ¾ cup 28.0
cube, bread, unseasoned *(Brownberry)*, 2 cups 51.0
garden and herb, country *(Pepperidge Farm)*, ½ cup 22.0
herb seasoned:
  (Arnold), 2 cups 48.0
  (Brownberry), 1 cup 41.0
  (Pepperidge Farm), ¾ cup 33.0
sage and onion:
  (Arnold), 2 cups 48.0
  (Brownberry 7 oz./14 oz.)*, 2 cups 49.0
  (Pepperidge Farm), ½ cup 49.0
Santa Fe *(Good Harvest)*, ½ cup 21.0
seasoned *(Arnold)*, 2 cups 49.0
sourdough, San Francisco *(Good Harvest)*, ½ cup 19.0
vegetable, harvest, and almond *(Pepperidge Farm)*, ½ cup 23.0
wild rice, mushroom *(Pepperidge Farm)*, ⅔ cup 22.0
wild rice, trio *(Good Harvest)*, ½ cup 27.0
Stuffing mix, ⅙ box dry, except as noted:
(Kellogg's Crouettes), 1 cup 25.0
for beef *(Stove Top)* 22.0
chicken flavor:
  (Stove Top) 20.0
  (Stove Top Lower Sodium)* 21.0
  (Stove Top Microwave)* 20.0
  with rice *(Rice-A-Roni)*, 1 cup* 20.0
corn bread:
  (Stove Top) 21.0
  homestyle *(Stove Top* Microwave)* 20.0
  with rice *(Rice-A-Roni)*, 1 cup* 21.0
herb *(Stove Top* Flexible Serve)*, 1 oz. 19.0
herb and butter *(Rice-A-Roni)*, 1 cup* 20.0
herbs, savory *(Stove Top)* 20.0
long grain and wild rice *(Stove Top)* 22.0
mushroom and onion *(Stove Top)* 20.0
for pork *(Stove Top)* 20.0
San Francisco style *(Stove Top)* 20.0
for turkey *(Stove Top)* 20.0
with wild rice *(Rice-A-Roni)*, 1 cup* 20.0

Sturgeon, without added ingredients 0
Subway, 1 serving:
sandwiches, deli style:
    bologna 38.0
    ham 37.0
    roast beef 38.0
    tuna 37.0
    tuna with lite mayo 38.0
    turkey breast, jumbo 38.0
cold submarines, 6":
    B.L.T. 44.0
    Classic Italian B.M.T. 45.0
    Classic Italian B.M.T. with lite mayo 45.0
    cold cut trio 46.0
    ham 45.0
    roast beef 45.0
    Subway Club 46.0
    Subway Seafood & Crab 45.0
    Subway Seafood & Crab with lite mayo 44.0
    tuna 44.0
    tuna with lite mayo 46.0
    turkey breast 46.0
    turkey breast & ham 46.0
    Veggie Delite 44.0
hot submarines, 6":
    chicken breast, roasted 47.0
    chicken taco sub 49.0
    meatball 51.0
    pizza sub 48.0
    steak and cheese 47.0
    Subway Melt 46.0
salads, without dressing:
    B.L.T. 10.0
    bread bowl 63.0
    chicken breast, roasted 13.0
    chicken taco 15.0
    Classic Italian B.M.T. 11.0
    cold cut trio 11.0
    meatball 16.0
    pizza 13.0
    roast beef 11.0
    steak and cheese 13.0

Subway Club 12.0
Subway Melt........................... 12.0
Subway Seafood & Crab 10.0
Subway Seafood & Crab with lite mayo 11.0
tuna 10.0
tuna with lite mayo 11.0
turkey breast 12.0
Veggie Delite.......................... 10.0

salad dressings, 1 tbsp.:
French 5.0
French, fat free 4.0
Italian, creamy 2.0
Italian, fat free 1.0
ranch 1.0
ranch, fat free 3.0
Thousand Island 2.0

sides and condiments:
bacon, 2 slices 0
cheese, 2 triangles 0
mayonnaise dressing, regular or lite, 1 tsp. 0
mustard, 2 tsp.......................... 1.0
olive oil blend, 1 tsp.................... 0
vinegar, 1 tsp.......................... 0

cookies, 1 piece:
chocolate, double, with Brazil nut 27.0
chocolate, white, with macadamias 28.0
chocolate chip, regular or with *M&M's* 29.0
chocolate chunk 29.0
oatmeal raisin 29.0
peanut butter 26.0
sugar 28.0

Succotash, ½ cup:
fresh, boiled, drained 23.4
canned:
cream-style corn 23.4
whole kernel corn 17.9
whole kernel corn *(S&W)* 19.0
whole kernel corn *(Seneca)* 18.0
whole kernel corn *(Stokely)* 14.0
frozen, boiled, drained 17.0
Sucker, without added ingredients 0

Sugar, beet or cane:
beet or cane, brown:
  1 oz. 27.6
  1 cup, not packed 141.0
  1 cup, packed 214.0
beet or cane, granulated:
  1 oz. 28.3
  1 cup 199.8
  1 tbsp. 12.0
  1 tsp. 4.0
beet or cane, powdered or confectioners':
  1 oz. 28.3
  1 cup, sifted 199.8
  1 tbsp., unsifted 12.0
  1 tsp. 4.0
cane *(Domino)*, ¼ cup, except as noted:
  brown, light or dark, 1 tsp. 4.0
  cube 3.0
  powdered 30.0
  powdered, lemon or strawberry flavored 27.0
  white, 1 tsp. or pkt. 4.0
Sugar, maple, 1 oz. 25.5
Sugar, substitute:
(Equal), 1 pkt. . . . . <1.0
(NutraSweet), 1 tsp. . . . . <1.0
(Sweet 'n Low), 1 pkt. 1.0
(Weight Watchers), 1 pkt. 1.0
Sugar apple:
untrimmed, 1 lb. 59.0
1 medium, 9.9 oz. 36.6
trimmed, ½ cup 29.6
Sugar loaf squash *(Frieda's)*, ¾ cup, 3 oz. 7.0
Sugar snap peas, see "Peas, edible-podded"
Summer sausage:
(Old Smokehouse), 1 oz. 1.0
(Oscar Mayer), 2 slices, 1.6 oz. 0
beef *(Oscar Mayer)*, 2 slices, 1.6 oz. 1.0
Summer squash *(Dole)*, ½ medium, 3.5 oz. 20.0
Sunburst squash, raw *(Frieda's)*, 1 oz. 9
Sunchoke, see "Jerusalem artichoke"
Sunfish, pumpkinseed, without added ingredients 0

Sunflower seed:
(Frito-Lay), ⅓ cup 12.0
dried, kernels, 1 oz. 5.3
dried, in shell (Arrowhead Mills), 1 cup, 1.3 oz. edible 6.0
dry-roasted, in shell:
    (Planters), 3-oz. bag, 1.5 oz. edible 8.0
    (Planters), ¾ cup, 1 oz. edible 5.0
    (Planters Original), ¾ cup, 1 oz. edible 5.0
    (Planters Munch 'N Go), .75 oz. edible 4.0
dry-roasted, kernels (Planters), ¼ cup 6.0
dry-roasted, kernels, salted or unsalted, 1 oz. 6.8
honey-roasted, kernels (Planters), 1.7 oz. 15.0
oil-roasted, kernels:
    (Planters), 1.7 oz. 9.0
    (Planters), 2 oz. 11.0
    (Planters Munch 'N Go), ¼ cup 6.0
    salted or unsalted, 1 oz. 4.2
barbecued kernels (Planters), 1.7 oz. 10.0
barbecued kernels (Planters Munch 'N Go), 3 tbsp. 6.0
salted kernels (Planters), 1 oz. 5.0
tamari-roasted (Eden), 1 oz. 9.0
toasted, kernels, 1 oz. 5.9
Sunflower seed butter:
(Roaster Fresh), 1 oz. 5.0
1 tbsp. 4.4
salted or unsalted, 1 oz. 7.8
Sunflower seed flour, partially defatted, 1 cup 28.7
Sunflower sprouts (Jonathan's), 1 cup 2.0
Surimi[1], 4 oz. 7.8
Swamp cabbage:
raw:
    untrimmed, 1 lb. 11.0
    .6-oz. shoot 4
    trimmed, 1 oz. or ½ cup chopped 9
boiled, drained, chopped, ½ cup 1.8
Sweet dumpling squash (Frieda's), ¾ cup, 3 oz. 7.0
Sweet peas, see "Peas, green"
Sweet potato:
raw:
    (Dole), 1 medium, 4.6 oz. 33.0

---

[1] Processed from walleye (Alaska) pollock.

Sweet potato, raw *(cont.)*
    untrimmed, 1 lb. 79.3
    1 medium, 5″ × 2″ diam. 31.6
baked in skin, 1 medium 27.7
baked in skin, mashed, ½ cup 24.3
boiled without skin, 4 oz. 27.5
boiled without skin, mashed, ½ cup 39.8
Sweet potato, canned, ½ cup, except as noted:
(Seneca Yams) 34.0
in syrup, with liquid 23.9
in syrup, drained 24.9
whole *(Royal Prince/Trappey's)*, 4 pieces 48.0
halves *(Royal Prince)*, 3 pieces, 5.7 oz. 46.0
cut, vacuum pack 21.1
cut or pieces *(Allens/Sugary Sam/Princella* Yams), ⅔ cup .. 40.0
mashed *(Princella/Sugary Sam)*, ⅔ cup 28.0
mashed, vacuum pack 26.9
candied *(Royal Prince)* 50.0
candied *(S&W)* 46.0
orange-pineapple *(Royal Prince)* 43.0
Sweet potato, frozen, candied:
(Mrs. Paul's), 5 fl. oz. 73.0
(Mrs. Paul's Sweets'n Apples), 1¼ cups 66.0
(Ore-Ida), 5 pieces 40.0
baked, cubed, ½ cup 20.6
Sweet potato chips, 1 oz.:
plain *(Terra* Chips) 18.0
cinnamon *(Terra* Chips) 17.0
Sweet potato leaf:
raw, untrimmed, 1 lb. 27.2
raw, chopped, ½ cup 1.1
steamed, ½ cup 2.3
Sweet and sour dinner mix *(La Choy)*, ¼ pkg. 22.0
Sweet and sour drink mixer *(Holland House/Mr & Mrs T/*
    Rose's), 4 fl. oz. 23.0
Sweet and sour entree, see "Entree mix, frozen" and
    specific entree listings
Sweet and sour sauce, 2 tbsp., except as noted:
(Chun King) 14.0
(Contadina) 8.0
(House of Tsang) 7.0
(House of Tsang), .5-oz. pkt. 4.0

(Ka•Me) 13.0
(Kikkoman) 9.0
(Kraft) 19.0
(La Choy) 14.0
(Sauceworks) 14.0
(Woody's) 17.0
(World Harbors Maui Mountain) 14.0
concentrate *(House of Tsang)*, 1 tsp. 3.0
chicken *(Gold's Dip'n Joy)*, 1 tbsp. 7.0
duck sauce:
   (Ka•Me) 20.0
   (La Choy) 15.0
   all varieties *(Gold's)* 14.0
Sweetbreads, see "Pancreas" and "Thymus"
Swiss chard:
raw:
   (Frieda's), 1 cup, 3 oz. 1.0
   untrimmed, 1 lb. 15.6
   chopped, ½ cup 7
boiled, drained, chopped, ½ cup 3.6
Swiss steak gravy mix *(Durkee)*, ¼ cup* 4.0
Swiss steak seasoning mix *(Durkee/French's* Roasting
   Bag), ⅑ pkg. 3.0
Swordfish:
fresh, without added ingredients 0
frozen, steaks *(Peter Pan)*, 4 oz. 0
Syrup, see specific listings
Szechuan entree, see "Entree mix, frozen" and specific
   entree listings
Szechwan sauce (see also "Stir-fry sauce"):
(Ka•Me), 1 tbsp. 2.0
cooking *(Kylin* Chili & Tomato), ¼ cup 11.0

T

FOOD AND MEASURE   **CARBOHYDRATE GRAMS**

Tabouli:
(Frieda's), ½ cup 17.0
salad (Cedar's Taboule), 2 tbsp. 3.0
Tabouli mix:
(Casbah), 1 oz. 20.0
(Fantastic), ¼ cup 26.0
Taco Bell, 1 serving:
breakfast items:
    burrito, bacon and egg 39.0
    burrito, country 26.0
    burrito, fiesta 25.0
    burrito, grande 43.0
    quesadilla, cheese 32.0
    quesadilla, with bacon or sausage 33.0
burritos:
    bacon cheeseburger 43.0
    bean 55.0
    big beef Burrito Supreme 52.0
    Burrito Supreme 50.0
    chicken 45.0
    chicken, light 41.0
    chicken Burrito Supreme 50.0
    chicken Burrito Supreme, light 52.0
    chicken club 43.0
    chili cheese 37.0
    7 layer 65.0
fajitas:
    chicken 49.0
    chicken Supreme 51.0
    steak 48.0
    steak Supreme 50.0
    veggie 51.0
    veggie Supreme 53.0
quesadilla, cheese 32.0
quesadilla, chicken 33.0

tacos and tostadas:

BLT soft taco	22.0
Double Decker Taco	37.0
Double Decker Taco Supreme	39.0
kid's soft taco, chicken	21.0
kid's soft taco, light chicken or roll-up	20.0
soft taco	20.0
soft taco, chicken	23.0
soft taco, chicken, light	21.0
soft taco, steak	18.0
soft *Taco Supreme*	22.0
taco	11.0
Taco Supreme	13.0
tostada	31.0

specialty items:

beef *MexiMelt*	21.0
cinnamon twists	19.0
Mexican pizza	41.0
Mexican rice	20.0
nachos	34.0
nachos *BellGrande*	83.0
nachos supreme, big beef	43.0
pintos 'n cheese	18.0
taco salad	62.0
taco salad without shell	29.0

sides and condiments:

cheese, cheddar	0
cheese, cheddar, nonfat	0
cheese, pepper jack	0
green sauce	1.0
guacamole	2.0
nacho cheese sauce	5.0
picante sauce	1.0
pico de gallo	1.0
red sauce	2.0
salsa	5.0
sour cream	1.0
sour cream, nonfat	2.0
taco sauce, hot or mild	0

Taco entree, frozen:

beef *(Schwan's Barquito),* 1 piece, 5 oz.	31.0
beef *(Schwan's Taquito),* 5 pieces, 5 oz.	44.0

Taco entree *(cont.)*

chicken *(Schwan's Taquito)*, 5 pieces, 5 oz. 41.0
mini, with cheese sauce *(Swanson Fun Feast)*, 1 pkg. 50.0
three meat *(Schwan's Barquito)*, 1 piece, 5 oz. 31.0

Taco John's, 1 serving:

burritos:
    bean 56.6
    beef 44.0
    combination 50.3
    meat and potato 53.0
    ranch 43.8
    smothered, platter 132.0
    super 53.0
chimichanga platter 127.0
enchilada platter, double 106.0
fajitas, chicken:
    burrito 45.1
    salad without dressing 44.3
    soft shell 20.5
Mexi Rolls with nacho cheese 71.7
nachos, super 72.1
sampler platter 156.0
Sierra chicken fillet sandwich 39.6
tacos:
    crispy 11.6
    kid's meal with crispy taco 53.8
    kid's meal with soft shell taco 63.7
    soft shell 22.6
    Taco Bravo 38.9
    taco burger 27.5
sides and condiments:
    beans, refried 52.6
    chili 19.0
    Mexican rice 39.9
    nachos 26.6
    nacho cheese 0
    Potato Oles 37.7
    Potato Oles, large 50.3
    Potato Oles, with nacho cheese 37.7
    salad dressing, house 2.9
    sour cream 1.0

desserts:

choco taco	38.0
churro	17.4
flauta, apple	18.8
flauta, cherry	26.7
flauta, cream cheese	26.5
Italian ice	19.0

Taco mix, dinner:

(Lawry's), ⅕ pkg.	19.0
(Old El Paso), 2 tacos*	21.0
(Pancho Villa), 2 tacos*	20.0
nacho cheese flavor *(Old El Paso One Skillet Mexican)*, 2 tacos*	55.0
salsa flavor *(Old El Paso One Skillet Mexican)*, 2 tacos*	57.0
soft *(Old El Paso)*, 2 tacos*	46.0
taco flavor *(Old El Paso One Skillet Mexican)*, 2 tacos*	53.0
vegetarian *(Natural Touch)*, 3 tbsp.	5.0

Taco sauce, 1 tbsp., except as noted:

(Chi-Chi's Thick & Chunky)	1.0
(Hunt's Manwich), ¼ cup	6.0
(Lawry's Chunky), 2 tbsp.	2.0
(Lawry's Sauce 'n Seasoner), 2 tbsp.	3.0
(Pancho Villa), 2 tbsp.	3.0
all varieties *(Old El Paso)*	1.0
green *(La Victoria)*	<1.0
red *(La Victoria)*	1.0

Taco seasoning *(Tone's)*, 2 tsp. 4.0

Taco seasoning mix:

(Durkee Pouch), ⅛ pkg.	2.0
(Durkee Pouch Family), 1/16 pkg.	2.0
(Lawry's), 1 tbsp.	5.0
(McCormick), 2 tsp.	3.0
(Old El Paso), 2 tsp.	0
(Old El Paso 40% Less Sodium), 2 tsp.	0
(Pancho Villa), 2 tsp.	5.0
chicken *(Lawry's)*, 2 tsp.	5.0
mild *(Durkee Pouch)*, ⅛ pkg.	3.0
salad *(Durkee Pouch)*, ⅙ pkg.	4.0
salad *(Lawry's)*, 1 tsp.	3.0

Taco shell:

(Gebhardt), 3 shells	19.0
(Lawry's), 2 shells	13.0

Taco shell *(cont.)*
(Lawry's Super Size), 2 shells 21.0
(Old El Paso Super), 2 shells 18.0
(Pancho Villa), 3 shells 19.0
(Rosarita), 3 shells 19.0
golden (Old El Paso), 3 shells 18.0
mini (Old El Paso), 7 shells 18.0
soft, see "Tortilla"
tostada:
   (Lawry's), 2 shells 13.0
   (Old El Paso), 3 shells 19.0
   (Rosarita), 2 shells 17.0
white corn (Chi-Chi's), 2 shells 22.0
white corn (Old El Paso), 3 shells 18.0
Tahini:
(Arrowhead Mills), 1 oz. 4.0
(Joyva), 2 tbsp. 2.0
(Krinos), 2 tbsp. 3.0
from unroasted kernels, 1 tbsp. 2.5
from roasted, toasted kernels, 1 tbsp. 3.2
Tahini sauce mix *(Casbah)*, 1 oz. 5.0
Tamale, canned:
(Derby), 3 pieces 21.0
(Gebhardt), 2 pieces 19.0
(Gebhardt Jumbo), 2 pieces 24.0
(Just Rite), 3 pieces 21.0
(Nalley), 3 pieces 25.0
(Van Camp's), 2 pieces 20.0
beef:
   (Hormel/Hormel Hot-Spicy), 3 pieces 20.0
   (Hormel), 7½-oz. can 20.0
   jumbo (Hormel), 2 pieces 18.0
chicken (Hormel), 3 pieces 23.0
in chile gravy (Old El Paso), 3 pieces 31.0
Tamale, frozen *(Goya)*, 1 piece 28.0
Tamale pie, Mexican, frozen *(Amy's)*, 8 oz. 41.0
Tamari, see "Soy sauce"
Tamarillo:
red (Frieda's), 2 pieces, 4¼ oz. 9.0
yellow (Frieda's), 2 pieces, 4¼ oz. 8.0

Tamarind:
fresh:
    (Frieda's Tamarindo), 1.1 oz. 19.0
    untrimmed, 1 lb. 96.4
    1 fruit, 3″ × 1″, .2 oz. 1.3
    pulp, ½ cup 37.5
frozen, chunks *(Goya),* ⅓ pkg. 15.0
Tamarind nectar, canned *(Goya),* 12 fl. oz. 59.0
Tandoori paste, mild *(Patak's),* 2 tbsp. 3.0
Tangerine:
fresh:
    (Dole), 2 fruits 19.0
    untrimmed, 1 lb. 36.6
    1 medium, 2⅜″ diam. 9.4
    sections, without membrane, ½ cup 10.9
canned:
    in juice, ½ cup 11.9
    in juice *(S&W* Mandarin), ⅔ cup 16.0
    in light syrup, ½ cup 20.4
    in light syrup *(Del Monte),* ½ cup 19.0
    in light syrup *(Dole),* ½ cup 19.0
    in light syrup *(S&W* Mandarin), ⅔ cup 23.0
    clementines, in light syrup *(Haddon House),* ½ cup 19.0
Tangerine juice, fresh, 8 fl. oz. 24.9
Tangerine juice beverage, frozen* *(Minute Maid),* 8 fl. oz. 30.0
Tangerine juice blend *(Dole* Mandarin), 8 fl. oz. 35.0
Tapenade, see "Tomato tapenade"
Tapioca, dry:
(Minute), 1½ tsp. 5.0
pearl, 1 oz. 25.1
Tapioca pudding, see "Pudding"
Tarama, see "Caviar"
Taramosalata, see "Caviar spread"
Taro:
raw, untrimmed, 1 lb. 103.2
raw, sliced, ½ cup 13.8
cooked *(Frieda's* Taro Root), 5 oz. 36.0
cooked, sliced, ½ cup 22.8
Taro, Tahitian:
raw, untrimmed, 1 lb. 31.3
raw, sliced, ½ cup 4.3
cooked, sliced, ½ cup 4.7

Taro chips:
1 oz.	19.3
½ cup	8.1
spiced *(Terra)*, 1 oz.	20.0

Taro leaf:
raw, untrimmed, 1 lb.	18.3
raw, ½ cup	.9
steamed, ½ cup	3.0

Taro shoots:
raw, untrimmed, 1 lb.	9.3
raw, sliced, ½ cup	1.0
cooked, sliced, ½ cup	2.0

Tarragon, dried:
(McCormick), ¼ tsp.	.1
ground, 1 tbsp.	2.4
ground, 1 tsp.	.8

Tart shell, see "Pastry shell"

Tartar sauce, 2 tbsp.:
(Bookbinder's)	4.0
(Hellmann's/Best Foods)	1.0
(Hellmann's/Best Foods Low Fat)	7.0
(Nalley)	1.0
(Sauceworks)	4.0
lemon herb flavor *(Sauceworks)*	<1.0

TCBY, ½ cup, except as noted:
nonfat yogurt:
apple pie alamode	27.0
banana split	25.0
cappuccino	26.0
chocolate, brown/white	26.0
chocolate sundae, chewy	28.0
peach cobbler	25.0
raspberry cheesecake	27.0
strawberry shortcake	26.0
vanilla caramel custard	29.0

soft-serve yogurt, all flavors:
regular	23.0
nonfat	23.0
nonfat, no sugar	20.0
sorbet, all flavors	24.0

Yog•A•Bar, 1 bar:
orange	18.0

raspberry swirl 18.0
vanilla, chocolate dipped 13.0
vanilla, with *Heath* toffee 22.0
vanilla, with toasted almonds 19.0
Tea (see also "Tea, iced"), 1 bag or 1 tbsp.:
plain, regular or instant, all varieties 0
black, all varieties *(Lipton Brisk/Lipton Iced Tea Brew)* 0
flavored, all varieties *(Lipton)* 0
green, plain or flavored *(Lipton)* 0
herbal, all varieties, except chamomile, iced collection, and
    lemon *(Lipton)* 0
herbal, chamomile, iced collection, or lemon *(Lipton)* . . . . . <1.0
Tea, iced, 8 fl. oz., except as noted:
(Lipton's Iced) 0
(Lipton's Iced Sweetened) 18.0
(Schweppes) 22.0
(Snapple) 18.0
(Veryfine Chillers) 19.0
all fruit flavors *(Apple & Eve)* 25.0
all fruit flavors, herbal *(R.W. Knudsen* Coolers) 23.0
Caribbean cooler *(Lipton Brisk)*, 12 fl. oz. 34.0
green tea and passion fruit *(Lipton's Iced)* 19.0
lemon/lemon flavor:
    (Lipton Brisk), 12 fl. oz. 33.0
    (Lipton Brisk Chilled Original/Sweetened) 20.0
    (Lipton's Iced) 21.0
    (Snapple) 25.0
    (Tropicana) 25.0
    (Veryfine Chillers) 23.0
    diet *(Lipton Brisk* Chilled) 0
    diet *(Lipton's Iced)* 0
    diet decaffeinated *(Lipton Brisk)*, 12 fl. oz. 1.0
    natural *(Lipton* Aseptic), 8.45 fl. oz. 25.0
and lemonade *(Lipton's Iced)* 26.0
mango *(Snapple)* 27.0
mint *(Snapple)* 29.0
passion fruit *(Snapple)* 27.0
peach:
    (Lipton Brisk Chilled) 20.0
    (Lipton's Iced) 26.0
    (Snapple) 26.0
    (Snapple), 11.5 fl. oz. 36.0

Tea, iced, peach *(cont.)*

    (Tropicana), 11.5 fl. oz.................................. 41.0

peach-kiwi *(Veryfine Chillers)* 18.0

raspberry:

    (Lipton Brisk Chilled) 20.0

    (Lipton's Iced) 26.0

    (Snapple) 26.0

    (Snapple), 11.5 fl. oz....................... 37.0

    (Tropicana), 11.5 fl. oz..................... 41.0

    (Veryfine Chillers) 24.0

    blast *(Lipton Brisk),* 12 fl. oz. 35.0

southern style:

    extra sweet *(Lipton's Iced)* 29.0

    lemon flavor *(Lipton's Iced)*................ 25.0

    sweetened *(Lipton's Iced)* 24.0

strawberry *(Snapple)*............................ 26.0

sweet *(Lipton Brisk* Chilled) 20.0

tangerine twist *(Lipton Brisk),* 12 fl. oz. 33.0

Tea, iced, mix, 1²/₃ tbsp., except as noted:

all varieties *(Lipton 100%),* 1½ tsp.................. 0

diet, all flavors *(Lipton/Lipton Natural Brew),* 1 tbsp. 1.0

lemon flavor:

    (Lipton/Lipton Decaffeinated/*Lipton Natural Brew)* 22.0

    (Lipton Envelopes), 1 envelope or 6 fl. oz.* 13.0

    (Lipton Natural Brew Unsweetened) .... <1.0

and lemonade *(Lipton Natural Brew)* 22.0

peach, raspberry, or tropical *(Lipton Natural Brew)* 22.0

Teff flour *(Arrowhead Mills),* 2 oz................. 41.0

Teff seed *(Arrowhead Mills),* 2 oz. 41.0

Tempeh:

1 oz. 4.8

½ cup 14.1

Tempura batter, mix *(Golden Dipt),* ¼ cup 15.0

Teriyaki entree (see also specific entree listings), frozen

    (Lean Cuisine Lunch Classics), 10 oz. 40.0

Teriyaki entree mix, see "Entree mix, frozen"

Teriyaki sauce, 1 tbsp., except as noted:

(Chun King) 3.0

(House of Tsang Korean Teriyaki) 6.0

(La Choy) 3.0

(Rice Road)................................... 4.0

barbecue *(Mary Rose Sumi)*...................... 7.0

baste and glaze *(Kikkoman)* 11.0
baste and glaze, with honey and pineapple *(Kikkoman)* 18.0
cooking, and marinade *(S&W/S&W Lite)* 5.0
hot:
    (Chun King) 3.0
    (La Choy) 3.0
    (Mountain Harbors Maui Mountain), 2 tbsp. 17.0
marinade *(Lawry's)* 5.0
marinade and:
    (Kikkoman) 2.0
    (Lea & Perrins) 4.0
    (World Harbors Maui Mountain), 2 tbsp. 17.0
    light *(Kikkoman)* 3.0
Teriyaki seasoning mix, beef *(Durkee)*, 1 tbsp. 6.0
Thai sauce *(World Harbors Nong Khai)*, 2 tbsp. 8.0
Thyme, dried: •
(McCormick), ¼ tsp. 2
ground, 1 tbsp. 2.6
ground, 1 tsp. 9
Thymus, beef or veal, without added ingredients 0
Tikka sauce, see "Curry sauce"
Tilefish, without added ingredients 0
Toaster muffins and pastries, 1 piece, except as noted:
apple *(Toaster Strudel)* 27.0
apple cinnamon *(Pop-Tarts)* 38.0
apple cinnamon *(Thomas' Toast-r-Cakes)* 18.0
banana nut *(Thomas' Toast-r-Cakes)* 16.0
blueberry:
    (Pop-Tarts) 36.0
    (Thomas' Toast-r-Cakes) 17.0
    (Toaster Strudel) 26.0
    frosted *(Pop-Tarts)* 37.0
    frosted *(Toastettes)* 35.0
brown sugar–cinnamon:
    (Pop-Tarts) 32.0
    frosted *(Pop-Tarts)* 34.0
    frosted *(Toastettes)* 35.0
cherry:
    (Pop-Tarts) 37.0
    (Toaster Strudel) 26.0
    frosted *(Pop-Tarts)* 37.0
    frosted *(Toastettes)* 35.0

Toaster muffins and pastries *(cont.)*

chocolate:

    (Pop-Tarts Minis), 1 pkt. 30.0

    fudge, frosted *(Pop-Tarts)* 37.0

    graham *(Pop-Tarts)* 36.0

chocolate-vanilla creme, frosted *(Pop-Tarts)* 37.0

cinnamon *(Toaster Strudel)* 26.0

corn *(Thomas' Toast-r-Cakes)* 19.0

cream cheese *(Toaster Strudel)* 23.0

cream cheese and blueberry, cherry, or strawberry *(Toaster
    Strudel)* 24.0

French toast style *(Toaster Strudel)* 28.0

fudge, frosted *(Toastettes)* 34.0

grape, frosted *(Pop-Tarts)* 38.0

grape, frosted *(Pop-Tarts Minis)*, 1 pkt. 32.0

raisin bran *(Thomas' Toast-r-Cakes)* 17.0

raspberry *(Toaster Strudel)* 26.0

raspberry, frosted *(Pop-Tarts)* 37.0

S'mores *(Pop-Tarts)* 37.0

strawberry:

    (Pop-Tarts Minis), 1 pkt. 37.0

    (Thomas' Toast-r-Cakes) 32.0

    (Toastettes) 35.0

    frosted *(Pop-Tarts)* 38.0

    frosted *(Toaster Strudel)* 26.0

    frosted *(Toastettes)* 35.0

Toffee baking bits *(Skor)*, 1 tbsp. 7.0

Tofu:

fresh:

    1 oz. 5

    ½ cup 2.3

    extra firm *(Nasoya)*, ⅕ of 1-lb. block 1.0

    firm, 1 oz. 1.2

    firm, ½ cup 5.4

    firm *(Frieda's)*, 3 oz. 2.0

    firm *(Nasoya)*, ⅕ of 1-lb. block 2.0

    silken *(Nasoya)*, ⅕ of 1-lb. block 2.0

    soft *(Nasoya)*, ⅙ of 1-lb. block 2.0

5-spice *(Nasoya)*, ¼ block 0

French *(Nasoya)*, ¼ block 0

fried, 1 oz. 3.0

okara, 1 oz. 3.6

okara, ½ cup 7.7
salted and fermented (fuyu), 1 oz. 1.5
Tofu dishes, mix, dry:
burger *(Fantastic* Classics), ⅛ cup 12.0
chow mein, Mandarin *(Fantastic* Classics), ⅝ cup 33.0
shells 'n curry *(Fantastic* Classics), ½ cup 40.0
Stroganoff, creamy *(Fantastic* Classics), ½ cup 35.0
Tofu seasoning mix, ¼ pkg., except as noted:
breakfast scramble *(Fantastic* Classics), 2½ tbsp. 12.0
breakfast scramble *(TofuMate)* 3.0
eggless *(TofuMate)* 3.0
Mandarin stir fry *(TofuMate)* 6.0
Mediterranean herb *(TofuMate)* 3.0
Szechwan stir fry *(TofuMate)* 3.0
Texas taco *(TofuMate)* 3.0
Tom Collins mixer, bottled *(Holland House)*, 3 fl. oz. 37.0
Tomatillo:
fresh, 1 medium, 1⅝″ diam. 2.0
fresh, chopped, ½ cup 3.8
in jars *(La Victoria* Entero), 5 pieces 7.0
in jars, crushed *(La Victoria)*, 4½ oz. 8.0
Tomato, ripe:
raw:
   (Dole), 1 medium, 3.5 oz. 7.0
   untrimmed, 1 lb. 19.2
   1 medium, 2⅗″ diam., 4¾ oz. 5.7
   chopped, ½ cup 4.2
boiled, ½ cup 7.0
dried, see "Tomato, dried"
Tomato, canned (see also "Tomato sauce"), ½ cup, except
  as noted:
(Contadina Pasta Ready) 5.0
(Contadina Recipe Ready) 5.0
whole:
   (Del Monte) 6.0
   Italian pear *(Contadina)*. 4.0
   Italian pear, with basil *(S&W)* 4.0
   pear *(Hunt's)* 4.0
   peeled *(Contadina)*. 4.0
   peeled *(Hunt's)*, 2 pieces 5.0
   peeled *(Hunt's* No Salt Added), 2 pieces 4.0
   peeled *(Progresso)*. 4.0

Tomato, canned, whole *(cont.)*
    peeled *(S&W/S&W No Salt)* 4.0
    with basil *(Progresso/Progresso Imported)* 4.0
    with green chilies *(Ro*Tel)* 4.0
aspic *(S&W)* 14.0
with cheeses, three *(Contadina Pasta Ready)* 8.0
chunky:
    chili *(Del Monte)* 8.0
    pasta *(Del Monte)* 11.0
    salsa *(Del Monte)* 8.0
crushed:
    (Contadina), 1/4 cup 4.0
    (Eden) 3.0
    (Progresso) 4.0
    (S&W), 1/4 cup 4.0
crushed or ground *(Hunt's)* 7.0
cut:
    (Hunt's Choice Cut) 5.0
    in juice *(S&W Ready-Cut/Ready-Cut No Salt)* 4.0
    in juice, Italian style *(S&W Ready-Cut)* 4.0
    in puree *(S&W Ready-Cut)* 6.0
    with Italian herb *(Hunt's Choice Cut)* 5.0
    with red pepper and basil *(Hunt's Choice Cut)* 6.0
    with roasted garlic *(Hunt's Choice Cut)* 5.0
diced:
    (Del Monte/Del Monte No Salt) 6.0
    (Eden Organic) 6.0
    in juice *(Hunt's)* 4.0
    in puree *(Hunt's)* 5.0
    with basil *(Master Choice)* 9.0
    with basil, garlic, and oregano *(Del Monte)* 11.0
    with onion and garlic *(Del Monte)* 7.0
with green chilies:
    (Eden Organic) 5.0
    (Hunt's Choice Cut), 2 tbsp. 0
    (Old El Paso), 1/4 cup 2.0
    whole or diced *(Ro*Tel)* 4.0
    diced *(Chi-Chi's)*, 1/4 cup 4.0
with jalapeños *(Old El Paso)*, 1/4 cup 2.0
with mushrooms *(Contadina Pasta Ready)* 9.0
with olives *(Contadina Pasta Ready)* 8.0
paste, see "Tomato paste"

primavera *(Contadina Pasta Ready)* 8.0
puree, see "Tomato puree"
with red pepper, crushed *(Contadina Pasta Ready)* 8.0
stewed:
    (Contadina) 8.3
    (Del Monte/Del Monte No Salt) 9.0
    (Green Giant Classic) 7.0
    (Hunt's/Hunt's No Salt Added) 7.0
    (S&W/S&W No-Salt) 7.0
    Cajun *(Del Monte)* 9.0
    Italian *(Contadina)* 8.0
    Italian *(Del Monte)* 8.0
    Italian *(Green Giant)* 7.0
    Italian *(S&W)* 7.0
    Mexican *(Contadina)* 9.0
    Mexican *(Del Monte)* 9.0
    Mexican *(Green Giant)* 7.0
wedges *(Del Monte)* 9.0
Tomato, dried:
(Frieda's No Salt), 1 oz. 21.2
1 oz. 15.8
1 piece, 32 pieces per cup 1.1
½ cup 15.1
bits *(Sonoma)*, 2–3 tsp. 3.0
flakes *(Christopher Ranch)*, 3 tbsp. 15.0
halves *(Sonoma)*, 2–3 pieces 3.0
julienne *(Sonoma)*, 7–9 strips 3.0
in oil, drained *(Sonoma Spice Medley)*, 1 tbsp. 3.0
pasta toss *(Sonoma)*, ½ cup 13.0
seasoning *(Sonoma Season It)*, 2–3 tsp. 3.0
Tomato, green, raw:
untrimmed, 1 lb. 21.1
2⅗″-diam. tomato 6.3
Tomato, green, pickled, 1 oz.:
(Claussen) 1.0
(Hebrew National/Shorr's) 1.0
half sour *(Rosoff)* 1.0
Tomato, sun-dried, see "Tomato, dried"
Tomato-chile cocktail:
(Snap-E-Tom), 6 oz. 8.0
(Snap-E-Tom), 10 oz. 13.0
Tomato chutney, see "Chutney"

Tomato dip, sun-dried *(Marie's)*, 2 tbsp. 2.0
Tomato juice, 8 fl. oz., except as noted:
(Campbell's/Campbell's Enhanced Flavor Low Sodium) 9.0
(Campbell's), 11.5 oz. 13.0
(Del Monte) 10.0
(Del Monte Not from Concentrate) 7.0
(Hunt's/Hunt's No Salt Added) 7.5
(R.W. Knudsen) 14.0
(S&W) 7.0
(Sacramento) 8.0
garlic *(R.W. Knudsen)* 13.0
Tomato paste, 2 tbsp.:
(Contadina) 6.0
(Del Monte) 7.0
(Goya) 6.0
(Hunt's/Hunt's No Salt Added) 6.0
(Progresso) 6.0
(S&W) 6.0
with garlic or Italian *(Hunt's)* 6.0
Italian *(Contadina)* 7.0
Tomato pesto, see "Pesto sauce"
Tomato powder *(AlpineAire)*, 2 oz. 22.0
Tomato puree, ¼ cup:
(Angelia Mia) 3.0
(Contadina) 4.0
(Hunt's) 5.0
(Progresso/Progresso Thick Style) 5.0
Tomato sauce, canned (see also "Pasta sauce" and
  "Tomato, canned"), ¼ cup, except as noted:
(Contadina) 4.0
(Contadina Thick & Zesty) 3.0
(Del Monte/Del Monte No Salt Added) 4.0
(Goya) 4.0
(Hunt's/Hunt's No Salt Added) 3.0
(Hunt's Special) 4.0
(Progresso) 4.0
(S&W) 4.0
chili, chunky *(Hunt's Ready Sauce)* 4.0
chunky *(Hunt's Ready Sauce)* 3.0
garden *(S&W* Original) 4.0
garden, Italian herb *(S&W)*, ½ cup 9.0
garden, mild Mexican *(S&W)* 4.0

garlic and herb *(Hunt's Ready Sauce)* 5.0
herb *(Hunt's)* 5.0
herb and garlic *(S&W Cooking Sauce)*, 1 tbsp. 0
Italian:
   (Contadina) 4.0
   (Hunt's) 5.0
   chunky *(Hunt's Ready Sauce)* 4.0
meat loaf *(Hunt's Ready Sauce Meatloaf Fixin's)* 4.0
Mexican, chunky *(Hunt's Ready Sauce)* 4.0
salsa, chunky *(Hunt's Ready Sauce)* 3.0
seasoned, lightly *(Eden)* 5.0
Tomato tapenade, dried *(Sonoma)*, 1 tbsp. 4.0
Tomato-beef cocktail *(Beefamato)*, 8 fl. oz. 20.0
Tomato-chile cocktail:
(Snap-E-Tom), 6 fl. oz. 8.0
(Snap-E-Tom), 10 fl. oz. 13.0
Tomato-clam cocktail, 8 fl. oz.:
(Clamato) 24.0
Caesar *(Clamato)* 24.0
Tongue:
beef, braised, 4 oz. 4
lamb, pork, or veal (calf), braised, without added ingredients . . 0
Tongue lunch meat, beef, corned *(Hebrew National)*, 2 oz. . . 0
Tortellini (see also "Tortelloni"), frozen or refrigerated:
cheese:
   (Contadina), ¾ cup 41.0
   (Di Giorno), ¾ cup 37.0
   (Schwan's), 1 cup 37.0
   three *(Contadina)*, ¾ cup 39.0
chicken *(Real Torino)*, 1 cup 49.0
chicken *(Schwan's)*, 1 cup 38.0
chicken, herb *(Contadina)*, ¾ cup 39.0
herb and garlic *(Real Torino)*, 1 cup 55.0
with meat *(Di Giorno)*, ¾ cup 40.0
spinach *(Contadina)*, ¾ cup 42.0
spinach *(Putney)*, 1 cup 49.0
tofu *(Soy-Boy)*, ⅞ cup 32.0
tofu *(Tofutti)*, 1 cup 54.0
Tortellini entree, canned, 1 cup, except as noted:
cheese *(Chef Boyardee)* 46.0
cheese *(Franco-American)* 44.0
ground beef *(Chef Boyardee)*, 7½ oz. 39.0

Tortellini entree, canned *(cont.)*
meat *(Chef Boyardee)* 48.0
meat *(Franco-American)* 36.0
Tortelloni, refrigerated, 1 cup, except as noted:
cheese, four *(Real Torino)* 44.0
cheese and basil *(Contadina)* 49.0
cheese and garlic *(Contadina)* 50.0
with chicken and herbs *(Di Giorno)* 40.0
chicken and prosciutto *(Contadina)* 46.0
hot red pepper and cheese *(Di Giorno)* 41.0
mozzarella garlic *(Di Giorno)* 40.0
mushroom *(Contadina)* 48.0
mushroom *(Di Giorno)* 42.0
pumpkin *(Tutta Pasta)*, 11 pieces, 3¼ oz. 36.0
sausage *(Contadina)* 48.0
tomato, dried *(Real Torino)* 44.0
Tortilla:
(Cedar's Boston), 1.1 oz. 18.0
(Cedar's Boston), 2.6 oz. 35.0
corn, white *(Goya)*, 2 pieces 26.0
flour, 1 piece:
    (Goya) 18.0
    (Mesa 6″) 15.0
    (Old El Paso) 24.0
    small *(Goya)* 14.0
    frozen *(Tyson)*, 1.9 oz. 30.0
    frozen *(Tyson)*, 1.4 oz. 21.0
    frozen *(Tyson* Heat Pressed), 2 oz. 30.0
    refrigerated *(Old El Paso)* 21.0
    refrigerated *(Old El Paso* Low Fat) 22.0
soft taco *(Old El Paso)*, 2 pieces 29.0
soft taco, refrigerated *(Old El Paso)*, 1 piece 17.0
Tortilla chips, see "Corn chips, puffs, and similar snacks"
Tortilla mix, flour *(Burris Light Crust)*, ⅓ cup 28.0
Tostaco or tostada shell, see "Taco shell"
Trail mix:
(Eden Fruit & Nuts), 1 oz. 10.0
(Sonoma), ¼ cup 24.0
California:
    (Dole), 1.2 oz. 23.0
    (Dole), 2 oz. 38.0
    (Eden Harvest), 1 oz. 14.0

Hawaiian *(Dole)*, 1.2 oz. 26.0
Hawaiian *(Dole)*, 2 oz. 44.0
Sierra:
   (Del Monte), .9 oz. 15.0
   (Del Monte), 1 oz. 16.0
   (Del Monte), ¼ cup 20.0
Tree fern, cooked:
1 frond, 6½″ long, 1.1 oz. 3.4
chopped, ½ cup 7.8
Triticale, whole-grain, 1 cup 138.5
Triticale flour, whole-grain, 1 cup 95.1
Tropical punch, see "Fruit drink blends" and "Fruit juice
  blends"
Trout, fresh or smoked, without added ingredients 0
Tuna:
fresh or frozen, without added ingredients 0
canned, in water or oil, 2 oz. 0
"Tuna," vegetarian, frozen *(Worthington Tuno)*, drained,
  ½ cup 2.0
Tuna casserole, frozen, noodle:
(Stouffer's), 10 oz. 37.0
(Swanson), 1 pkg. 38.0
(Weight Watchers), 9.5 oz. 39.0
Tuna entree mix, dry, except as noted:
au gratin *(Tuna Helper)*, ½ cup 33.0
au gratin *(Tuna Helper)*, 1 cup* 36.0
broccoli, creamy *(Tuna Helper)*, ⅔ cup 33.0
broccoli, creamy *(Tuna Helper)*, 1 cup* 35.0
cheddar, garden *(Tuna Helper)*, ⅔ cup 33.0
cheddar, garden *(Tuna Helper)*, 1 cup* 35.0
fettuccine Alfredo *(Tuna Helper)*, ¾ cup 30.0
fettuccine Alfredo *(Tuna Helper)*, 1 cup* 32.0
pasta, cheesy *(Tuna Helper)*, ¾ cup 29.0
pasta, cheesy *(Tuna Helper)*, 1 cup* 32.0
pasta, creamy *(Tuna Helper)*, ¾ cup 29.0
pasta, creamy *(Tuna Helper)*, 1 cup* 31.0
pasta salad *(Tuna Helper)*, ⅓ cup 25.0
pasta salad *(Tuna Helper)*, ⅔ cup* 26.0
pasta salad, low-fat recipe *(Tuna Helper)*, ⅔ cup* 46.0
potpie *(Tuna Helper)*, ½ cup 35.0
potpie *(Tuna Helper)*, 1 cup* 40.0
Romanoff *(Tuna Helper)*, ⅔ cup or 1 cup* 38.0

Tuna entree mix *(cont.)*
tetrazzini *(Tuna Helper)*, ⅔ cup 32.0
tetrazzini *(Tuna Helper)*, 1 cup* 33.0
Tuna spread:
(Underwood), ¼ cup 2.0
light or white, in water, with 6 crackers *(StarKist Lunch
    Kit)*, 1 pkg. 17.0
salad:
    (Bumble Bee), 2.75-oz. can 10.0
    (Libby's Spreadables), ⅓ cup 6.0
    with 6 crackers *(Bumble Bee)*, 2.75-oz. can 25.0
    with 6 crackers *(StarKist Tuna Salad)*, 1 can 25.0
Turban squash *(Frieda's)*, ¾ cup, 3 oz. 7.0
Turbot, without added ingredients 0
Turkey, without added ingredients 0
Turkey, canned, chunk, 2 oz., ¼ cup:
(Hormel) 0
(Swanson Premium*)* 2.0
white *(Hormel)* 0
white *(Swanson* Premium*)* 4.0
Turkey, frozen or refrigerated, 4 oz., except as noted:
all cuts, unseasoned:
    (Empire Kosher*)* 0
    (Hebrew National) 0
    (Norbest) 0
    (Perdue) 0
breast:
    raw, fillet, skinless and boneless *(Schwan's)*, 3 oz. 1.0
    honey roasted *(Louis Rich)*, 2.8-oz. slice 3.0
    oven roasted *(Louis Rich)*, 2.8-oz. slice 1.0
    smoked *(Hormel Light & Lean 97)*, 3 oz. 1.0
    smoked *(Louis Rich)*, 2.8-oz. slice 1.0
ground, see "Turkey, ground"
meatballs, Italian style *(Shady Brook Farms)*, 3 meatballs . . . 5.0
maple glaze *(Boar's Head Honey Coat)*, 3 oz. 3.0
Turkey, ground:
raw, 4 oz.:
    (Norbest) 0
    (Perdue) 0
    (Shady Brook Farms) 0
    all varieties *(Louis Rich)* 0
cooked, 4 oz. 0

cooked, all varieties *(Perdue)*, 3 oz. 0
"Turkey," vegetarian:
canned *(Worthington Turkee)*, 3 slices 3.0
frozen, smoked *(Worthington)*, 3 slices 3.0
Turkey bacon *(Louis Rich)*, .5-oz. slice 0
Turkey bologna:
(Empire), 3 slices 3.0
(Louis Rich), 1-oz. slice 1.0
(Norbest), 2 oz. 0
Turkey dinner, frozen:
breast:
    (Healthy Choice), 10.5 oz. 40.0
    with gravy *(Schwan's)*, 1 pkg. 40.0
    with pasta *(Swanson)*, 1 pkg. 31.0
    stuffed *(The Budget Gourmet)*, 11 oz. 34.0
mostly white meat *(Swanson)*, 1 pkg. 42.0
mostly white meat *(Swanson Hungry Man)*, 1 pkg. 59.0
and gravy, with dressing:
    (Banquet Extra Helping), 18.8 oz. 63.0
    (Freezer Queen Meal), 9.2 oz. 31.0
    (Marie Callender's), 14 oz. 51.0
roast *(Healthy Choice Country Inn)*, 10 oz. 29.0
Turkey entree, canned:
gravy and dressing *(Dinty Moore American Classics)*, 10 oz. 32.0
gravy and dressing *(Libby's Diner)*, 7 oz. 17.0
stew *(Dinty Moore)*, 1 cup 20.0
stew *(Dinty Moore)*, Cup), 7.5 oz. 17.0
Turkey entree, freeze-dried, tetrazzini *(Mountain House)*,
    1 cup 20.0
Turkey entree, frozen:
(Lean Cuisine Homestyle), 9⅜ oz. 27.0
breast, with gravy *(Schwan's)*, 4 oz. 1.0
breast, stuffed *(Weight Watchers)*, 9 oz. 28.0
croquettes, gravy and *(Freezer Queen Family)*, 1 patty and
    gravy, 4.65 oz. 13.0
glazed *(The Budget Gourmet Light)*, 9 oz. 38.0
glazed *(Lean Cuisine Cafe Classics)*, 9 oz. 36.0
and gravy, with dressing:
    (Banquet Homestyle), 9¼ oz. 31.0
    (Freezer Queen Deluxe Family), ¼ of 28-oz. pkg. 33.0
    (Freezer Queen Homestyle), 9 oz. 27.0
    (Swanson), 1 pkg. 30.0

Turkey entree, frozen *(cont.)*
gravy and:
 (Banquet Family), 2 slices, 4.8 oz. 5.0
 (Banquet Toppers), 5-oz. bag 7.0
 (Freezer Queen Family), 4.5 oz. 6.0
 with dressing *(Morton)*, 9 oz. 27.0
medallions *(Smart Ones)*, 8.5 oz. 34.0
pie or potpie:
 (Banquet), 7-oz. pie 38.0
 (Empire Kosher), 1 pkg. 46.0
 (Lean Cuisine), 9.5 oz. 38.0
 (Marie Callender's), 10-oz. pie 57.0
 (Marie Callender's), 1 cup, 8.5 oz. 52.0
 (Stouffer's), 10-oz. pie 36.0
 (Swanson), 1 pkg. 44.0
 (Swanson Hungry Man), 1 pkg. 65.0
 (Tyson), 8.9 oz. 51.0
roast:
 breast, and stuffing *(Lean Cuisine)*, 9¾ oz. 50.0
 with mushrooms *(Healthy Choice* Country), 8.5 oz. 28.0
 and stuffing *(Stouffer's* Homestyle), 9⅝ oz. 31.0
sliced, gravy and *(Freezer Queen* Cook-in-Pouch), 5-oz. pkg. . 6.0
tetrazzini *(Stouffer's)*, 10 oz. 33.0
and vegetables *(Healthy Choice* Hearty Handfuls), 6.1 oz. . . 51.0
Turkey fat 0
Turkey frankfurter, 1 link:
(Empire Kosher) . . . . <1.0
and beef *(Oscar Mayer* Fat Free) 2.0
and chicken:
 (Louis Rich 8 links, 12 oz.), 1.5 oz. 2.0
 (Louis Rich 10 links, 16 oz.), 1.6 oz. 2.0
 (Louis Rich Bun-Length) 3.0
 cheese *(Louis Rich)* 2.0
Turkey giblets:
simmered, 4 oz. 2.4
simmered, chopped or diced, 1 cup 3.0
Turkey gravy, ¼ cup:
(Franco-American) 3.0
roasted *(Heinz* Home Style) 3.0
seasoned, with turkey *(Pepperidge Farm)* 4.0
mix*:
 (Durkee/French's) 4.0

    (McCormick) 4.0
    roasted *(Knorr)* 4.0
Turkey ham, 2 oz., except as noted:
(Healthy Deli) 2.0
(Louis Rich), 1-oz. slice 0
(Louis Rich Chunk) 1.0
(Louis Rich Deli-Thin), 4 slices 1.0
canned *(Hormel)* 0
chopped *(Louis Rich),* 1-oz. slice 1.0
honey cured *(Louis Rich),* 1-oz. slice 1.0
Turkey hash, roast, canned *(Mary Kitchen),* 1 cup 23.0
Turkey lunch meat (see also "Turkey ham," etc.), breast,
    2 oz., except as noted:
(Boar's Head Premium Lower Sodium) . . . . <1.0
(Boar's Head Ovengold) 1.0
(Boar's Head Ovengold Skinless) 0
(Boar's Head Salsalito) 1.0
(Hormel Deli No Salt/Deli Premium) 0
(Hormel Light & Lean 97) 1.0
(Hormel Light & Lean 97), 1-oz. slice 0
(Hormel Sandwich Maker) 2.0
(Norbest Bronze Label/Silver Label) 2.0
(Norbest Gold Label/Gold Label Golden Browned) 0
barbecued *(Louis Rich)* 2.0
Black Forest *(Healthy Deli)* 1.0
cured *(Norbest* Gourmet) 0
honey roasted:
    (Healthy Deli) 3.0
    (Hormel Light & Lean 97) 1.0
    (Louis Rich) 3.0
    and white *(Louis Rich),* 1-oz. slice 1.0
lemon garlic *(Hebrew National),* 5 thin slices 0
maple honey *(Boar's Head)* 2.0
oven roasted:
    (Alpine Lace) 0
    (Boar's Head Golden/Golden Skinless) 0
    (Empire), 3 slices . . . . <1.0
    (Healthy Deli Gourmet/Gourmet Brick Oven) 1.0
    (Healthy Deli Less Sodium/Natural Shape) 1.0
    (Hebrew National), 5 thin slices 0
    (Louis Rich) 1.0
    (Louis Rich Fat Free), 1-oz. slice 1.0

Turkey lunch meat, oven roasted *(cont.)*

    (Louis Rich Carving Board Thin), 6 slices 1.0

    (Louis Rich Carving Board Traditional), 2 slices 0

    (Louis Rich Deli-Thin Fat Free), 4 slices 2.0

    (Oscar Mayer Fat Free), 4 slices 2.0

    glazed *(Healthy Deli* Gourmet) 1.0

    Italian *(Healthy Deli)* 4.0

    white *(Oscar Mayer)*, 1-oz. slice 2.0

    and white *(Louis Rich)*, 1-oz. slice 1.0

    and white *(Louis Rich* Chunk) 2.0

roast, and white *(Oscar Mayer Deli-Thin)*, 4 slices, 1.8 oz. . . . 2.0

rotisserie flavor *(Louis Rich)* 1.0

rotisserie flavor *(Louis Rich Carving Board)*, 2 slices 0

skinless *(Hormel)* 1.0

skinless *(Hormel* Deli) 0

smoked:

    (Boar's Head Hickory) . . . . <1.0

    (Boar's Head Cracked Pepper Mill) 0

    (Empire), 3 slices 0

    (Healthy Deli Mesquite) 1.0

    (Hebrew National), 5 thin slices 0

    (Hebrew National Hickory) 0

    (Hormel Mesquite) 1.0

    (Hormel Light & Lean 97 Mesquite), 1 oz. 0

    (Louis Rich Fat Free Hickory), 1-oz. slice 1.0

    (Louis Rich Hickory) 1.0

    (Louis Rich Carving Board), 2 slices 0

    (Louis Rich Deli-Thin Hickory), 4 slices 1.0

    (Norbest Gold Label) 0

    (Oscar Mayer Fat Free), 4 slices, 1.8 oz. 2.0

    white *(Louis Rich)*, 1-oz. slice 0

    white *(Oscar Mayer)* 1.0

    and white, honey roasted *(Oscar Mayer Deli-Thin)*,

        4 slices, 1.8 oz. 2.0

Turkey nuggets, breaded *(Louis Rich)*, 4 pieces, 3.25 oz. . . . 15.0

Turkey pastrami, 2 oz., except as noted:

(Boar's Head) 0

(Empire), 3 slices 0

(Healthy Deli) 2.0

(Hebrew National) 0

(Louis Rich), 1-oz. slice 0

(Louis Rich Chunk) 1.0

(Norbest) 0
Turkey patty, breaded, 1 piece:
(Empire Kosher) 14.0
(Louis Rich) 13.0
Turkey pie, see "Turkey entree"
Turkey salami:
(Empire), 3 slices 1.0
(Louis Rich), 1-oz. slice 0
(Louis Rich Chunk), 2 oz. 1.0
(Norbest), 2 oz. 2.0
cooked, 1 oz. 2
cotto *(Louis Rich)*, 1-oz. slice 0
Turkey sandwich, frozen:
with broccoli *(Mrs. Paterson's Aussie Pie)*, 1 piece 42.0
with broccoli and cheese *(Lean Pockets)*, 4.5-oz. piece 35.0
and ham with cheese:
    (Hot Pockets), 4.5-oz. piece 38.0
    (Lean Pockets), 4.5-oz. piece 37.0
    Swiss *(Croissant Pockets)*, 4.5-oz. piece 40.0
Turkey sausage, raw, except as noted:
(Shady Brook Farms Old World), 4 oz. 3.0
breakfast, raw *(Shady Brook Farms)*, 4 oz. 1.0
breakfast, raw or cooked *(Perdue)*, 2 links 0
Italian, hot or sweet:
    (Louis Rich), 2.5 oz. 1.0
    (Shady Brook Farms), 4 oz. 1.0
    raw or cooked *(Perdue)*, 1 link 1.0
smoked:
    (Louis Rich), 2 oz. 2.0
    (Louis Rich Polska), 2 oz. 1.0
    and duck, precooked *(Gerhard's Sausage)*, 2.5 oz. 2.0
Turkey seasoning, with gravy *(McCormick Bag 'n Season)*,
    1 tsp. 2.0
Turkey spread:
chunky *(Underwood)*, ¼ cup 2.0
salad *(Libby's Spreadables)*, ⅓ cup 6.0
Turkey sticks, breaded *(Louis Rich)*, 3 pieces 12.0
Turmeric, dried:
(McCormick), ¼ tsp. 4
ground, 1 tbsp. 4.4
ground, 1 tsp. 1.4

Turnip:
fresh or stored, ½ cup, except as noted:

 raw, untrimmed, 1 lb. 22.9
 raw, cubed 4.1
 boiled, drained, cubed 3.8
 ⚘ boiled, drained, mashed 5.6
frozen, boiled, drained, 4 oz. 4.9

Turnip greens:
fresh:

 raw, untrimmed, 1 lb. 18.2
 raw, chopped, ½ cup 1.6
 boiled, drained, chopped, ½ cup 3.1
canned, ½ cup:

 (Allens/Sunshine) 3.0
 (Stubb's Harvest) 3.0
 chopped, with diced turnips *(Allens/Sunshine)* 5.0
 with liquid 2.8
frozen, boiled, drained, with diced turnips, 4 oz. 3.3
frozen, with diced turnips *(Seabrook)*, ½ cup 2.0

Turnover, frozen or refrigerated, 1 piece, except as noted:
apple:

 (Pepperidge Farm) 48.0
 (Pillsbury), 2 pieces 46.0
 iced *(Pepperidge Farm)*. 53.0
 mini *(Pepperidge Farm)* 15.0
blueberry *(Pepperidge Farm)* 45.0
cherry:

 (Pepperidge Farm) 46.0
 (Pillsbury), 2 pieces 48.0
 iced *(Pepperidge Farm)*. 51.0
 mini *(Pepperidge Farm)* 16.0
peach *(Pepperidge Farm)* 47.0
peach cobbler, mini *(Pepperidge Farm)* 21.0
raspberry *(Pepperidge Farm)* 47.0
raspberry, iced *(Pepperidge Farm)*. 53.0
strawberry, mini *(Pepperidge Farm)*. 18.0
Tzatziki *(Western Creamy),* 2 tbsp. 1.0

V

FOOD AND MEASURE   **CARBOHYDRATE GRAMS**

Vanilla flavor drink:
canned, 10 fl. oz.:
(Sego) 37.0
(Sego Lite) 18.0
creme (Sweet Success) 38.0
French (Sego Lite) 18.0
mix, 1 pkt.:
creamy (Sweet Success) 20.0
French (Carnation Instant Breakfast) 27.0
French (Carnation Instant Breakfast No Sugar) 12.0
Vanilla shake:
(Nestlé Killer), 14 oz. 65.0
(Nestlé Quik), 9 oz. 42.0
Veal, without added ingredients 0
"Veal," vegetarian, frozen (Worthington Veelets), 1 patty   10.0
Veal parmigiana dinner, frozen:
(Freezer Queen Meal), 10.2 oz. 44.0
(Swanson), 1 pkg. 40.0
(Swanson Hungry Man), 1 pkg. 74.0
Veal parmigiana entree, frozen:
(Banquet), 9 oz. 35.0
(Freezer Queen Deluxe Family), 1 patty, 4.9 oz. 15.0
(Morton), 8.75 oz. 30.0
(Swanson), 1 pkg. 33.0
breaded, with tomato sauce (Freezer Queen Cook-in-Pouch),
  5 oz. 18.0
with spaghetti (Stouffer's Homestyle), 11⅞ oz. 49.0
patties (Banquet Family), 1 patty, 4.7 oz. 19.0
Vegetable antipasto, in jars (Paesana), 3¾ oz. 3.0
Vegetable burger, see "'Hamburger,' vegetarian"
Vegetable chips:
(Eden), 50 chips, 1.1 oz. 24.0
sea (Eden), 50 chips, 1.1 oz. 23.0
Vegetable dinner, frozen:
(Amy's Country), 11 oz. 60.0

Vegetable dinner *(cont.)*
loaf *(Amy's)*, 10 oz. 47.0
Vegetable dishes, frozen (see also specific listings),
samosa *(Deep* Indian Cuisine), 2 pieces 15.0
Vegetable entree, in jars, curry *(Patak's)*, ½ cup 18.0
Vegetable entree, frozen (see also "Vegetarian entree,
　　frozen"):
Chinese, and chicken *(The Budget Gourmet* Special
　　Selections), 9 oz. 42.0
chow mein *(La Choy)*, 1 cup, 9 oz. 20.0
country, and beef *(Lean Cuisine)*, 9 oz. 32.0
Italian, and chicken *(The Budget Gourmet* Special
　　Selections), 9 oz. 47.0
kofta curry *(Deep)*, 5 oz. 20.0
pilaf, Indian *(Deep)*, 1 cup 45.0
potpie:
　　(Amy's), 7.5 oz. 44.0
　　(Amy's Nondairy), 7.5 oz. 50.0
　　with beef *(Morton)*, 7 oz. 34.0
　　with cheese *(Banquet)*, 7-oz. pie 49.0
　　with chicken *(Morton)*, 7 oz. 18.0
　　with turkey *(Morton)*, 7 oz. 18.0
　　shepherd's pie, nondairy *(Amy's)*, 8 oz. 27.0
Szechuan style, and chicken *(The Budget Gourmet* Special
　　Selections), 10 oz. 46.0
Vegetable entree, mix, stew *(Knorr)*, 1 pkg. 32.0
Vegetable entree, mix, frozen, see "Entree mix, frozen"
Vegetable juice:
(V-8 Plus 100%), 5.5 fl. oz. 7.0
(V-8 Plus 100%), 8 fl. oz. 10.0
(V-8 Plus 100%), 10 fl. oz. 13.0
all flavors *(R.W. Knudsen Very Veggie)*, 8 fl. oz. 10.0
cocktail *(Hunt's)*, 5.5-oz. can 7.0
low sodium *(V-8)*, 5.5 fl. oz. 7.0
low sodium *(V-8)*, 8 fl. oz. 11.0
picante:
　　(V-8), 5.5 fl. oz. 7.0
　　(V-8), 8 fl. oz. 10.0
　　(V-8), 10.75 fl. oz. 13.0
　　(V-8), 11.5 fl. oz. 14.0
spicy hot:
　　(V-8 100%), 5.5 fl. oz. 7.0

(V-8 100%), 8 fl. oz. 10.0
(V-8 100%), 10.75 fl. oz. 13.0
(V-8 100%), 11.5 fl. oz. 15.0
tangy *(V-8* 100%), 8 fl. oz. 11.0
tangy *(V-8* 100%), 11.5 fl. oz. 16.0
Vegetable oyster, see "Salsify"
Vegetable pie, see "Vegetable entree"
Vegetable pocket (see also specific vegetable listings),
    frozen, 1 piece:
Bar-B-Q *(Ken & Robert's Veggie Pockets)* 45.0
Greek *(Ken & Robert's Veggie Pockets)* 37.0
Indian or Oriental *(Ken & Robert's Veggie Pockets)* 40.0
potpie *(Amy's Pocketfuls),* 5 oz. 37.0
potpie *(Ken & Robert's Veggie Pockets)* 38.0
Tex-Mex *(Ken & Robert's Veggie Pockets)* 46.0
Vegetables, see specific vegetable listings
Vegetables, mixed, fresh, 3 oz.:
California style *(Dole)* 5.0
garden style *(Dole)* 4.0
Italian style *(Dole)* 3.0
New England style *(Dole)* 9.0
Oriental style *(Dole)* 4.0
stir-fry *(Frieda's* Asian) 3.0
Vegetables, mixed, canned, ½ cup, except as noted:
(Del Monte/Del Monte No Salt) 8.0
(Goya) 7.0
(Green Giant) 12.0
(Green Giant Garden Medley) 9.0
(S&W) 7.0
(Seneca/Seneca No Salt) 9.0
(Stokely/Stokely No Salt) 7.0
Chinese *(La Choy* Fancy), ⅔ cup 1.0
chop suey *(La Choy)* 2.0
chow mein *(Chun King),* ⅔ cup 3.0
and sauce *(House of Tsang* Cantonese Classic) 14.0
and sauce, hot and spicy *(House of Tsang* Szechuan) 14.0
and sauce, sweet and sour *(House of Tsang* Hong Kong) . . 40.0
and sauce, teriyaki *(House of Tsang* Tokyo) 23.0
stew *(Seneca)* 9.0
stew *(Stokely)* 10.0
Vegetables, mixed, freeze-dried, ½ cup:
(AlpineAire) 16.0

Vegetables, mixed, freeze-dried *(cont.)*
garden *(AlpineAire)* 17.0
Vegetables, mixed, frozen:
(Birds Eye), ⅓ cup 12.0
(Goya), ⅔ cup 11.0
(Green Giant), ¾ cup 11.0
(Green Giant Harvest Fresh), ⅔ cup 10.0
(Stilwell), ½ cup 11.0
butter sauce *(Green Giant)*, ¾ cup 11.0
California *(Stilwell)*, ½ cup 4.0
Capri *(Stilwell)*, ½ cup 4.0
soup *(Birds Eye)*, ⅔ cup 9.0
stew *(Ore-Ida)*, ⅔ cup 11.0
stir-fry *(Schwan's)*, 1 cup 5.0
tropical:
    (Goya Pasteles de Masa)*, 1 pouch 21.0
    (Goya Viando Sancocho)*, 3 oz. . . . . , ... 23.0
    (Goya Yautia Malanga)*, ⅛ pkg. 30.0
Vegetables, mixed, pickled:
(Krinos Gardiniera)*, 3 oz. 0
(Zorba Gardiniera)*, ½ cup 2.0
Vegetarian burger, see " 'Hamburger,' vegetarian"
Vegetarian entree, canned (see also specific listings):
(Loma Linda Swiss Stake), 1 piece 8.0
(Worthington Numete), ⅜" slice 5.0
(Worthington Protose), ⅜" slice 5.0
choplet *(Worthington)*, 2 pieces 3.0
cutlet *(Worthington)*, 1 piece 3.0
cutlet, multigrain *(Worthington* 20 oz.)*, 2 pieces 5.0
cuts, dinner *(Loma Linda)*, 2 pieces 3.0
Vegetarian entree, frozen (see also "Vegetable entree,
    frozen" and specific listings):
(Worthington FriPats), 1 patty 4.0
(Worthington Stakelets), 1 piece 6.0
croquettes *(Worthington* Golden)*, 4 pieces 14.0
dinner entree *(Natural Touch)*, 3-oz. patty 2.0
fillets *(Worthington)*, 2 slices 8.0
nuggets, with rice *(Hain* Hawaiian)*, 10 oz. 55.0
roast, dinner *(Worthington)*, ¾" slice 5.0
Vegetarian entree, mix, dry, ⅓ cup:
dinner loaf *(Loma Linda)* 7.0
patty *(Loma Linda)* 7.0

Vegetarian foods, see specific listings
Venison, meat only, roasted, 4 oz. 0
Vienna sausage, canned:
(Goya), 4 links 1.0
(Hormel), 2 oz. 1.0
(Libby's), 3 links 1.0
with barbecue sauce *(Libby's* BBQ), 3 links 1.0
with hot sauce *(Goya),* 3 links 1.0
chicken *(Hormel),* 2 oz. 1.0
chicken *(Libby's),* 3 links 0
Vindaloo sauce, see "Curry sauce"
Vine spinach, raw, untrimmed, 1 lb. 15.4
Vinegar, 1 tbsp.:
all varieties:
    (Progresso) 0
    (Regina) 0
    (S&W) 0
balsamic *(Pastorelli Italian Chef)* 2.0
red wine *(Pastorelli Italian Chef)* 0
Vodka sour mixer, instant *(Bar-Tenders),* 2 pouches, 1.1 oz. 26.0

W

FOOD AND MEASURE	CARBOHYDRATE GRAMS

Waffle, frozen, 2 pieces, except as noted:
(Aunt Jemima Original) 29.0
(Aunt Jemima Low Fat) 33.0
(Belgian Chef), 1 piece 34.0
(Downyflake Homestyle) 26.0
(Downyflake Homestyle Low Fat) 34.0
(Eggo Homestyle) 30.0
(Eggo Minis Homestyle),* 3 sets 34.0
(Eggo Nutri-Grain) 30.0
(Eggo Special K) 29.0
(Schwan's), 4 pieces 40.0
apple cinnamon *(Downyflake)* 30.0
apple cinnamon *(Eggo)* 33.0
blueberry:
    (Aunt Jemima) 29.0
    (Downyflake) 30.0
    (Eggo) 33.0
    (Eggo Minis), 3 sets 37.0
buttermilk:
    (Aunt Jemima) 28.0
    (Downyflake) 26.0
    (Eggo) 30.0
cinnamon toast *(Eggo),* 3 sets 44.0
multibran *(Eggo Nutri-Grain)* 32.0
nut and honey *(Eggo)* 32.0
oat bran *(Eggo Common Sense)* 27.0
oat bran, with fruit and nut *(Eggo Common Sense)* 32.0
raisin and bran *(Eggo Nutri-Grain)* 36.0
strawberry *(Eggo)* 32.0
Waffle breakfast, frozen *(Swanson Kids Breakfast Blast),*
    1 pkg. 39.0
Waffle mix, see "Pancake mix"
Walnut, dried, shelled, except as noted:
(Paradise/Wild Swan), ¼ cup, 1 oz. 3.0

black:
　　(Planters), 2-oz. pkg. 8.0
　　in shell, 1 lb. 13.2
　　1 oz. 3.4
　　chopped, 1 cup 15.1
English or Persian:
　　in shell, 1 lb. 37.4
　　1 oz. 5.2
　　pieces, 1 cup 22.0
　　halves, 1 cup 18.3
halves *(Planters)*, 1/3 cup 5.0
halves *(Planters Gold Measure)*, 2-oz. pkg. 8.0
pieces *(Planters)*, 1/4 cup 4.0
Walnut topping, syrup *(Smucker's)*, 2 tbsp. 23.0
Wasabi chips *(Eden)*, 50 pieces, 1.1 oz. 24.0
Water chestnut, Chinese:
fresh:
　　(Frieda's), 1 tbsp., 1.1 oz. 7.0
　　untrimmed, 1 lb. 83.6
　　4 medium, 2″ diam., 1.7 oz. 8.6
　　sliced, 1/2 cup 14.8
canned:
　　4 medium or 1 oz. 3.5
　　with liquid, sliced, 1/2 cup 8.7
　　whole *(Chun King/La Choy)*, 2 pieces 2.0
　　sliced *(Chun King/La Choy)*, 2 tbsp. 3.0
　　sliced *(Sun Luck)*, 1/4 cup 4.0
　　chopped *(La Choy)*, 2 tbsp. 2.0
Watercress:
(Frieda's), 1 cup, 3 oz. 1.0
untrimmed, 1 lb. 5.4
10 sprigs, 11 1/4″ 3
chopped, 1/2 cup 2
Watermelon:
(Dole), 1/18 medium melon, 10 oz. 26.0
untrimmed, 1 lb. 16.9
1 slice, 10″ diam. × 1″ thick 34.6
diced, 1/2 cup 5.7
seedless *(Frieda's)*, 2 cups, approx. 10 oz. 23.0
Watermelon drink:
(Hi-C Watermelon Rapids Box), 8.45 fl. oz. 33.0
(R.W. Knudsen Cooler), 8 fl. oz. 29.0

Watermelon juice *(After the Fall)*, 8 fl. oz. 22.0
Watermelon seed, dried, 1 oz. 4.4
Wax beans, cut:
canned:
  (S&W), ½ cup 4.0
  (Seneca/Seneca No Salt), ½ cup 5.0
  (Stokely/Stokely No Salt), ½ cup 4.0
  golden *(Del Monte)*, ½ cup 4.0
frozen *(Seabrook)*, ⅔ cup 4.0
Wax gourd:
raw, untrimmed, 1 lb. 9.7
raw, cubed, ½ cup 2.0
boiled, drained, cubed, ½ cup 2.6
Welsh rarebit, frozen *(Stouffer's)*, 2.2 oz. 5.0
Wendy's, 1 serving:
sandwiches:
  bacon cheeseburger, Jr. 34.0
  Big Bacon Classic 46.0
  cheeseburger, Jr. 34.0
  cheeseburger deluxe, Jr. 36.0
  cheeseburger, Kid's Meal 33.0
  chicken, breaded 44.0
  chicken, grilled 35.0
  chicken, spicy 43.0
  chicken club 44.0
  hamburger, single, plain 31.0
  hamburger, single, with everything 37.0
  hamburger, Jr. 34.9
  hamburger, Kid's Meal 33.0
sandwich components:
  American cheese 1.0
  American cheese, Jr. 0
  bacon, 1 slice 0
  bun, kaiser 36.0
  bun, sandwich 29.0
  burger patty, ¼ lb. 0
  chicken patty, breaded 10.0
  chicken patty, grilled 0
  chicken patty, spicy 10.0
  honey mustard, reduced calorie, 1 tsp. 2.0
  ketchup, 1 tsp. 2.0
  lettuce, 1 leaf 0

   mayonnaise, 1½ tsp. 1.0
   mustard, ½ tsp. 0
   onion, 4 rings 1.0
   pickles, 4 slices 0
   tomato, 1 slice 1.0
chicken nuggets, 5 pieces 7.0
nuggets sauces, 1 oz.:
   barbecue 11.0
   honey mustard 6.0
   spicy buffalo wing 4.0
   sweet and sour 12.0
chili:
   small, 8 oz. 21.0
   large, 12 oz. 32.0
   cheddar cheese, shredded, 2 tbsp. 1.0
   saltine crackers, 2 pieces 4.0
baked potato:
   plain 71.0
   bacon and cheese 78.0
   broccoli and cheese 80.0
   cheese 78.0
   chili and cheese 83.0
   sour cream and chive 74.0
   sour cream, 1 pkt. 1.0
   whipped margarine, 1 pkt. 0
fries:
   small, 3.2 oz. 33.0
   medium, 4.6 oz. 47.0
   Biggie, 5.6 oz. 58.0
salads-to-go, fresh, without dressing:
   deluxe garden 10.0
   grilled chicken 10.0
   grilled chicken Caesar 17.0
   side salad 5.0
   side salad, Caesar 8.0
   taco salad 53.0
   soft breadstick, 1 piece 24.0
salad dressing, 2 tbsp., except as noted:
   blue cheese 0
   French 6.0
   French, fat free 8.0
   French, sweet red 9.0

Wendy's, salad dressing *(cont.)*

Italian, reduced fat and calorie	2.0
Italian Caesar	1.0
ranch, *Hidden Valley*	1.0
ranch, *Hidden Valley,* reduced fat and calorie	2.0
salad oil, 1 tbsp.	0
Thousand Island	3.0
wine vinegar, 1 tbsp.	0

Garden Spot salad bar:

applesauce, 2 tbsp.	7.0
bacon bits, 2 tbsp.	0
banana and strawberry glaze, ¼ cup	8.0
broccoli, ¼ cup	1.0
cantaloupe, 1 slice	4.0
carrots, ¼ cup	2.0
cauliflower, ¼ cup	1.0
cheese, shredded, imitation, 2 tbsp.	1.0
chicken salad, 2 tbsp.	2.0
chow mein noodles, ¼ cup	4.0
coleslaw, 2 tbsp.	5.0
cottage cheese, 2 tbsp.	1.0
croutons, 2 tbsp.	4.0
cucumbers, 2 slices	0
eggs, hard-cooked, 2 tbsp.	0
green peas, 2 tbsp.	3.0
green pepper, 2 pieces	1.0
honeydew, 1 slice	5.0
lettuce, 1 cup	2.0
mushrooms, ½ cup	1.0
orange, 2 slices	4.0
Parmesan blend, grated, 2 tbsp.	5.0
pasta salad, 2 tbsp.	3.0
peaches, 1 slice	4.0
pepperoni, 6 slices	0
pineapple chunks, 4 pieces	5.0
potato salad, 2 tbsp.	5.0
pudding, chocolate or vanilla, ¼ cup	10.0
red onion, 3 rings	1.0
seafood salad, ¼ cup	5.0
sesame breadstick, 1 piece	2.0
strawberries, 1 piece	2.0
sunflower seeds and raisins, 2 tbsp.	5.0

tomato wedges, 1 piece 1.0
turkey ham, diced, 2 tbsp.......................... 0
watermelon, 1 wedge 4.0
desserts:
  chocolate chip cookie, 1 piece 38.0
  Frosty, small 57.0
  Frosty, medium 76.0
  Frosty, large 95.0
Western-style entree, frozen *(Banquet* Country), 9.5 oz.... 28.0
Wheat, whole-grain, 1 cup, except as noted:
durum 136.6
hard red:
  spring 130.6
  winter *(Arrowhead Mills),* ¼ cup 34.0
  winter 136.7
soft red winter 124.7
hard white 145.7
soft white 126.6
Wheat, parboiled, see "Bulgur"
Wheat, sprouted, 1 cup 45.9
Wheat bran (see also "Cereal"):
(Arrowhead Mills), ¼ cup 7.0
(Shiloh Farms), ¼ cup 7.0
crude, 1 oz. 18.3
crude, 2 tbsp. 4.5
toasted *(Kretschmer),* ¼ cup 10.0
unprocessed *(Quaker),* ⅓ cup 11.0
Wheat flakes *(Arrowhead Mills),* ⅓ cup 24.0
Wheat flour, ¼ cup, except as noted:
(All Trump) 22.0
(Gladiola HD) 24.0
(La Pina) 23.0
(Wondra), 1 oz., approx. ¼ cup 22.0
all varieties *(Robin Hood)* 22.0
all-purpose, white:
  (Gold Medal) 22.0
  (Goya) 23.0
  (Red Brand) 23.0
  1 cup 95.4
  bleached *(Burris Light Crust/Dixie Lily/Gladiola/Light
    Crust/Omega/Martha White/Mother's Best)* 23.0
  bleached *(Pillsbury)* 23.0

Wheat flour, all-purpose, white *(cont.)*

unbleached *(Arrowhead Mills)*, ⅓ cup	33.0
unbleached *(Gold Medal)*	22.0
unbleached *(Pillsbury)*	21.0
unbleached, whole-grain *(Arrowhead Mills)*	24.0
bread, wheat blend *(Gold Medal)*	21.0
bread, white *(Gold Medal)*	22.0
bread, white *(Pillsbury)*	22.0
cake, white:	
(Betty Crocker Softasilk)	23.0
(Martha White)	23.0
(Swan's Down)	22.0
1 cup	85.1
gluten *(Arrowhead Mills)*, 3 tbsp.	15.0
gluten *(General Mills Supreme Hygluten)*	22.0
pastry, soft:	
white, unbleached *(Arrowhead Mills)*	23.0
whole grain *(Arrowhead Mills)*, ⅓ cup	22.0
presifted, white *(Pillsbury Shake & Blend)*	23.0
self-rising, white:	
(Gold Medal)	22.0
(Red Brand)	22.0
1 cup	92.8
bleached *(Dixie Lily/Gladiola/Hollyhock/Omega/Martha White/Mother's Best)*	23.0
bleached or unbleached *(Pillsbury)*	22.0
tortilla mix, 1 cup	74.5
whole-grain, 1 cup	87.1
whole-grain, stone ground *(Arrowhead Mills)*	25.0
whole wheat:	
(Gold Medal)	21.0
(Martha White)	24.0
(Pillsbury)	22.0
Wheat germ:	
(Kretschmer), 2 tbsp.	6.0
crude, 1 oz.	14.7
honey crunch *(Kretschmer)*, 1⅔ tbsp.	8.0
raw *(Arrowhead Mills)*, 3 tbsp.	10.0
toasted, 1 oz.	14.1
Wheat grass *(Pines)*, 3 servings	4.0
Wheat nuts *(Sonoma)*, 2 tbsp.	8.0
Wheat pilaf mix *(Near East)*, 1 cup*	42.0

Whelk, meat only, raw, 4 oz. 8.8
Whey:
acid, dry, 1 oz. 20.8
acid, fluid, 1 cup 12.6
sweet, dry, 1 oz. 21.1
sweet, fluid, 1 cup 12.6
Whipped topping, see "Cream topping"
Whiskey, see "Liquor"
Whiskey sour mixer:
bottled *(Holland House)*, 4 fl. oz. 34.0
bottled *(Mr & Mrs T)*, 4 fl. oz. 23.0
mix:
   (Bar-Tenders), 2 pkt. 30.0
   (Bar-Tenders Lite), 3 pkt. 2.0
   (Bar-Tenders Slightly Sour), 2 pkt. 28.0
White beans:
dried:
   uncooked, ¼ cup. 30.5
   uncooked, small, ¼ cup 33.6
   boiled, ½ cup 22.6
   boiled, small, ½ cup 23.2
canned, ½ cup:
   (Goya). 18.0
   (S&W Small) 19.0
   with liquid 28.7
   in tomato sauce *(Goya* Guisados) 19.0
White Castle, hamburger or cheeseburger, 2 pieces 23.0
White sauce mix:
(Knorr), ⅛ pkg. 4.0
1¾-oz. pkt. 25.1
Whitefish, fresh or smoked, without added ingredients 0
Whiting, without added ingredients 0
Wiener, see "Frankfurter"
Wild rice:
raw:
   (Fantastic), ¼ cup 28.0
   (Frieda's), ¼ cup 26.0
   1 oz. 21.2
cooked, 1 cup 35.0
blends, see "Rice"
Wild rice dishes, see "Rice dishes"

Wine, 1 fl. oz.:
dessert or aperitif[1] 2.3
dry or table[2] 1.2
Wine, cooking, 2 tbsp.:
(La Vina Gold/Red/White) 0
all varieties except Marsala, red, and sherry *(Holland House)* . . 0
Marsala *(Holland House)* 2.0
red *(Holland House)* 1.0
sherry *(Holland House)* 2.0
Wine cooler, 12-oz. bottle:
(Bartles & Jaymes Original) 29.0
berry *(Bartles & Jaymes)* 32.0
black cherry *(Bartles & Jaymes)* 31.0
Fuzzy Navel *(Bartles & Jaymes)* 41.0
Long Island iced tea *(Bartles & Jaymes)* 42.0
mai tai *(Bartles & Jaymes)* 41.0
Margarita *(Bartles & Jaymes)* 45.0
peach *(Bartles & Jaymes)* 34.0
piña colada *(Bartles & Jaymes)* 48.0
strawberry *(Bartles & Jaymes)* 32.0
strawberry daiquiri *(Bartles & Jaymes)* 36.0
tropical *(Bartles & Jaymes)* 37.0
Winged beans:
fresh:
    raw, untrimmed, 1 lb. 19.2
    raw, sliced, ½ cup 1.0
    boiled, drained, ½ cup 1.0
dried, uncooked, ½ cup 38.0
dried, boiled, ½ cup 12.8
Winged bean leaves, trimmed, 1 oz. 4.0
Winged bean tuber, trimmed, 1 oz. 8.0
Winter radish, see "Radish, black"
Wolffish, without added ingredients 0
Wonton wrapper:
(Frieda's), 4 pieces 17.0
(Nasoya), 5 pieces 18.0

[1]*Includes fortified wines containing more than 15% alcohol (port, sherry, vermouth, etc.).*
[2]*Includes wines containing less than 15% alcohol (red, white, or rosé; Burgundy, Chablis, champagne, etc.).*

Worcestershire sauce, 1 tsp.:
(French's) . . . . <1.0
(Lea & Perrins) 1.0
white wine (Lea & Perrins) 0
wine and pepper (Try Me) 1.0

Y

FOOD AND MEASURE	CARBOHYDRATE GRAMS

Yam:
raw, untrimmed, 1 lb. 108.8
raw, cubed, ½ cup 20.9
baked or boiled, ½ cup 18.8
canned or frozen, see "Sweet potato"
Yam, mountain, Hawaiian:
raw:
    untrimmed, 1 lb. 61.4
    1 medium, 8¼″ × 2½″ diam., 1.1 lb. 68.5
    cubed, ½ cup 11.1
steamed, cubed, ½ cup 14.4
Yam, name (Frieda's), 3 oz. 24.0
Yam bean tuber:
raw:
    (Frieda's Jicama), ¾ cup, 3 oz. 7.0
    untrimmed, 1 lb. 36.8
    sliced, ½ cup 5.3
boiled, drained, 4 oz. 10.0
Yard-long beans:
fresh:
    raw (Frieda's), ¾ cup, 3 oz. 7.0
    raw, untrimmed, 1 lb. 36.0
    raw, sliced, ½ cup 3.8
    boiled, drained, ½ cup 4.8
dried, raw, ½ cup 52.0
dried, boiled, ½ cup 18.1
Yeast, baker's, all varieties (Fleischmann's), ¼ tsp. 0
Yellow beans, dried:
uncooked, ¼ cup 29.8
boiled, ½ cup 22.2
Yellow-eye beans:
dried (Frieda's), ½ cup 22.0
canned, baked (B&M), ½ cup 30.0
Yellow squash:
fresh or frozen, see "Crookneck squash"

canned *(Allens/Sunshine)*, ½ cup 5.0
Yellowtail, without added ingredients 0
Yogurt:
plain:
    (Breyers), 8 oz. 15.0
    (Dannon Lowfat/Nonfat), 8 oz. 16.0
    (Dannon Lowfat/Nonfat 16/32 oz.), 1 cup 17.0
    (Friendship), 8 oz. 13.0
    (Ultimate 90), 8 oz. 14.0
    (Yoplait), 6 oz. 14.0
    (Yoplait Extra Creamy Non-Fat), 8 oz. 19.0
all flavors:
    (Colombo Light), 8 oz. 16.0
    (Dannon Natural Flavored), 8 oz. 36.0
    (Dannon Natural Flavored 16/32 oz.), 1 cup 39.0
    (Dannon Sprinkl'ins Magic Crystals), 4.1 oz. 21.0
    (Dannon Sprinkl'ins Rainbow Sprinkles), 4.1 oz. 24.0
    (Weight Watchers Nonfat), 8 oz. 14.0
    (Yoplait Custard Style), 6 oz. 32.0
    (Yoplait Light), 6 oz. 16.0
    except coconut cream pie *(Yoplait)*, 6 oz. 33.0
all fruit flavors:
    (Light n'Lively Free 50 Cal), 4.4 oz. 8.0
    (Yoplait/Yoplait Custard Style), 4 oz. 22.0
    (Yoplait Fat Free Fruit-on-the-Bottom), 6 oz. 34.0
    (Yoplait Trix), 6 oz. 28.0
    (Yoplait Trix), 4 oz. 19.0
    except banana-strawberry *(Colombo Fat Free)*, 8 oz. . . . 41.0
apple cinnamon *(Dannon Chunky Fruit)*, 6 oz. 33.0
apple cinnamon *(Dannon Fruit on Bottom)*, 8 oz. 46.0
apple crisp *(Yoplait Crunch 'n Yogurt Light)*, 7 oz. 24.0
apple crunch, caramel *(Dannon Light 'n Crunchy)*, 8 oz. . . . 26.0
banana *(Tropifruita)*, 6 oz. 30.0
banana cream pie *(Dannon Light)*, 8 oz. 15.0
banana creme/strawberry *(Dannon Double Delights)*, 6 oz. . . 32.0
banana-strawberry *(Colombo Fat Free)*, 8 oz. 45.0
Bavarian creme/raspberry *(Dannon Double Delights)*, 6 oz. . 34.0
berry, mixed:
    (Breyers), 8 oz. 48.0
    (Dannon Fruit on Bottom), 8 oz. 45.0
    (Dannon Fruit on Bottom), 4.4 oz. 25.0
    (Knudsen Free), 6 oz. 33.0

Yogurt, berry, mixed *(cont.)*

(*Light n'Lively Free*), 6 oz. 34.0

blueberry:

(*Breyers*), 8 oz. 48.0

(*Dannon* Chunky Fruit), 6 oz. 32.0

(*Dannon* Fruit on Bottom), 8 oz. 46.0

(*Dannon* Light), 8 oz. 18.0

(*Dannon* Nonfat), 4.4 oz. 25.0

(*Dannon Danimals*), 4.4 oz. 24.0

(*Knudsen Cal 70*), 6 oz. 12.0

(*Light n'Lively* Multi), 4.4 oz. 27.0

(*Light n'Lively Free*), 6 oz. 38.0

(*Light n'Lively Free* 70 Cal), 6 oz. 11.0

and creme (*Ultimate 90*), 8 oz. 14.0

boysenberry (*Dannon* Fruit on Bottom), 8 oz. 45.0

cappuccino, 8 oz., except as noted:

(*Dannon* Light) 16.0

(*Ultimate 90*) 14.0

(*Yoplait* Crunch 'n Yogurt Light), 7 oz. 22.0

all flavors (*Colombo* Fat Free) 32.0

mocha (*Dannon Light 'n Crunchy*) 26.0

cheesecake, cherry (*Yoplait* Crunch 'n Yogurt Light), 7 oz. . . 22.0

cheesecake/cherry (*Dannon Double Delights*), 6 oz. 34.0

cheesecake/strawberry (*Dannon Double Delights*), 6 oz. . . . 33.0

cherry (*Dannon* Fruit on Bottom), 8 oz. 46.0

cherry (*Dannon* Nonfat), 4.4 oz. 24.0

cherry, black:

(*Breyers*), 8 oz. 50.0

(*Knudsen Cal 70*), 6 oz. 12.0

(*Light n'Lively Free* 70 Cal), 6 oz. 11.0

cherry jubilee (*Ultimate 90*), 8 oz. 14.0

chocolate, mint cream pie (*Dannon* Light), 8 oz. 17.0

chocolate chip, mint (*Dannon Light 'n Crunchy*), 8 oz. 27.0

coconut cream pie (*Dannon* Light), 8 oz. 16.0

coconut cream pie (*Yoplait*), 6 oz. 35.0

coffee (*Breyers*), 8 oz. 38.0

cranberry-raspberry (*Dannon* Natural Flavored), 8 oz. 36.0

cranberry-raspberry (*Ultimate 90*), 8 oz. 14.0

creme caramel (*Dannon* Light), 8 oz. 15.0

grape-lemonade (*Dannon Danimals*), 4.4 oz. 22.0

guava (*Tropifruita*), 6 oz. 29.0

lemon:

   (Knudsen Cal 70), 6 oz. 11.0

   (Knudsen Free), 6 oz. 33.0

   (Light n'Lively Free), 6 oz. 35.0

   (Light n'Lively Free 70 Cal), 6 oz. 12.0

   chiffon *(Dannon Light)*, 8 oz. 15.0

   chiffon *(Ultimate 90)*, 8 oz. 14.0

   chiffon, with blueberry *(Dannon Light 'n Crunchy)*, 8 oz. 25.0

   creamy *(Breyers)*, 8 oz. 38.0

   creme *(Yoplait Crunch 'n Yogurt Light)*, 7 oz. 22.0

   ice *(Dannon Danimals)*, 4.4 oz. 22.0

mango *(Tropifruita)*, 6 oz. 31.0

orange *(Dannon Fruit on Bottom)*, 8 oz. 45.0

orange-banana *(Dannon Danimals)*, 4.4 oz. 24.0

papaya-pineapple *(Tropifruita)*, 6 oz. 30.0

peach:

   (Breyers), 8 oz. 48.0

   (Dannon Chunky Fruit), 6 oz. 33.0

   (Dannon Fruit on Bottom), 8 oz. 45.0

   (Dannon Light), 8 oz. 16.0

   (Dannon Nonfat), 4.4 oz. 23.0

   (Knudsen Cal 70), 6 oz. 11.0

   (Knudsen Free), 6 oz. 33.0

   (Light n'Lively Multi), 4.4 oz. 27.0

   (Light n'Lively Free), 6 oz. 35.0

   (Light n'Lively Free 70 Cal), 6 oz. 12.0

   (Ultimate 90), 8 oz. 14.0

   (Yoplait Crunch 'n Yogurt Light), 7 oz. 22.0

piña colada *(Tropifruita)*, 6 oz. 30.0

pineapple:

   (Breyers), 8 oz. 49.0

   (Knudsen Cal 70), 6 oz. 11.0

   (Light n'Lively Multi), 4.4 oz. 27.0

raspberry:

   (Breyers), 8 oz. 48.0

   (Dannon Fruit on Bottom), 8 oz. 45.0

   (Dannon Light), 8 oz. 17.0

   (Dannon Nonfat), 4.4 oz. 24.0

   (Dannon Danimals), 4.4 oz. 22.0

   (Knudsen Cal 70), 6 oz. 11.0

   (Knudsen Free), 6 oz. 31.0

Yogurt, raspberry *(cont.)*
    (Light n'Lively Multi), 4.4 oz. 24.0
    (Light n'Lively Free), 6 oz. 36.0
    (Light n'Lively Free 70 Cal), 6 oz. 11.0
    creme *(Ultimate 90)*, 8 oz. 14.0
    granola *(Dannon Light 'n Crunchy)*, 8 oz. 26.0
strawberry:
    (Breyers), 8 oz. 47.0
    (Dannon Chunky Fruit), 6 oz. 32.0
    (Dannon Fruit on Bottom), 8 oz. 46.0
    (Dannon Fruit on Bottom), 4.4 oz. 25.0
    (Dannon Light), 8 oz. 17.0
    (Dannon Nonfat), 4.4 oz. 23.0
    (Dannon Danimals), 4.4 oz. 24.0
    (Knudsen Cal 70), 6 oz. 11.0
    (Knudsen Free), 6 oz. 32.0
    (Light n'Lively Multi), 4.4 oz. 26.0
    (Light n'Lively Free), 6 oz. 36.0
    (Light n'Lively Free 70 Cal), 6 oz. 11.0
    (Tropifruita), 6 oz. 31.0
    (Ultimate 90), 8 oz. 14.0
    (Yoplait), 6 oz. 33.0
    (Yoplait Crunch 'n Yogurt Light), 7 oz. 25.0
    fruit basket *(Knudsen Cal 70)*, 6 oz. 11.0
    fruit cup *(Light n'Lively* Multi), 4.4 oz. 27.0
    fruit cup *(Light n'Lively Free)*, 6 oz. 35.0
    fruit cup *(Light n'Lively Free* 70 Cal), 6 oz. 11.0
    wild *(Light n'Lively* Kidpack), 4.4 oz. 28.0
strawberry-banana:
    (Breyers), 8 oz. 50.0
    (Dannon Chunky Fruit), 6 oz. 32.0
    (Dannon Fruit on Bottom), 8 oz. 43.0
    (Dannon Light), 8 oz. 17.0
    (Dannon Nonfat), 4.4 oz. 23.0
    (Knudsen Cal 70), 6 oz. 11.0
    (Light n'Lively Multi), 4.4 oz. 28.0
    (Light n'Lively Free 70 Cal), 6 oz. 11.0
    (Tropifruita), 6 oz. 31.0
    (Ultimate 90), 8 oz. 14.0
    (Yoplait), 6 oz. 33.0
strawberry-kiwi *(Dannon* Light), 8 oz. 16.0

strawberry-kiwi *(Tropifruita)*, 6 oz. 30.0
tangerine chiffon *(Dannon Light)*, 8 oz. 15.0
toffee crunch *(Yoplait Crunch 'n Yogurt Light)*, 7 oz. 24.0
tropical punch *(Dannon Danimals)*, 4.4 oz. 25.0
vanilla:
    (Breyers), 8 oz. 38.0
    (Dannon Light), 8 oz. 15.0
    (Dannon Danimals), 4.4 oz. 23.0
    (Knudsen Cal 70), 6 oz. 11.0
    (Knudsen Free), 6 oz. 32.0
    (Light n'Lively Free), 6 oz. 32.0
    (Ultimate 90), 8 oz. 14.0
    (Yoplait Custard Style), 4 oz. 21.0
    (Yoplait Extra Creamy Non-Fat), 8 oz. 41.0
    cherry *(Dannon Chunky Fruit)*, 6 oz. 31.0
    cherry *(Dannon Light)*, 8 oz. 18.0
    chocolate crunch *(Dannon Light 'n Crunchy)*, 8 oz. 23.0
    with chocolate nuggets *(Yoplait Crunch 'n Yogurt Light)*,
      7 oz. 22.0
    with vanilla wafers *(Yoplait Crunch 'n Yogurt Light)*,
      7 oz. 22.0
vanilla/peach and apricot *(Dannon Double Delights)*, 6 oz. . . 33.0
vanilla/strawberry *(Dannon Double Delights)*, 6 oz. 33.0
Yogurt, frozen, ½ cup, except as noted:
all flavors:
    (Colombo Cooler) 19.0
    (Colombo Slender Sensations) 11.0
    except blueberry pie and chocolate *(Dannon Fat Free*
      Soft) 20.0
    except Old World chocolate and peanut butter
      (Colombo Lowfat) 21.0
apple pie *(Colombo Nonfat)* 20.0
banana *(Colombo Nonfat)* 20.0
banana cream pie *(Dannon Light 'n Crunchy)* 23.0
banana pudding, homestyle *(TCBY)* 24.0
blueberry *(Colombo Nonfat)* 20.0
blueberry pie *(Dannon Fat Free Soft)* 21.0
butter pecan *(Breyers)*. 25.0
cappuccino:
    (Ben & Jerry's No Fat) 30.0
    (Breyers Fat Free) 22.0

Yogurt, frozen, cappuccino *(cont.)*
    (Colombo Nonfat) 20.0
caramel praline crunch *(Breyers* Fat Free) 27.0
caramel praline crunch *(Edy's/Dreyer's* Fat Free) 21.0
caramel toffee crunch *(Dannon Light 'n Crunchy)* 26.0
cheesecake *(Colombo* Nonfat) 20.0
cherry, black:
    (Colombo Nonfat) 20.0
    (Schwan's) 21.0
    vanilla swirl *(Edy's/Dreyer's* Fat Free) 18.0
cherry chocolate chunk *(Edy's/Dreyer's)* 18.0
cherry vanilla:
    (Colombo Nonfat) 20.0
    (Häagen-Dazs) 30.0
    chocolate chip *(Ben & Jerry's Cherry Garcia)* 31.0
chocolate:
    (Breyers) 24.0
    (Breyers Fat Free) 23.0
    (Dannon Fat Free Light Soft) 16.0
    (Dannon Fat Free/Lowfat Soft) 22.0
    (Häagen-Dazs) 28.0
    (Schwan's) 20.0
    all chocolate flavors except German chocolate fudge
       (Colombo Nonfat) 22.0
    Dutch *(TCBY)* 20.0
    German chocolate fudge *(Colombo* Nonfat) 23.0
    Old World *(Colombo* Lowfat) 22.0
    peanut crunch *(Dannon Light 'n Crunchy)* 24.0
    triple *(Dannon Light 'n Crunchy)* 25.0
chocolate brownie chunk *(Edy's/Dreyer's)* 17.0
chocolate chip:
    cookie dough *(Ben & Jerry's)* 39.0
    cookie dough *(Breyers)* 27.0
    mint *(Breyers)* 26.0
chocolate fudge *(Edy's/Dreyer's* Fat Free) 21.0
chocolate fudge brownie *(Ben & Jerry's)* 36.0
chocolate silk mousse *(Edy's/Dreyer's* Fat Free) 19.0
coconut *(Colombo* Nonfat) 20.0
coffee:
    (Häagen-Dazs) 29.0
    fudge *(Ben & Jerry's* No Fat) 31.0
    fudge sundae *(Edy's/Dreyer's* Fat Free) 21.0

cone crunch, crispy *(TCBY)* 22.0
cookie dough *(Edy's/Dreyer's)* 22.0
cookies and cream:
   (Breyers Fat Free) 25.0
   (Edy's/Dreyer's) 19.0
   (TCBY) 23.0
eggnog *(Colombo Nonfat)* 20.0
honey almond *(Colombo Nonfat)* 20.0
Irish creme *(Colombo Nonfat)* 20.0
lemon *(Schwan's)* 25.0
marble fudge *(Edy's/Dreyer's Fat Free)* 21.0
mocha *(Colombo Nonfat)* 20.0
mocha chocolate chunk *(Dannon Light 'n Crunchy)* 23.0
peach:
   (Breyers) 23.0
   (Breyers Fat Free) 22.0
   (Colombo Nonfat) 20.0
   (Schwan's) 22.0
   (TCBY) 21.0
   raspberry trifle *(Ben & Jerry's)* 37.0
peanut butter:
   (Colombo Lowfat) 20.0
   (Dannon Lowfat Soft) 19.0
   fudge sundae *(TCBY)* 23.0
pecan praline *(Colombo Nonfat)* 20.0
pecan praline, crisp *(TCBY)* 23.0
peppermint stick *(Colombo Nonfat)* 20.0
piña colada *(Colombo Nonfat)* 20.0
pineapple *(Colombo Nonfat)* 20.0
pumpkin *(Colombo Nonfat)* 20.0
raspberry, black, swirl *(Ben & Jerry's No Fat)* 32.0
raspberry, mountain or royal *(Colombo Nonfat)* 20.0
raspberry sorbet 'n cream *(Edy's/Dreyer's Fat Free)* 21.0
(Starburst), 1 cup 14.0
rocky road *(Dannon Light 'n Crunchy)* 27.0
strawberry:
   (Breyers) 23.0
   (Breyers Fat Free) 22.0
   (Colombo Nonfat) 20.0
   (Schwan's) 22.0
   cheesecake *(Breyers)* 25.0

Yogurt, frozen, strawberry *(cont.)*
  summertime *(TCBY)* 20.0
toffee crunch:
  (Edy's/Dreyer's Heath) 18.0
  bar *(Breyers)* 26.0
  English *(Ben & Jerry's)* 32.0
vanilla:
  (Breyers) 23.0
  (Breyers Fat Free) 21.0
  (Colombo Nonfat) 22.0
  (Dannon Fat Free Light Soft) 16.0
  (Dannon Lowfat Soft) 19.0
  (Edy's/Dreyer's) 17.0
  (Edy's/Dreyer's Fat Free) 18.0
  (Häagen-Dazs) 29.0
  (Schwan's) 19.0
  classic *(TCBY)* 21.0
  French *(Breyers)* 21.0
vanilla chocolate swirl *(Edy's/Dreyer's Fat Free)* 18.0
vanilla and chocolate *(Breyers Take Two Fat Free)* 21.0
vanilla, chocolate, and strawberry combination *(Breyers)* . . . 23.0
vanilla, chocolate, and strawberry combination *(Breyers Fat
  Free)* 22.0
vanilla fudge:
  (Häagen-Dazs) 34.0
  swirl *(Ben & Jerry's No Fat)* 31.0
  twirl *(Breyers)* 22.0
  twirl *(Breyers Fat Free)* 24.0
vanilla raspberry swirl *(Häagen-Dazs)* 28.0
vanilla raspberry truffle *(Dannon Pure Indulgence)* 25.0
vanilla streusel *(Dannon Light 'n Crunchy)* 25.0
white chocolate *(Colombo Nonfat)* 20.0
Yogurt bar, frozen, 1 piece:
(Creamsicle) 13.0
all flavors *(Schwan's Push-Ems)* 17.0
all flavors *(Starburst)* 13.0
cherry chocolate chip *(Ben & Jerry's Cherry Garcia)* 31.0
chocolate almond *(Frozfruit)* 23.0
peach *(Frozfruit)* 22.0
strawberry or strawberry-banana *(Frozfruit)* 22.0
Yogurt cup, frozen, chocolate chip *(Breyers)*, 1 cup 38.0

Youngberry juice *(Ceres)*, 8 fl. oz. 30.0
Yow choy sum *(Frieda's)*, 1 cup 3.0
Yuca:
boiled, drained *(Frieda's)*, 4 oz. 38.6
frozen *(Goya)*, ½ cup 44.0

Z

FOOD AND MEASURE	CARBOHYDRATE GRAMS

Ziti, see "Pasta"
Ziti entree, frozen:
mozzarella *(Weight Watchers),* 9 oz. 45.0
Parmesano *(The Budget Gourmet* Value Classics), 9 oz. . . . 52.0
Zucchini, ½ cup, except as noted:
fresh:
    raw, untrimmed, 1 lb. 12.5
    raw, sliced 1.9
    raw, baby, 1 large, 3⅛" long, ⅝" diam. 5
    boiled, drained, sliced 3.5
    boiled, drained, mashed 4.7
canned, Italian style:
    (Del Monte) 7.0
    (Progresso) 7.0
    with tomato juice 7.8
frozen, sliced *(Stilwell),* ⅔ cup 2.0
Zucchini, breaded, frozen *(Empire),* 1 piece 18.0
Zucchini, sun-dried, in olive oil and balsamic vinegar
    (Antica Italia), 1 oz. 2.0

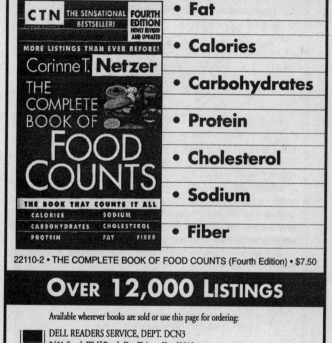

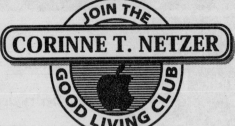